Digital innovation in Multiple Sclerosis Management

Digital innovation in Multiple Sclerosis Management

Editors

Tjalf Ziemssen
Rocco Haase

MDPI • Basel • Beijing • Wuhan • Barcelona • Belgrade • Manchester • Tokyo • Cluj • Tianjin

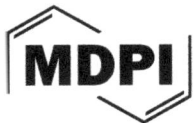

Editors
Tjalf Ziemssen
Center of Clinical Neuroscience
TU Dresden
Dresden
Germany

Rocco Haase
Center of Clinical Neuroscience
TU Dresden
Dresden
Germany

Editorial Office
MDPI
St. Alban-Anlage 66
4052 Basel, Switzerland

This is a reprint of articles from the Special Issue published online in the open access journal *Brain Sciences* (ISSN 2076-3425) (available at: www.mdpi.com/journal/brainsci/special_issues/ Digital_innovation_Multiple_Sclerosis_Management).

For citation purposes, cite each article independently as indicated on the article page online and as indicated below:

LastName, A.A.; LastName, B.B.; LastName, C.C. Article Title. *Journal Name* **Year**, *Volume Number*, Page Range.

ISBN 978-3-0365-2889-2 (Hbk)
ISBN 978-3-0365-2888-5 (PDF)

© 2022 by the authors. Articles in this book are Open Access and distributed under the Creative Commons Attribution (CC BY) license, which allows users to download, copy and build upon published articles, as long as the author and publisher are properly credited, which ensures maximum dissemination and a wider impact of our publications.

The book as a whole is distributed by MDPI under the terms and conditions of the Creative Commons license CC BY-NC-ND.

Contents

About the Editors vii

Preface to "Digital Innovation in Multiple Sclerosis Management" ix

Tjalf Ziemssen and Rocco Haase
Digital Innovation in Multiple Sclerosis Management
Reprinted from: *Brain Sci.* **2021**, *12*, 40, doi:10.3390/brainsci12010040 1

Rocco Haase, Isabel Voigt, Maria Scholz, Hannes Schlieter, Martin Benedict, Marcel Susky, Anja Dillenseger and Tjalf Ziemssen
Profiles of eHealth Adoption in Persons with Multiple Sclerosis and Their Caregivers
Reprinted from: *Brain Sci.* **2021**, *11*, 1087, doi:10.3390/brainsci11081087 5

Isabel Voigt, Christine Stadelmann, Sven G. Meuth, Richard H. W. Funk, Franziska Ramisch, Joachim Niemeier and Tjalf Ziemssen
Innovation in Digital Education: Lessons Learned from the Multiple Sclerosis Management Master's Program
Reprinted from: *Brain Sci.* **2021**, *11*, 1110, doi:10.3390/brainsci11081110 17

Jana Mäcken, Marie Wiegand, Mathias Müller, Alexander Krawinkel and Michael Linnebank
A Mobile App for Measuring Real Time Fatigue in Patients with Multiple Sclerosis: Introducing the Fimo Health App
Reprinted from: *Brain Sci.* **2021**, *11*, 1235, doi:10.3390/brainsci11091235 31

Anneke van der Walt, Helmut Butzkueven, Robert K. Shin, Luciana Midaglia, Luca Capezzuto, Michael Lindemann, Geraint Davies, Lesley M. Butler, Cristina Costantino and Xavier Montalban
Developing a Digital Solution for Remote Assessment in Multiple Sclerosis: From Concept to Software as a Medical Device
Reprinted from: *Brain Sci.* **2021**, *11*, 1247, doi:10.3390/brainsci11091247 41

Katrin Trentzsch, Benjamin Melzer, Heidi Stölzer-Hutsch, Rocco Haase, Paul Bartscht, Paul Meyer and Tjalf Ziemssen
Automated Analysis of the Two-Minute Walk Test in Clinical Practice Using Accelerometer Data
Reprinted from: *Brain Sci.* **2021**, *11*, 1507, doi:10.3390/brainsci11111507 55

Anja Dillenseger, Marie Luise Weidemann, Katrin Trentzsch, Hernan Inojosa, Rocco Haase, Dirk Schriefer, Isabel Voigt, Maria Scholz, Katja Akgün and Tjalf Ziemssen
Digital Biomarkers in Multiple Sclerosis
Reprinted from: *Brain Sci.* **2021**, *11*, 1519, doi:10.3390/brainsci11111519 71

Sonja Cloosterman, Inez Wijnands, Simone Huygens, Valérie Wester, Ka-Hoo Lam, Eva Strijbis, Bram den Teuling and Matthijs Versteegh
The Potential Impact of Digital Biomarkers in Multiple Sclerosis in The Netherlands: An Early Health Technology Assessment of MS Sherpa
Reprinted from: *Brain Sci.* **2021**, *11*, 1305, doi:10.3390/brainsci11101305 97

Diana M. Sima, Giovanni Esposito, Wim Van Hecke, Annemie Ribbens, Guy Nagels and Dirk Smeets
Health Economic Impact of Software-Assisted Brain MRI on Therapeutic Decision-Making and Outcomes of Relapsing-Remitting Multiple Sclerosis Patientsmdash;A Microsimulation Study
Reprinted from: *Brain Sci.* **2021**, *11*, 1570, doi:10.3390/brainsci11121570 111

Maria Scholz, Rocco Haase, Dirk Schriefer, Isabel Voigt and Tjalf Ziemssen
Electronic Health Interventions in the Case of Multiple Sclerosis: From Theory to Practice
Reprinted from: *Brain Sci.* **2021**, *11*, 180, doi:10.3390/brainsci11020180 131

Bruno Bonnechère, Aki Rintala, Annemie Spooren, Ilse Lamers and Peter Feys
Is mHealth a Useful Tool for Self-Assessment and Rehabilitation of People with Multiple Sclerosis? A Systematic Review
Reprinted from: *Brain Sci.* **2021**, *11*, 1187, doi:10.3390/brainsci11091187 145

Michael Lang, Daniela Rau, Lukas Cepek, Fia Cürten, Stefan Ringbauer and Martin Mayr
An ID-Associated Application to Facilitate Patient-Tailored Management of Multiple Sclerosis
Reprinted from: *Brain Sci.* **2021**, *11*, 1061, doi:10.3390/brainsci11081061 169

Wim Van Hecke, Lars Costers, Annabel Descamps, Annemie Ribbens, Guy Nagels, Dirk Smeets and Diana M. Sima
A Novel Digital Care Management Platform to Monitor Clinical and Subclinical Disease Activity in Multiple Sclerosis
Reprinted from: *Brain Sci.* **2021**, *11*, 1171, doi:10.3390/brainsci11091171 179

About the Editors

Tjalf Ziemssen

Prof. Dr. Tjalf Ziemssen graduated in medicine from the medical schools of Bochum, Bern and London in 1998. Between 1998 and 2000, he finished his postgraduate neurological training in the Department of Neurology, University Clinic Dresden, Germany. In 1999, he completed his doctoral thesis in the laboratory of Prof. Michael Krieg (Institute of Clinical Chemistry, Laboratory Medicine and Transfusion Medicine, University of Bochum.). Between 2000 and 2003, Dr. Ziemssen was post-doctoral fellow of the Deutsche Forschungsgemeinschaft (DFG) and Max-Planck-Society (MPG) at the Max-Planck Institute of Neurobiology, Department of Neuroimmunology, within the groups of Prof. Reinhard Hohlfeld, Prof. Hartmut Wekerle and Dr. Antonio Iglesias. He is currently director of the Center of Clinical Neuroscience and vice-director and consultant at the Neurological University Clinic in Dresden, head of the Autonomic Lab and MS center in Dresden. He has published more than 350 papers up to now and received several awards (e.g., of the European Charcot foundation, of the German Ophthalmological Society, of the German Parkinson Society). In 2011, he received the professorship for clinical neuroscience at a new established Center at Technische Universität Dresden. One important research area is personalized medicine and digital neurology applying the use case of multiple sclerosis. Multidimensional patient phenotyping applying AI has been introduced into the concept of MS digital twin to predict disease course and treatment response, which is component of several ongoing projects.

Rocco Haase

Rocco Haase graduated in psychology from Technische Universität Dresden in 2014. Already as a student, he joined the Center of Clinical Neuroscience at the Neurological University Clinic Dresden. At the moment, he is heading the research group "eHealth and analytics" and has published more than 50 papers. His multi-professional research team works on solutions to simplify patient, treatment and study management using software approaches. An eHealth portal solution is adapted to the medical requirements of the patient, integrates various participants in health care, supports necessary care models and thus makes medical and supplementary care services efficiently usable. In addition, his research is directed to the still unexplained aspects of neurological diseases using elaborated statistical and psychometric methods.

Preface to "Digital innovation in Multiple Sclerosis Management"

Multiple sclerosis (MS) is one of the world's most common neurologic diseases, causing most non-traumatic neurologic disability in young adults. MS is a lifelong unpredictable disability that can affect the different functional systems of the central nervous system (CNS), with symptoms such as fatigue, visual disturbances, altered sensation, and motor difficulties with mobility.

Therefore, the chronic, heterogenic, and multifocal "disease of a thousand faces" requires a complex, ubiquitous, differentiated, and adaptive monitoring and treatment strategy. This strategy should be personalized and tailored to the individual needs and disease course of the patient and be continuous. Due to innovation in technology, a new type of patient has been created, the e-patient, characterized by the use of electronic communication tools and commitment to participate in their own care. The extent to which the world of digital health has changed during the COVID-19 pandemic has been widely recognized. Remote medicine has become part of the new normal for patients and clinicians, introducing innovative care delivery models that are likely to endure even if the pendulum swings back to some degree in a post-COVID age.

The development of digital applications and remote communication technologies for patients with multiple sclerosis has increased rapidly in recent years. For patients, eHealth apps have been shown to improve outcomes and increase access to care, disease information, and support. For HCPs, eHealth technology may facilitate the assessment of clinical disability, analysis of lab and imaging data, and remote monitoring of patient symptoms, adverse events, and outcomes. It may allow time optimization and more timely intervention than is possible with scheduled face-to-face visits. The way we measure the impact of MS on daily life has remained relatively unchanged for decades, and is heavily reliant on clinic visits that may only occur once or twice each year.

These benefits are important because multiple sclerosis requires ongoing monitoring, assessment, and management. In this Special Issue, screening and assessment, disease monitoring and self-management, treatment and rehabilitation, and advice and education using digital tools are discussed. The aim of this Special Issue is to cover the state of knowledge and expertise in the field of eHealth technology applied to multiple sclerosis, from clinical evaluation to patient education.

Tjalf Ziemssen, Rocco Haase
Editors

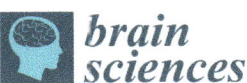

Editorial

Digital Innovation in Multiple Sclerosis Management

Tjalf Ziemssen * and Rocco Haase

Multiple Sclerosis Center Dresden, Center of Clinical Neuroscience, Department of Neurology, University Clinic Carl-Gustav Carus, Dresden University of Technology, Fetscherstrasse 74, 01307 Dresden, Germany; rocco.haase@uniklinikum-dresden.de
* Correspondence: tjalf.ziemssen@uniklinikum-dresden.de; Tel.: +49-351-458-4465; Fax: +49-351-458-5717

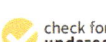

Citation: Ziemssen, T.; Haase, R. Digital Innovation in Multiple Sclerosis Management. *Brain Sci.* 2022, 12, 40. https://doi.org/10.3390/brainsci12010040

Received: 20 December 2021
Accepted: 24 December 2021
Published: 29 December 2021

Publisher's Note: MDPI stays neutral with regard to jurisdictional claims in published maps and institutional affiliations.

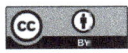

Copyright: © 2021 by the authors. Licensee MDPI, Basel, Switzerland. This article is an open access article distributed under the terms and conditions of the Creative Commons Attribution (CC BY) license (https://creativecommons.org/licenses/by/4.0/).

The development of digital applications and remote communication technologies for people with multiple sclerosis (pwMS) has increased rapidly in recent years. eHealth apps have been shown to improve outcomes and facilitate access to care, disease information, and support. On the patient side, pwMS facing a disease onset in their early adulthood are often seen as the ideal target group for new trends in digital healthcare because of their demand for a more personalized and tailored disease management that results from the complexity and heterogeneity of multiple sclerosis (MS). For healthcare professionals (HCPs) treating MS, eHealth technologies can facilitate clinical disability assessment; analysis of laboratory and imaging data; and the remote monitoring of patient symptoms, adverse events, and outcomes. They can enable time optimization and more timely intervention than is possible with scheduled in-person visits.

This Special Issue addresses screening and assessment; disease surveillance; self-management, treatment, and rehabilitation; and counseling and education using digital tools for MS. In particular, we collected research that paints a more detailed picture of pwMS and their practitioners as eHealth users, and research that shows progress in measuring and diagnosing MS as well in the treatment and rehabilitation through digital innovations.

Haase et al. continued their investigation of active stakeholders in the process of digital MS management in a multi-survey study [1]. They took a close look at the attitudes, needs, and behaviors of pwMS, as well as at their relatives and caregivers regarding electronically assisted disease management. There was broad and robust enthusiasm among various subgroups. For pwMS, the focus was on eHealth services that connect information already collected and make it easily accessible and understandable. HCP preferred digital solutions that provided aid in the preparation of future visits and adherence.

During the COVID-19 pandemic, remote medicine and education has become part of the new normal for patients and clinicians, introducing innovative care delivery models that are likely to endure. The master's program "Multiple Sclerosis Management", a digital program for HCPs at Dresden International University, was evaluated by Voigt et al., confirming feasibility and acceptability of a highly specialized study program that focuses solely on the management of one disease and delivers best-practice knowledge in digital form in 90% of lessons over a course of two years [2].

Due to the heterogeneous phenotype of the disease and large time intervals between neurologic examinations, measuring MS remains a complex task. Digital innovations may provide a solution to the problem of how we can avoid missing disease activity. Mäcken et al. developed a digital solution for one of the most common symptoms of MS, fatigue [3]. They included patient-reported outcomes, cognitive tests, and sensor data in a smartphone app applying a transtheoretical model of health behavior change that manifests in a training course for pwMS facing fatigue. Both patients and HCPs may benefit from objective fatigue assessments that can be easily administered by the patients themselves. In another article, van der Walt et al. explored the development pathway for a software as a medical device in MS, leveraging lessons learned from the development of Floodlight™ MS, an evolving app for MS functional assessment [4]. The strength of this solution is the integration of hand motor testing, gait tests, as well as cognitive and affective assessment under highest regulatory standards. With a special focus on gait testing, Trentzsch et al. developed a digitally assisted measurement system that uses accelerometers and multiple algorithms to assess the distance of a 2-min walk test [5]. The benefit of such a system is the simultaneous realization of standardization as well as objectification of measurement, which can be applied independently of human resources.

Towards a holistic approach to digital measurement of pwMS, Dillenseger et al. provided a comprehensive introduction into digital biomarkers in MS [6]. Digital biomarkers have the potential to close temporal gaps in diagnostics, to capture problem areas not addressed in clinical practice, to compile separate data sources in a timely manner, and thus to pave the way to personalized medicine at the pace of a clinical decision conversation. Therefore, digital biomarkers may include data from various sensors, tablets, medical devices. as well as video- and audio-based data and lead directly to the use of complex (big data) analyses that are largely based on machine learning approaches. A digital twin is a clinically useful representation of the knowledge gained in this way [7], which allows the treatment concept to be more data-driven at the individual longitudinal level as well as at the normative population level.

Cloosterman et al. presented a study on the potential impact of such a digital biomarker approach by assessing costs and benefits of the MS Sherpa app and online portal [8]. In this case, they performed an early health technology assessment that simulates the added value of digital biomarker-based eHealth interventions to the standard MS care path. Cost-effectiveness was demonstrated in all simulated scenarios, suggesting that digital biomarkers can be a valuable addition to routine clinical practice even with a small reduction in progression. With the software-assisted assessment of brain magnet resonance imaging (MRI) data, Sima et al. evaluated another digital biomarker and its impact on therapeutic decision-making [9]. A simulation on the effectiveness of an MRI-triggered switch of the disease-modifying therapy resulted in an increase in quality-adjusted life years and reduced societal costs due to MS.

A switch of treatments may be one result of the use of innovative digital technologies to treat MS. Beyond this, however, there are more facets and constellations in which eHealth can offer a contribution to improved treatment. In their review, Scholz et al. discussed the different types of interventions, standards, and advantages of quality eHealth approaches for pwMS [10]. They laid out several MS-specific use cases, such as single-use, social, integrated, and complex eHealth solutions, and collected factors of success for eHealth interventions in MS. In a second review, Bonnechère et al. focused on the existing clinical evidence of mobile health (mHealth) technologies in the rehabilitation and self-assessment of pwMS [11]. They reported small benefits of mHealth for cognitive functioning and moderate benefits for fatigue. For quality of life, further evidence on the level of activity and motor function was requested.

To promote an easy-to-access platform for interoperable data sharing and disease management across several HCPs, Lang et al. developed a CE-certified mobile application that provides risk management plans of current disease modifying therapies for MS [12]. Its use is not restricted to MS but already 3000 pwMS have used this integrative system that includes clinical information, patient-reported-outcomes, and functional and laboratory assessment in an electronic-health-record-like environment.

A complex management solution for MS was presented by Van Hecke et al., which combines functions of an online portal for HCPs, a web/mobile application for pwMS, and an elaborated solution for brain MRI analyses [13]. For its digital biomarkers, a notable increase in sensitivity to detect disease activity was reported. To underline the market readiness and the will to translate into clinical practice, the developers acquired a CE mark and a FDA clearance.

Overall, the twelve articles in this Brain Science Special Issue demonstrated what pwMS and HCPs expect from digital innovations for the treatment of MS, what contribution these technologies can make in everyday practice, and which areas of MS assessment can benefit from these new approaches in particular. The opportunity to focus simultaneously on technical development and clinical relevance in a selected and somewhat predisposed disease, such as MS, has provided valuable insights for neurologists, epidemiologists, and developers of eHealth solutions working on chronic neurological diseases.

Funding: This research received no external funding.

Conflicts of Interest: T.Z. received personal compensation from Biogen, Bayer, Celgene, Novartis, Roche, Sanofi and Teva for consulting services and additional financial support for the research activities from Bayer, BAT, Biogen, Novartis, Teva and Sanofi. R.H. received personal compensation by Sanofi and travel grants by Celgene and Sanofi.

References

1. Haase, R.; Voigt, I.; Scholz, M.; Schlieter, H.; Benedict, M.; Susky, M.; Dillenseger, A.; Ziemssen, T. Profiles of eHealth Adoption in Persons with Multiple Sclerosis and Their Caregivers. *Brain Sci.* **2021**, *11*, 1087. [CrossRef] [PubMed]
2. Voigt, I.; Stadelmann, C.; Meuth, S.G.; Funk, R.H.W.; Ramisch, F.; Niemeier, J.; Ziemssen, T. Innovation in Digital Education: Lessons Learned from the Multiple Sclerosis Management Master's Program. *Brain Sci.* **2021**, *11*, 1110. [CrossRef] [PubMed]
3. Macken, J.; Wiegand, M.; Muller, M.; Krawinkel, A.; Linnebank, M. A Mobile App for Measuring Real Time Fatigue in Patients with Multiple Sclerosis: Introducing the Fimo Health App. *Brain Sci.* **2021**, *11*, 1235. [CrossRef] [PubMed]
4. van der Walt, A.; Butzkueven, H.; Shin, R.K.; Midaglia, L.; Capezzuto, L.; Lindemann, M.; Davies, G.; Butler, L.M.; Costantino, C.; Montalban, X. Developing a Digital Solution for Remote Assessment in Multiple Sclerosis: From Concept to Software as a Medical Device. *Brain Sci.* **2021**, *11*, 1247. [CrossRef] [PubMed]
5. Trentzsch, K.; Melzer, B.; Stolzer-Hutsch, H.; Haase, R.; Bartscht, P.; Meyer, P.; Ziemssen, T. Automated Analysis of the Two-Minute Walk Test in Clinical Practice Using Accelerometer Data. *Brain Sci.* **2021**, *11*, 1507. [CrossRef] [PubMed]
6. Dillenseger, A.; Weidemann, M.L.; Trentzsch, K.; Inojosa, H.; Haase, R.; Schriefer, D.; Voigt, I.; Scholz, M.; Akgun, K.; Ziemssen, T. Digital Biomarkers in Multiple Sclerosis. *Brain Sci.* **2021**, *11*, 1519. [CrossRef] [PubMed]
7. Voigt, I.; Inojosa, H.; Dillenseger, A.; Haase, R.; Akgün, K.; Ziemssen, T. Digital Twins for Multiple Sclerosis. *Front. Immunol.* **2021**, *12*, 1556. [CrossRef] [PubMed]
8. Cloosterman, S.; Wijnands, I.; Huygens, S.; Wester, V.; Lam, K.H.; Strijbis, E.; den Teuling, B.; Versteegh, M. The Potential Impact of Digital Biomarkers in Multiple Sclerosis in The Netherlands: An Early Health Technology Assessment of MS Sherpa. *Brain Sci.* **2021**, *11*, 1305. [CrossRef] [PubMed]
9. Sima, D.M.; Esposito, G.; Van Hecke, W.; Ribbens, A.; Nagels, G.; Smeets, D. Health Economic Impact of Software-Assisted Brain MRI on Therapeutic Decision-Making and Outcomes of Relapsing-Remitting Multiple Sclerosis Patients—A Microsimulation Study. *Brain Sci.* **2021**, *11*, 1570. [CrossRef] [PubMed]
10. Scholz, M.; Haase, R.; Schriefer, D.; Voigt, I.; Ziemssen, T. Electronic Health Interventions in the Case of Multiple Sclerosis: From Theory to Practice. *Brain Sci.* **2021**, *11*, 180. [CrossRef] [PubMed]
11. Bonnechere, B.; Rintala, A.; Spooren, A.; Lamers, I.; Feys, P. Is mHealth a Useful Tool for Self-Assessment and Rehabilitation of People with Multiple Sclerosis? A Systematic Review. *Brain Sci.* **2021**, *11*, 1187. [CrossRef] [PubMed]
12. Lang, M.; Rau, D.; Cepek, L.; Curten, F.; Ringbauer, S.; Mayr, M. An ID-Associated Application to Facilitate Patient-Tailored Management of Multiple Sclerosis. *Brain Sci.* **2021** *11*, 1061. [CrossRef] [PubMed]
13. Van Hecke, W.; Costers, L.; Descamps, A.; Ribbens, A.; Nagels, G.; Smeets, D.; Sima, D.M. A Novel Digital Care Management Platform to Monitor Clinical and Subclinical Disease Activity in Multiple Sclerosis. *Brain Sci.* **2021**, *11*, 1171. [CrossRef] [PubMed]

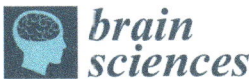

Article

Profiles of eHealth Adoption in Persons with Multiple Sclerosis and Their Caregivers

Rocco Haase [1,*], Isabel Voigt [1], Maria Scholz [1], Hannes Schlieter [2], Martin Benedict [2], Marcel Susky [2], Anja Dillenseger [1] and Tjalf Ziemssen [1]

1 Center of Clinical Neuroscience, Department of Neurology, University Hospital Carl Gustav Carus, Technical University of Dresden, 01307 Dresden, Germany; isabel.voigt@ukdd.de (I.V.); maria.scholz@uniklinikum-dresden.de (M.S.); anja.dillenseger@ukdd.de (A.D.); Tjalf.Ziemssen@uniklinikum-dresden.de (T.Z.)
2 Faculty of Business and Economics, Technical University of Dresden, 01062 Dresden, Germany; hannes.schlieter@tu-dresden.de (H.S.); martin.benedict@gmail.com (M.B.); marcel.susky@tu-dresden.de (M.S.)
* Correspondence: rocco.haase@uniklinikum-dresden.de

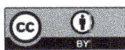

Citation: Haase, R.; Voigt, I.; Scholz, M.; Schlieter, H.; Benedict, M.; Susky, M.; Dillenseger, A.; Ziemssen, T. Profiles of eHealth Adoption in Persons with Multiple Sclerosis and Their Caregivers. *Brain Sci.* **2021**, *11*, 1087. https://doi.org/10.3390/brainsci11081087

Academic Editor: Damiano Paolicelli

Received: 22 July 2021
Accepted: 16 August 2021
Published: 19 August 2021

Publisher's Note: MDPI stays neutral with regard to jurisdictional claims in published maps and institutional affiliations.

Copyright: © 2021 by the authors. Licensee MDPI, Basel, Switzerland. This article is an open access article distributed under the terms and conditions of the Creative Commons Attribution (CC BY) license (https://creativecommons.org/licenses/by/4.0/).

Abstract: (1) Background: Persons with multiple sclerosis (pwMS) are often characterized as ideal adopters of new digital healthcare trends, but it is worth thinking about whether and which pwMS will be targeted and served by a particular eHealth service like a patient portal. With our study, we wanted to explore needs and barriers for subgroups of pwMS and their caregivers when interacting with eHealth services in care and daily living. (2) Methods: This study comprises results from two surveys: one collecting data from pwMS and their relatives (as informal caregivers) and another one providing information on the opinions and attitudes of healthcare professionals (HCPs). Data were analyzed descriptively and via generalized linear models. (3) Results: 185 pwMS, 25 informal caregivers, and 24 HCPs in the field of MS participated. Nine out of ten pwMS used information technology on a daily base. Individual impairments like in vision and cognition resulted in individual needs like the desire to actively monitor their disease course or communicate with their physician in person. HCPs reported that a complete medication overview, additional medication information, overview of future visits and a reminder of medication intake would be very helpful eHealth features for pwMS, while they themselves preferred features organizing and enriching future visits. (4) Conclusions: A closer look at the various profiles of eHealth adoption in pwMS and their caregivers indicated that there is a broad and robust enthusiasm across several subgroups that does not exclude anyone in general, but constitutes specific areas of interest. For pwMS, the focus was on eHealth services that connect previously collected information and make them easily accessible and understandable.

Keywords: multiple sclerosis; eHealth; patient empowerment; health information seeking; user-centered design; patient portal

1. Introduction

Persons with multiple sclerosis (pwMS) are often characterized as early or ideal adopters of new digital healthcare trends [1]. They are faced with a disease that usually starts in early adulthood and warrants the attention of pwMS, their relatives, and several types of healthcare professionals (HCPs) for the rest of patients' life. The disease itself is complex and may result in a multitude of different symptoms [2,3]. Overall, every person involved has to put a lot of effort in treatment management and associated multimodal monitoring, which will generate large numbers of multidimensional data [4]. Modern standardized disease management of multiple sclerosis (MS) should therefore include time- and cost-saving health information technology (HIT) that improves the conditions for and the connections between pwMS, HCPs, and informal caregivers [5,6].

We know from cross-domain research that younger patients and patients who are more active IT users are particularly interested in and have established skills with using eHealth services [7,8]. With the understanding that these characteristics are connected to pwMS [1], research on eHealth in the domain of MS has focused on creating a variety of new technologies to aid in the diagnostic and monitoring process and treatment of MS [6,9,10]. One focus is on providing new methods for networked generation of data, particularly to address symptom domains underrepresented in the standard MS assessment and temporal gaps in data collection. These approaches include self-monitoring via mobile health technologies, new (wearable) sensor systems like accelerometers, as well as extended and adapted electronic health records (EHR). All these efforts are aimed at preventing the disease from progressing unnoticed and unanswered [11].

A second major area of research on eHealth in MS deals with sharing and retrieving health-related information and experiences. In recent years, the availability of high-quality information about MS for pwMS and the ways to disseminate this knowledge have increased steadily [9]. Research on patient networks, professionally curated websites, and how patients find and process information online have gained much attention [9,12–15].

The goal of almost all of these eHealth services was to address all pwMS in a similar manner, or at least all within a given language area, which maintains the assumption that all pwMS are potential eHealth adopters, or at least that they all are to a similar degree. The low age at onset [16] and the general trend toward more digital devices [17] may suggest this conclusion, but it is also contradicted by the wide range of possible symptoms, the growing age of patients under treatment, the large number of HCPs involved, and the dispersion of those affected by MS within a society [5,16]. However, there is evidence that it is worth thinking about whether and which pwMS will be targeted and served by a particular eHealth service [15,18–20].

User-centered design (UCD) in the development of eHealth services represents an important principle for the differentiated consideration of attitudes and wishes of designated users like patients and HCPs [21,22]. For a development according to UCD, the following questions arise. Are all potential users identified as both information sources and target users? What are key needs, barriers and success factors for these individuals? Are differentiating factors such as a priori usage behavior, socio-demographic, and motivational characteristics considered? Are quantitative and qualitative methods used to capture outcomes and factors?

In a mixed-method study of Giunti et al., twelve pwMS and twelve HCPs from Switzerland were interviewed and assessed with questionnaires to gain insights into the needs of pwMS when using a mobile app to increase physical activity [22]. While pwMS and HCPs were used as a source of information in this regard, HCPs were not seen as active partners in the process of optimizing patients' physical activity through an app. As Giunti et al. themselves noted, the results of the study were based on a relatively small number of cases and a prelimited study population, which significantly reduced overall representativeness and did not allow for systematic multifactorial analyses. Marrie et al. contributed a very large study on usage behavior of pwMS in North America, which also systematically looked for differences in subgroups of pwMS. With more than 6400 pwMS, a very broad data set was created and numerous important factors were used in multivariate analyses, but the outcomes collected were often only binary and mostly addressed the general IT use of the pwMS. This is due to the epidemiological approach, which, unlike the UCD-based development process of a specific application, does not target a specific application purpose and thus provides less detail, especially for attitudes and needs.

In our study, we aimed to combine the strengths of these two approaches by asking detailed questions about current and potential usage patterns of eHealth services for MS and linking them to various factors so that systematic associations with subgroups are revealed. Since this study was designed in the context of a UCD-based software development, many involved perspectives should be considered both as information providers and as participants in the usage process. Specifically, this study sought to explore how willing pwMS (and their caregivers) would be to interact with their electronic health record, use alternative communication channels, and incorporate mobile devices and eHealth apps into care and their daily lives.

2. Materials and Methods

The research was conducted as part of the joint project "Integrated Care Portal for Multiple Sclerosis" by the Multiple Sclerosis Center (MSC) at University Hospital Carl Gustav Carus Dresden, the Technical University of Dresden (TUD), Chair of Wirtschaftsinformatik, Systems Engineering, and the Carus Consilium Sachsen GmbH between October 2017 and November 2019 [23]. This study comprises results from two surveys that were created by a team of neurologists, psychologists, and computer scientists at the MSC and TUD to enable a user-entered development process for an integrative care portal for MS including the perspectives of the most important persons involved.

The first survey collected data from pwMS and their relatives (as informal caregivers) and the second survey provided information on the opinions and attitudes of the neurologists treating MS. In both surveys, we gathered information concerning the use of information technology, disease-related barriers, requirements and needs for adopting eHealth solutions for MS.

2.1. Participants

PwMS and their relatives were enrolled during routine visits at the MSC and events like an information day and via support groups of the German Multiple Sclerosis Society. Questionnaires should only be given to persons with a verified diagnosis of MS and their relatives. No further restrictions were made to include a representative range of patients. The paper-based questionnaire could be filled in during the visit/event or later be submitted at the next appointment, by post or electronically by email as a scan. All submitted questionnaires were processed anonymously.

HCPs from Germany treating MS were contacted by mail and email through a network list of neurological practices to answer questions of the second survey anonymously online via web link. Experts must have treated pwMS regularly and have at least two years of personal experience in the field to provide appropriate answers for the analyses, which was ensured with initial items on these aspects.

2.2. Data Collection
2.2.1. Patient Survey

The questionnaire assessing pwMS and their relatives consisted of 65 items including information about their background and their condition as well as their attitudes and behavior regarding the eHealth in the context of MS. To include relevant patient characteristics in the analyses, we asked the patients with ordinal and bivariate items about their age, the distance to their treating neurologist, whether they suffered from symptoms of fatigue, depression, pain, spasticity, impaired cognition, walking ability, vision, bladder and bowel function, or other symptoms due to their MS. We added up the presence of these symptoms to estimate a severity index ranging from 0 to 10 for further analyses. Further questions concerned the frequency and purpose of use of digital devices and reasons for not using such tools for health-related tasks, especially to manage their MS. Answers were provided on a 5-point Likert scale or as dichotomous outcome. The second part of this survey focused on expectations and needs regarding the use of a common eHealth infrastructure that is accessible for pwMS and their caregivers as well.

2.2.2. Physician Survey

With a second survey for HCPs in the field of MS, we wanted to address their attitudes towards eHealth for treating MS, their current use of HIT and their needs and requirements for a an eHealth environment that connects pwMS as well as their respective formal and informal caregivers. In total, 100 items were used to assess HCPs basic characteristics

(8 items), their current way of using HIT (13 items), information about processes in the clinical practice (32 items), needs and opinions about a patient portal for MS (40 items), and electronic health records for MS (7 items). Responses were given as free text, 5-point Likert scale or multiple-choice option. HCPs could skip items if they did not feel qualified to answer.

2.3. Statistical Analyses

Absolute and relative numbers, median and interquartile range were used to describe the study variables. Percentages based only on complete answers. When recoding of ordinal data was required, the two most favorable outcomes on a 5-point Likert scale were coded as favorable binary outcome. For a deeper understanding of the patterns in which subgroups in both surveys may differ, generalized linear models (GLMs) with binomial and multinomial link function were applied to analyze responses with respect to individual characteristics. A p-value < 0.05 was considered significant. For analyses of the patient survey, the model factors included age, type of participant, distance to and type of treating neurologist, disease severity (via index), and major symptom classes (fatigue, depression, cognition, pain, spasticity, walk, vision, bladder, bowel). Wilcoxon tests were used to compare ordinal ratings. Kendall's tau–b (τ) was used to estimate agreement for ordinal ratings.

3. Results

3.1. Participants

Overall, 185 pwMS, 25 informal caregivers, and 24 healthcare professionals in the field of MS participated in our surveys.

In the first survey, the age of pwMS and their relatives ranged from 18 to over 60 years with a median of 31 to 40 years. Most cases were treated at the MSC (74.3%) while 25.7% were treated in general neurological practices and clinics. The median distance pwMS had to travel to treat HCP was between 5 to 15 km. Major self-reported symptoms were fatigue (58.6), impairment of walking (51.0%), vision (35.2%), cognition (31.9%), as well as pain (31.9%), bladder problems (28.6%), other symptoms (22.4%), depression (20.5%), and bowel problems (11.9%) with an average of 3.14 symptoms per patient.

In the second survey, 20 neurologists, 2 radiologists, and 2 specialized MS nurses answered our questions with a median experience of 11 to 25 years in the field of MS. Participating HCPs working in neurological practices (50%) and clinics (41.7%) treated an average of 901 patients per quarter with 15.5% of these patients being pwMS (range between 1% and 100%).

3.2. Patient Survey

Overall, 89.0% of pwMS and their caring relatives used information technology on a daily base (Table 1). Only 5.7% of them did not use or rarely used devices such as a smartphone or a computer with the smartphone being the most used device.

Typical health-related tasks that include the use of HIT were accessing health information on the Internet and self-tracking (Table 2). Finding a new physician and contacting physicians were the least common use cases for our subjects. The most common reasons for not using HIT solutions were the lack of knowledge about existing services (17.6%), concerns about the usefulness of a service (11.4%), low familiarity with the technology (9.5%), a lack of trust in existing services (5.7%), and other reasons (21.9%).

Table 1. Frequencies of information technology use in persons with multiple sclerosis and their relatives (N = 210).

Use of Device	Parameter	Daily	Weekly	Less than Weekly	Unknown
Computer or Notebook	n	110	51	29	20
	%	57.9	26.8	15.3	
Tablet	n	61	24	47	78
	%	46.2	18.2	35.6	
Smartphone	n	158	3	12	37
	%	91.3	1.7	6.9	
Smartwatch	n	10	2	66	132
	%	12.8	2.6	84.6	
Any of These Devices	n	187	11	12	0
	%	89.0	5.2	5.7	

Percentages based on complete answers.

Table 2. Purpose of use of information technology use in persons with multiple sclerosis and their relatives (N = 210).

Use of Device	Parameter	Daily or Weekly	Monthly	Rarely or Never	Unknown
Access General Information on Health	n	59	62	54	35
	%	33.7	35.4	30.9	
Access Information on Multiple Sclerosis	n	45	65	70	30
	%	25.0	36.1	38.9	
Find a New Physician	n	12	56	102	40
	%	7.1	32.9	60.0	
Self-Tracking	n	22	10	113	65
	%	15.2	6.9	77.9	
Organize Appointments	n	44	43	77	49
	%	27.3	26.7	47.8	
Exchange with Other Patients	n	22	17	114	57
	%	14.4	11.1	74.5	
Contact Physicians	n	10	51	101	48
	%	6.2	31.5	62.3	

Percentages based on complete answers.

When being asked whether they had ever accessed information about MS from a specific source, 76.2% of the participants answered that they had used the Internet, 75.2% contacted a specialized physician, 41.0% read books and magazines, 21.4% visited MS-related events, 20.5% talked to other patients, 2.9% used an app for MS, and 7.6% accessed other sources. Barriers for accessing information about MS were the general lack of understandability (76.3%) as well as the accessing (53.4%), overviewing (51.0%), and understanding (38.7%) of personal health records and the unavailability of suitable information (13.9%) and other patients to communicate with (43.0%). A patient portal for MS was welcomed by 93.1% of the participants. At the MS Day event of the MSC in 2019, we also asked our attending pwMS whether they would be willing to pay for the use of such a portal (N = 60) and 61.7% of them were willing to do so in principle. Most desired features of such a portal were the access to personal EHRs (85.9%), an overview of the medication schedule (82.6%), additional information about the current treatment (86.9%), and an overview of past (74.0%) and future visits (87.3%). Also of interest to some degree were the options to remind patients for taking their medication (57.7%), as well as to mail (81.1%), call (49.2%), and video chat (35.3%) with physicians.

In analyses with GLMs, we found several significant associations between distinct subject characteristics and their behaviors and attitudes toward eHealth for MS (Table 3).

Table 3. Associations between subgroups of participants and their behaviors and attitudes toward eHealth for multiple sclerosis (MS) ($N = 210$).

Characteristic	Association	p
Younger Participants	Used any Modern Communication Device More Often	0.001
	Used Tablets More Often	0.028
	Used Smartphones More Often	0.031
	Looked More Often for a New Physician Online	<0.001
	Participated Less Often in Live Events about MS [1]	0.004
	Were More Interested in an Overview of Future Visits	0.013
Participants with Lower Distance to the Treating Physician	Received More Often MS-Related Information Directly from Their Specialized Physician	0.040
Participants being Treated in a Highly Specialized MS Unit	Were More Likely to Use Modern Communication Devices for Retrieving Health Information	<0.001
	Were Less Likely to Attend Live Events about MS	0.034
	Were More Interested in an Overview of Future Visits [1]	0.013
	Were More Interested in Filling in Questionnaires and Tests [1]	0.030
	Were More Interested in Managing Visits [1]	0.004
Participants with an Increased Number of MS Symptoms	Were More Interested in Accessing their Electronic Health Record [1]	0.026
Persons with MS in Comparison with Friends and Relatives of Persons with MS	Were More Likely to Use Modern Communication Devices for Retrieving Health Information	0.006
	Were More Interested in MS-Related Reminders [1]	0.001
	Were More Interested in an Overview of Past Visits [1]	0.044
	Were More Interested in an Overview of Future Visits [1]	0.012
	Were More Interested in Managing Visits [1]	0.009
Participants with Fatigue	Used any Modern Communication Device Less Often	0.001
	Used Computers and Notebooks Less Often	0.032
	Looked More Often for a New Physician Online	0.005
Participants with Cognition Problems	Used Computers and Notebooks Less Often	0.043
	Were More Likely to Look for Information on MS Online	0.006
	Were More Interested in Filling in Questionnaires and Tests [1]	0.047
Participants with Walking Problems	Looked Less Often for a New Physician Online	0.030
Participants with Vision Problems	Received more Often MS-Related Information Directly from their Specialized Physician	0.016
	Were Less Interested in in Accessing their Electronic Health Record [1]	0.036

Generalized linear models were used with binomial and multinomial link function and age, type of participant, distance to and type of treating neurologist, number of symptoms, and major symptom classes (fatigue, depression, cognition, pain, spasticity, walk, vision, bladder, bowel) as factors. Only significant associations are displayed ($p < 0.050$). [1] Via an online portal for persons with multiple sclerosis and their caregivers.

Individual impairments like in vision and cognition resulted in individual interests like the desire to actively monitor their disease course or communicate with their physician in person. As expected, pwMS were more interested in actively managing their disease than their informal caregivers who were nevertheless interested in many aspects of the disease. Participants who were associated to a highly specialized MS care unit like the MSC showed an increased interest in interactive possibilities of eHealth for MS like the possibility to do tests and questionnaires online and via a mobile accessible platform like a patient portal for pwMS. Also as expected, younger participants presented with an increased frequency of using modern communication devices. The general interest in a patient portal for MS did not differ between subgroups.

3.3. Physician Survey

All HCPs had already used HIT-like specific software on computers (100%) and mobile devices (65%) in their practices and clinics. Only a minority of them processed imaging data via the Internet (31.8%), which is a typical use case for diagnostics in MS. Another 55% already provided additional educational programs to their patients. Median number of contacts between HCPs and their patients was up to two times per quarter. Among common problems that HCPs were facing during disease management, the lack of forwarding of information by the patient (31.6%) the need for the patient to visit on site for inquiries (21.1%), a missing overview of treatments including those from other HCPs, and poor general reachability of patients (15.8%) were the most prominent ones.

Seen from the HCPs' point of view, a complete medication overview, additional medication information, overview of future visits, and a reminder of medication intake would be very helpful portal features for pwMS (Table 4, Appendix A). Helpful portal features for HCPs themselves were medication overview, overview of future visits, and preparing appointments so that pwMS know what to expect and what to bring with them. For most of the tasks of a common online portal for MS, a trend towards having more benefits for patients was observed, but only the contact via text message was rated significantly more favorable for pwMS ($p = 0.016$) than for HCPs. No differences were found for the ratings with respect to the HCPs' characteristics like working in clinics vs. in practices, their occupation (neurologist, radiologist, MS nurse), their professional experience, and or the share of pwMS among all treated patients.

Table 4. Healthcare professionals' ratings for useful features of an online portal for persons with multiple sclerosis and their caregivers ($N = 24$).

Task	Parameter	Useful for the Patient	Useful for the Physician	Unknown	τ
Access Electronic Health Record	n	9	5	7	0.631 [1]
	%	52.9	29.4		
Medical Overview	n	16	15	7	0.713 [1]
	%	94.1	88.2		
Patient Inquiries	n	13	10	7	0.548 [1]
	%	76.5	58.8		
Treatment Information	n	14	13	7	0.487 [1]
	%	82.4	76.5		
Reminder for Treatment	n	13	13	7	0.786 [1]
	%	76.5	76.5		
Overview of Past Visits	n	9	9	7	0.882 [1]
	%	52.9	52.9		
Overview of Future Visits	n	14	14	7	0.659 [1]
	%	82.4	82.4		
Contact via Text Message	n	9	4	7	0.550 [1]
	%	52.9	23.5		
Contact via Audio Call	n	7	5	7	0.663 [1]
	%	41.2	29.4		
Contact Via Video Call	n	6	5	7	0.825 [1]
	%	35.3	29.4		
Questionnaires and Tests	n	13	12	7	0.235
	%	76.5	70.6		
Prepare Visits	n	12	13	7	0.652 [1]
	%	70.6	76.5		
Post-Visit Tasks and Control	n	9	12	7	0.704 [1]
	%	52.9	70.6		

Percentages and correlations based on complete answers. Kendall's tau–b (τ) was used for correlations between rated usefulness for the patient and the physician. [1] Significant correlation on a at least 5% level.

The highest level of agreement for perceived use rated for patients and physicians was found in the systematic overview of past visits ($\tau = 0.882$), followed by video chats ($\tau = 0.825$), reminders for patients ($\tau = 0.786$), and medical overview ($\tau = 0.713$). The only non-significant correlation was detected for doing questionnaires and tests via patient portal ($\tau = 0.235$).

4. Discussion

In our study, we assessed the current and potential use of HIT by pwMS as well as by their formal and informal caregivers from a unified perspective and connected their answers with disease and treatment specific characteristics to promote a more detailed view on different profiles of eHealth adoption in MS.

We found that it was of particular importance for pwMS to get an effective access to their own medical data, especially treatment-related and visit-related data. This perspective was shared with HCPs treating MS. While there were high levels of use of modern communication technologies among all participating groups, we were able to identify significant differences in usage patterns as well as needs and experienced barriers to the use of eHealth technologies for MS.

As expected, younger pwMS were more receptive to modern communication technologies, but also pwMS and their relatives who had already experienced additional eHealth services in routine practice were more open towards the possibilities of a complex solution like an integrative patient portal for MS [6]. PwMS and their relatives shared many attitudes and knowledge about the disease and its treatment, but pwMS themselves were more interested in actively supporting disease management through electronically aided visit management. Patients with specific problems such as cognitive functional deficits were more interested in options to cope with these symptoms via a mobile-available assessment.

Research on the use of HIT in MS has evolved in the last ten years. In a number of studies, device use patterns and online search behavior for health information in pwMS [1,14,15,24,25] were assessed in several countries around the world. Our current study followed that tradition and updated previously established numbers with actual insights from a society that adopted a widespread use of smartphones across all subgroups [1]. For pwMS, we found that nine out of ten patients could be reached through modern communication devices, which extends the trend of previous studies [19,26]. Our numbers correspond to 90% of people in the general German population using a smartphone in 2020 [27]. Daily and weekly usage of HIT-ready devices and the Internet in general were the desired levels at which responsive disease management could be started [28]. For many routine tasks, access of eHealth services on a weekly or monthly base seemed sufficient for our pwMS, for example, to contact caregivers or to receive new information on MS. Therefore, a very high frequency in the use of HIT was not necessary for a successful adoption of eHealth services. Mobile applications that offer self-tracking and optimization options such as physical or cognitive trainings may be seen as one option that justifies a more frequent use of web-based services for MS [11,29].

Another approach that we wanted to take with this study is the multi-perspective research on needs and barriers that pwMS and caregivers face while managing MS, and that should be met and overcome by technical solutions [18,22]. To achieve this, patients and caregivers should be understood both as a source of information and as a target group for the development of eHealth solutions, and disease management itself as an interaction between these parties to be supported. Therefore, it was necessary to gather detailed requirements that should be met by a common web portal for pwMS and their caregivers, and to investigate whether these apply equally to subgroups. There was an increased need to access their EHR in pwMS with a large number of different functional deficits. However, in pwMS with impaired vision, we found less interest in accessing their EHR online. Instead, they contacted their specialized physician more often to get MS-related information directly from them, which was also seen in pwMS that lived near their treating HCPs. Here, we also see the potential that eHealth has for the care landscape in rural areas, which generally have a lower density of HCPs. Where face-to-face contact is rarely possible, more demand for information on MS can be served online. Optimizing readability may also promote the use of eHealth apps among pwMS with visual impairments. While younger pwMS and their relatives reported a more frequent use of modern communication devices, we also noted an increased interest in eHealth solutions in pwMS having already used such applications at their treating neurologist. While we cannot influence the age of pwMS, a high-quality offer of new eHealth methods like a patient portal by the practitioner may increase openness to them.

From HCPs, we learned that eHealth services can be equally important to patients and their caregivers when both were able to access them. For a common online portal for MS, features to overcome organizational and communicational deficits were most anticipated by HCPs. The benefits of this solution may also include improved patient education and networking and data sharing with other participating HCPs. Features that had already been implemented elsewhere, such as HCP's access to EHR and the ability to take mail and calls from patients, were met with less interest. This underlines the need for clear additional benefits for all stakeholders that should come with the use of new HIT.

In a study by Nielsen et al., pwMS that were already using an online portal focusing on patient–physician communication and accessing EHRs at the Beth Israel Deaconess Medical Center were assessed [20]. Like in our study, recommendations like font size adjustments were provided to overcome barriers related to physical disabilities. Further, younger age and normal vision were factors that predicted portal use. As this was a retrospective study, no specific questions could be answered. Atreja et al. used focus groups to get insights into needs and barriers of an Internet portal for MS [25]. Both studies have in common that they saw only patients as beneficiaries of the portal, yet envisioned HCPs using it for communication without primarily considering them in the portal design. Common recommendations from these studies and our findings include consideration of differential accessibility for patients with special impairments, integration of PROs and tests, and the objective that a patient portal must directly support shared physician–patient decision making, but certainly in ways that are different for physicians and patients.

Nevertheless, we have to address some limitations of our surveys. Since recruitment was on a voluntary basis, selection bias could have been present. The survey addressing HCPs achieved only a small sample size, which may have limited the representativeness of the findings and the power for statistical tests. In the survey directed to pwMS, we had to use binary surrogate items for assessing clinical symptoms. The use of a standard clinical instrument like the Expanded Disability Status Scale was prohibited due to the anonymous survey process [30]. Further, the use of the category "other symptoms" may have limited insights into further symptom areas like sensory impairment. A proportion of unanswered items reduced the amount of information available and may have reduced the number of responses in the "rarely or never" category, as participants may have omitted questions primarily when they did not apply to them personally.

5. Conclusions

Overall, pwMS as well as their formal and informal caregivers showed high interest in eHealth solutions for MS. A closer look at the various profiles of eHealth adoption indicated that there is a broad and robust enthusiasm across several subgroups of pwMS that does not exclude anyone in general, but constitutes specific areas of interest.

For pwMS, the main focus was on MS care portal options that connect previously collected information and make them easily accessible and understandable. For HCPs, organizing and enriching future visits was an important aspect.

Overall, a well-established, multilingual, standardized questionnaire on the usage behavior of modern communication devices and platforms would be a welcomed starting point for cross-domain comparable research on the topic.

With our integrated care portal and the vision of digital twins for MS, patient involvement will be strengthened by a purposeful assistance in organizing and caring [23,31]. In addition, context-sensitive information for patients and their relatives as well as concrete recommendations and options for action based on this information will be provided.

Author Contributions: Conceptualization R.H. and T.Z.; Methodology, R.H., I.V., M.S. (Maria Scholz), H.S., M.B., M.S. (Marcel Susky), A.D. and T.Z.; Formal analysis, R.H.; Data curation, M.B., M.S. (Marcel Susky) and R.H.; Writing—original draft preparation, R.H.; Writing—review and editing, R.H., I.V., M.S., H.S., M.B., M.S. (Marcel Susky), A.D. and T.Z.; Supervision, H.S. and T.Z.; Project administration, I.V., H.S., M.B. and T.Z. All authors have read and agreed to the published version of the manuscript.

Funding: This research is funded by the European Regional Development Fund (ERDF) and the Free State of Saxony.

Institutional Review Board Statement: Ethical review and approval were waived for this study according to local legislation and national guidelines.

Informed Consent Statement: Written informed consent was obtained from all subjects involved in the study.

Data Availability Statement: The data presented in this study are available on reasonable request from the corresponding author.

Conflicts of Interest: T.Z. received personal compensation from Biogen, Bayer, Celgene, Novartis, Roche, Sanofi, and Teva for consulting services and additional financial support for the research activities from Bayer, BAT, Biogen, Novartis, Teva, and Sanofi. R.H. received travel grants by Celgene and Sanofi.

Appendix A

Table A1. Standardized regression coefficients for significant associations in generalized linear models from Table 3 ($N = 210$).

Outcome	Factor	B1	B2	B3	B4	B5
Used of Any Modern Communication Device	Age	−1.670	−1.181	−0.485	0.298	0^2
	Fatigue	−1.512	0^2	−	−	−
Use of Computers and Notebooks	Fatigue	−0.817	0^2	−	−	−
	Cognition	−0.879	0^2	−	−	−
Use of Tablets	Age	−0.480	−1.005	0.167	0.397	0^2
Use of Smartphones	Age	−0.953	−0.707	0.156	0.762	0^2
Use Modern Communication Devices for Retrieving Health Information	Type of Participant	2.043	0^2	−	−	−
	Being Treated in a Highly Specialized MS Unit	−2.700	0^2	−	−	−
Look for a New Physician Online	Age	−2.266	−0.756	−1.156	0.233	0^2
	Fatigue	−1.426	0^2	−	−	−
	Walking	2.444	0^2	−	−	−
Look for Information on MS Online	Cognition	1.957	0^2	−	−	−
Participated in Live Events About MS [1]	Age	2.439	2.493	1.440	0.651	0^2
	Being Treated in a Highly Specialized MS Unit	0.979	0^2	−	−	−
Receive Information on MS Directly from a Specialized Physician	Distance to Physician	−1.149	−0.988	0.016	0^2	−
	Vision	1.371	0^2	−	−	−
Accessing Electronic Health Records [1]	Disease Severity	0.716	−	−	−	−
	Vision	−0.939	0^2	−	−	−
Medication Reminder [1]	Type of Participant	1.678	0^2	−	−	−
	Age	−1.882	−2.127	−1.749	−0.882	0^2
Overview of Past Visits [1]	Type of Participant	1.001	0^2	−	−	−

Table A1. *Cont.*

Outcome	Factor	B1	B2	B3	B4	B5
Overview of Future Visits [1]	Type of Participant	1.488	0^2	–	–	–
	Age	−1.223	−1.210	−0.843	0.090	0^2
	Being Treated in a Highly Specialized MS Unit	−0.897	0^2	–	–	–
Filling in Questionnaires and Tests [1]	Being Treated in a Highly Specialized MS Unit	−0.750	0^2	–	–	–
	Cognition	0.931	0^2	–	–	–
Manage Visits [1]	Type of Participant	1.437	0^2	–	–	–
	Being Treated in a Highly Specialized MS Unit	−0.987	0^2	–	–	–

Generalized linear models were used with binomial and multinomial link function and age, type of participant, distance to and type of treating neurologist, number of symptoms, and major symptom classes (fatigue, depression, cognition, pain, spasticity, walk, vision, bladder, bowel) as factors. Only significant associations are displayed ($p < 0.050$). [1] Via an online portal for persons with multiple sclerosis and their caregivers. [2] Reference category.

References

1. Haase, R.; Schultheiss, T.; Kempcke, R.; Thomas, K.; Ziemssen, T. Use and Acceptance of Electronic Communication by Patients with Multiple Sclerosis: A Multicenter Questionnaire Study. *J. Med. Internet Res.* **2012**, *14*, e135. [CrossRef]
2. Ziemssen, T. Symptom management in patients with multiple sclerosis. *J. Neurol. Sci.* **2011**, *311*, S48–S52. [CrossRef]
3. Compston, A.; Coles, A. Multiple sclerosis. *Lancet* **2008**, *372*, 1502–1517. [CrossRef]
4. Ziemssen, T.; Kern, R.; Thomas, K. Multiple sclerosis: Clinical profiling and data collection as prerequisite for personalized medicine approach. *BMC Neurol.* **2016**, *16*, 124. [CrossRef]
5. Hobart, J.; Bowen, A.; Pepper, G.; Crofts, H.; Eberhard, L.; Berger, T.; Boyko, A.; Boz, C.; Butzkueven, H.; Celius, E.G.; et al. International consensus on quality standards for brain health-focused care in multiple sclerosis. *Mult. Scler. J.* **2019**, *25*, 1809–1813. [CrossRef]
6. Scholz, M.; Haase, R.; Schriefer, D.; Voigt, I.; Ziemssen, T. Electronic Health Interventions in the Case of Multiple Sclerosis: From Theory to Practice. *Brain Sci.* **2021**, *11*, 180. [CrossRef] [PubMed]
7. Tennant, B.; Stellefson, M.; Dodd, V.; Chaney, B.; Chaney, D.; Paige, S.; Alber, J. eHealth Literacy and Web 2.0 Health Information Seeking Behaviors Among Baby Boomers and Older Adults. *J. Med. Internet Res.* **2015**, *17*, e70. [CrossRef]
8. Neter, E.; Brainin, E. eHealth Literacy: Extending the Digital Divide to the Realm of Health Information. *J. Med. Internet Res.* **2012**, *14*, e19. [CrossRef]
9. Lavorgna, L.; Brigo, F.; Moccia, M.; Leocani, L.; Lanzillo, R.; Clerico, M.; Abbadessa, G.; Schmierer, K.; Solaro, C.; Prosperini, L.; et al. e-Health and multiple sclerosis: An update. *Mult. Scler. J.* **2018**, *24*, 1657–1664. [CrossRef]
10. Marziniak, M.; Brichetto, G.; Feys, P.; Meyding-Lamadé, U.; Vernon, K.; Meuth, S.G. The Use of Digital and Remote Communication Technologies as a Tool for Multiple Sclerosis Management: Narrative Review. *JMIR Rehabil. Assist. Technol.* **2018**, *5*, e5. [CrossRef] [PubMed]
11. Aller-Philbey, K.; Middleton, R.; Tuite-Dalton, K.; Baker, E.; Stennett, A.; Albor, C.; Schmierer, K. Can We Improve the Monitoring of People with Multiple Sclerosis Using Simple Tools, Data Sharing, and Patient Engagement? *Front. Neurol.* **2020**, *11*, 464. [CrossRef] [PubMed]
12. Wicks, P.; Massagli, M.; Kulkarni, A.; Dastani, H.; Jacobs, D.; Jongen, P. Use of an Online Community to Develop Patient-Reported Outcome Instruments: The Multiple Sclerosis Treatment Adherence Questionnaire (MS-TAQ). *J. Med. Internet Res.* **2011**, *13*, e12. [CrossRef]
13. Jongen, P.J.; Sinnige, L.G.; Van Geel, B.M.; Verheul, F.; Verhagen, W.I.; Van Der Kruijk, R.A.; Haverkamp, R.; Schrijver, H.M.; Baart, J.C.; Visser, L.H.; et al. The interactive web-based program MSmonitor for self-management and multidisciplinary care in multiple sclerosis: Concept, content, and pilot results. *Patient Prefer. Adherence* **2015**, *9*, 1741–1750. [CrossRef]
14. Lejbkowicz, I.; Paperna, T.; Stein, N.; Dishon, S.; Miller, A. Internet Usage by Patients with Multiple Sclerosis: Implications to Participatory Medicine and Personalized Healthcare. *Mult. Scler. Int.* **2010**, *2010*, 640749. [CrossRef]
15. Marrie, R.A.; Salter, A.R.; Tyry, T.; Fox, R.J.; Cutter, G.R. Preferred Sources of Health Information in Persons with Multiple Sclerosis: Degree of Trust and Information Sought *J. Med. Internet Res.* **2013**, *15*, e67. [CrossRef]
16. Koch-Henriksen, N.; Sorensen, P.S. The changing demographic pattern of multiple sclerosis epidemiology. *Lancet Neurol.* **2010**, *9*, 520–532. [CrossRef]
17. Pew Research Center. Internet/Broadband Fact Sheet. 2021. Available online: https://www.pewresearch.org/internet/fact-sheet/internet-broadband/ (accessed on 4 August 2021).
18. Kern, R.; Haase, R.; Eisele, J.C.; Thomas, K.; Ziemssen, T.; Neter, E.; Mosconi, P.; Colombo, C. Designing an Electronic Patient Management System for Multiple Sclerosis: Building a Next Generation Multiple Sclerosis Documentation System. *Interact. J. Med. Res.* **2016**, *5*, e2. [CrossRef]

19. Marrie, R.A.; Leung, S.; Tyry, T.; Cutter, G.R.; Fox, R.; Salter, A. Use of eHealth and mHealth technology by persons with multiple sclerosis. *Mult. Scler. Relat. Disord.* **2019**, *27*, 13–19. [CrossRef]
20. Nielsen, A.S.; Halamka, J.D.; Kinkel, R.P. Internet portal use in an academic multiple sclerosis center. *J. Am. Med. Inform. Assoc.* **2012**, *19*, 128–133. [CrossRef]
21. Dabbs, A.D.V.; Myers, B.A.; MC Curry, K.R.; Dunbar-Jacob, J.; Hawkins, R.P.; Begey, A.; Dew, M.A. User-Centered Design and Interactive Health Technologies for Patients. *Comput. Inform. Nurs.* **2009**, *27*, 175–183. [CrossRef] [PubMed]
22. Giunti, G.; Kool, J.; Romero, O.R.; Zubiete, E.D.; Salcedo, V.T.; Jongerius, C.; Lyons, E.; Corbett, T. Exploring the Specific Needs of Persons with Multiple Sclerosis for mHealth Solutions for Physical Activity: Mixed-Methods Study. *JMIR mHealth uHealth* **2018**, *6*, e37. [CrossRef]
23. Voigt, I.; Benedict, M.; Susky, M.; Scheplitz, T.; Frankowitz, S.; Kern, R.; Müller, O.; Schlieter, H.; Ziemssen, T. A Digital Patient Portal for Patients with Multiple Sclerosis. *Front. Neurol.* **2020**, *11*, 400. [CrossRef]
24. Hay, M.C.; Strathmann, C.; Lieber, E.; Wick, K.; Giesser, B. Why patients go online: Multiple sclerosis, the internet, and physician-patient communication. *Neurologist* **2008**, *14*, 374–381. [CrossRef]
25. Atreja, A.; Mehta, N.; Miller, D.; Moore, S.M.; Nichols, K.; Miller, H.; Harris, C.M. One size does not fit all: Using qualitative methods to inform the development of an Internet portal for multiple sclerosis patients. *AMIA Annu. Symp. Proc.* **2005**, *2005*, 16–20.
26. Haase, R.; Schultheiss, T.; Kempcke, R.; Thomas, K.; Ziemssen, T. Modern communication technology skills of patients with multiple sclerosis. *Mult. Scler. J.* **2013**, *19*, 1240–1241. [CrossRef] [PubMed]
27. Statista. Persönliche Gerätenutzung für den Medienkonsum in Deutschland in den Jahren 2014 bis 2020. 2021. Available online: https://de.statista.com/statistik/daten/studie/476467/umfrage/persoenliche-geraetenutzung-fuer-den-medienkonsum-in-deutschland/ (accessed on 4 August 2021).
28. Potemkowski, A.; Brola, W.; Ratajczak, A.; Ratajczak, M.; Zaborski, J.; Jasińska, E.; Pokryszko-Dragan, A.; Gruszka, E.; Dubik-Jezierzańska, M.; Podlecka-Piętowska, A.; et al. Internet Usage by Polish Patients with Multiple Sclerosis: A Multi-center Questionnaire Study. *Interact. J. Med. Res.* **2019**, *8*, e11146. [CrossRef] [PubMed]
29. Giunti, G.; Rivera-Romero, O.; Kool, J.; Bansi, J.; Sevillano, J.L.; Granja-Dominguez, A.; Izquierdo-Ayuso, G.; Giunta, D. Evaluation of More Stamina, a Mobile App for Fatigue Management in Persons with Multiple Sclerosis: Protocol for a Feasibility, Acceptability, and Usability Study. *JMIR Res. Protoc.* **2020**, *9*, e18196. [CrossRef] [PubMed]
30. Kurtzke, J.F. Rating neurologic impairment in multiple sclerosis: An expanded disability status scale (EDSS). *Neurology* **1983**, *33*, 1444–1452. [CrossRef]
31. Voigt, I.; Inojosa, H.; Dillenseger, A.; Haase, R.; Akgün, K.; Ziemssen, T. Digital Twins for Multiple Sclerosis. *Front. Immunol.* **2021**, *12*, 669811. [CrossRef] [PubMed]

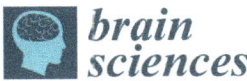

Article

Innovation in Digital Education: Lessons Learned from the Multiple Sclerosis Management Master's Program

Isabel Voigt [1], Christine Stadelmann [2], Sven G. Meuth [3], Richard H. W. Funk [4], Franziska Ramisch [4], Joachim Niemeier [4] and Tjalf Ziemssen [1,*]

1. Center of Clinical Neuroscience, Department of Neurology, University Clinic Carl Gustav Carus, Dresden University of Technology, 01307 Dresden, Germany; isabel.voigt@ukdd.de
2. Institute of Neuropathology, University Medical Center Göttingen, 37075 Göttingen, Germany; cstadelmann@med.uni-goettingen.de
3. Department of Neurology, Medical Faculty, University Clinic Düsseldorf, 40225 Düsseldorf, Germany; meuth@uni-duesseldorf.de
4. Institute of Anatomy, Medical Faculty Carl Gustav Carus, Technische Universität (TU) Dresden, 01307 Dresden, Germany; richard.funk@di-uni.de (R.H.W.F.); franziska.ramisch@di-uni.de (F.R.); joachim.niemeier@di-uni.de (J.N.)
* Correspondence: Tjalf.Ziemssen@ukdd.de

Abstract: Since 2020, the master's program "Multiple Sclerosis Management" has been running at Dresden International University, offering structured training to become a multiple sclerosis specialist. Due to the COVID-19 pandemic, many planned teaching formats had to be changed to online teaching. The subject of this paper was the investigation of a cloud-based digital hub and student evaluation of the program. Authors analyzed use cases of computer-supported collaborative learning and student evaluation of courses and modules using the Gioia method and descriptive statistics. The use of a cloud-based digital hub as a central data platform proved to be highly successful for learning and teaching, as well as for close interaction between lecturers and students. Students rated the courses very positively in terms of content, knowledge transfer and interaction. The implementation of the master's program was successful despite the challenges of the COVID-19 pandemic. The resulting extensive use of digital tools demonstrates the "new normal" of future learning, with even more emphasis on successful online formats that also increase interaction between lecturers and students in particular. At the same time, there will continue to be tailored face-to-face events to specifically increase learning success.

Keywords: multiple sclerosis; master's program; education; multiple sclerosis management; Dresden International University; digitization

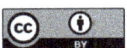

Citation: Voigt, I.; Stadelmann, C.; Meuth, S.G.; Funk, R.H.W.; Ramisch, F.; Niemeier, J.; Ziemssen, T. Innovation in Digital Education: Lessons Learned from the Multiple Sclerosis Management Master's Program. *Brain Sci.* **2021**, *11*, 1110. https://doi.org/10.3390/brainsci11081110

Academic Editor: Elisabeth Gulowsen Celius

Received: 28 July 2021
Accepted: 20 August 2021
Published: 23 August 2021

Publisher's Note: MDPI stays neutral with regard to jurisdictional claims in published maps and institutional affiliations.

Copyright: © 2021 by the authors. Licensee MDPI, Basel, Switzerland. This article is an open access article distributed under the terms and conditions of the Creative Commons Attribution (CC BY) license (https://creativecommons.org/licenses/by/4.0/).

1. Introduction

In neurology, there have been significant innovations in diagnosis and treatment of multiple sclerosis (MS) in the recent years [1]. Therefore, MS specialists need to be familiar with the "state of the art management" of chronic inflammatory diseases of the central nervous system. To date, however, there are no structured and industry-independent education programs for MS. Thus, a panel of MS experts and the experienced team of Dresden International University (DIU) developed the concept of the four-semester master's program "Multiple Sclerosis Management" (MSM), which was accredited in 2019 and started in German language in 2020 [2].

This is the first time that a master's degree program has been designed and launched around one single disease entity—a situation that does not yet exist in medical study programs or in further education studies. In addition, to date, there is no comparable study program on the market today. Either existing courses concentrate on a broader area such as neuroscience and neurodegeneration [3], immunology and inflammatory disease, neuroimmunology [4] or they address a specific target audience, such as physiotherapists [5] or MS nurses [6], or only partial aspects of MS are covered in webinars and single lectures [7]. Some specific advanced training programs are sponsored by pharmaceutical companies and are therefore not independent. The MSM master's program offers a full and industry-independent complete package around MS, unlike scientific journals or papers for further education that usually cover only a very small aspect of pathology, symptoms or treatment and care.

In the set-up phase of the program, experts developed a variety of modules focusing on basics, clinical and diagnostic aspects, studies and statistics, therapy and rehabilitation as well as monitoring and documentation of MS. The MSM master's program spans four semesters and is divided into six modules and a master's thesis (Table 1).

Table 1. Modules and topics in MSM master's program.

	Modules	Topics
1	Theoretical Principles	- basics and epidemiology of MS - factors of diagnosis and therapy - immunological basics - basics of pathology and pathophysiology - therapeutic interventions - methods for disease monitoring
2	Clinical & Diagnostic Aspects	- differential diagnostics - cerebrospinal fluid and blood tests - image diagnostic procedures - functional effects of demyelination - neurophysiological, neuropsychological and neuro-urological examination procedures
3	Studies & Statistics	- evaluation and application of study designs - selection of statistical tests - interpretation of results - analysis of real-world data in the context of MS practice
4	Therapy I	- differences between the therapy of acute relapses and a disease-modifying or progression-modifying therapy of MS - weighing of indications and patient profiles - successful therapy strategies for individual patients
5	Therapy II	- non-drug procedures to treat disease-associated symptoms - goals and implementation of symptomatic and complemetary therapies - neurocognitive and psychological interventions - rehabilitative and palliative medical measures
6	Monitoring & Documentation	- patient documentation - individual monitoring according to standards and therapy goals - health economic aspects - new possibilities in the field of e-health - MS-specific networks - associations and registers - big data
	Master's Thesis	- Master's thesis or scientific paper in a peer-reviewed or PubMed-listed journal (thematic review, meta-analysis, original scientific paper) - topic is submitted by the student and finalized by the scientific director of the program

The chronological sequence, the classification of the modules into semesters and the ECTS points to be earned in each case can be seen in Figure 1.

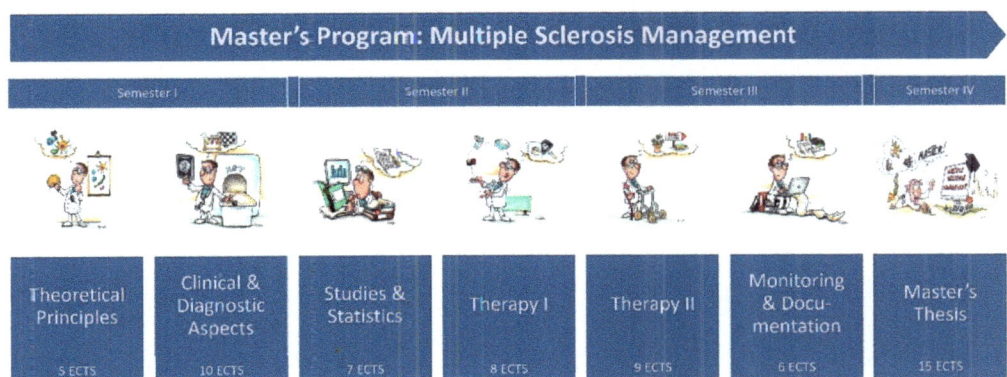

Figure 1. Timetable for modules in MSM master's program with indication of ECTS credits. The MSM cartoons were created by Phil Hubbe.

The module coordinators appointed for the content development of the individual modules exchanged ideas with all lecturers on the content and conceptual design of the study program several times in person and online. They selected as a team the lecturers, specified the course topics and assigned them to the teaching formats. Together with the program management of the master's program, they also worked out the concrete time and lesson planning. In addition to the traditional knowledge transfer through lectures and tutorials by experienced MS experts, the contents of the Master's program are to be taught with a particularly high practical component. For this purpose, preceptorships in specially selected MS centers, excursions and regular journal clubs as well as digital case conferences serve the direct practical implementation of the learned contents on site.

However, the start of the Master's program coincided with the beginning of the COVID-19 pandemic, so that it had to be conducted online to an even greater extent than planned. The existing plans could not be applied and new concepts had to be designed and implemented at short notice in an "emergency mode". Due to the COVID-19 pandemic situation the problem arose to shift all modules where it was possible from face-to-face learning to digital format. Although in the meantime many studies exist comparing digitally presented lectures and courses vs. face-to-face learning [8–13], DIU has been intensely concerned with the acceptability of a "digital only" education.

What remains of the creative digitization push, born out of necessity that has changed the image of universities so much? This paper provides an introduction and examines the innovative use of a cloud based digital hub (Microsoft Teams) for computer-supported collaborative learning in the MSM master's program as well as student evaluation of the program. In addition, the authors consider the extent to which the predominantly online master's program can successfully teach the complex, dynamically changing scientific work content in a way that is adapted to different levels of knowledge. Specifically, the authors take a look at the use cases of computer-assisted collaborative learning, the technical support provided by the organizers and the course instructor, the quality of the master's program content transferred to the virtual version, the performance of the instructors, and the students' interactions with the instructors are considered.

2. Materials and Methods

2.1. Use Case Analysis of Computer-Supported Collaborative Learning

Microsoft Teams [14,15] is used as a technological basis for the MSM Master's program in learning, teaching, collaboration, and cooperation processes, which has proven particularly effective during the COVID-19 pandemic. Since the services are cloud-based and software updates are provided automatically in the so-called "evergreen mode", there is no need for technicians and IT teams to support the platform itself after the initial setup.

Microsoft Teams serves as a digital hub that brings together conversations, content, tasks and apps in one place. The digital hub provides extensive security and compliance-specific features that will not be discussed here. Rather, the focus is on the analysis of innovative use cases that have been implemented within the MSM Master's program: one central data platform for highly effective organization of the Master's program, online classrooms in a distance learning environment for synchronous and self-directed asynchronous learning, flexible knowledge transfer in the learning video portal, and establishment of special learning areas for peer-to-peer learning. The use cases present possible applications of certain tools for students and lecturers in the pandemic situation and show how they were implemented.

2.2. Systematic Evaluation of Teaching and Student's Feedback

2.2.1. Participants

DIU program managers conducted the evaluation on a qualitative and quantitative level and asked the participants of the MSM master's program to share their experiences with module 1 ("Theoretical Principles", details see Table 1) in the form of qualitative feedback and to complete a standardized evaluation questionnaire (quantitative feedback) after module 2 ("Clinical & Diagnostic Aspects", details see Table 2). Participation was voluntary in both cases.

Table 2. Categories of evaluation questionnaire and the corresponding items.

Category	Questions
Content, structure and organization of the event	- The goals of the event were clearly identifiable. - The content structure ("red thread") of the overall event was sensible. - The relevance of the contents covered for practice became clear. - Course time was used in a way that was conducive to learning. - Students were able to appropriately contribute their personal competencies and prior experience.
Lecturer	- The lecturer has stimulated the discussion of the topics. - The lecturer emphasized active participation of the students. - The lecturer is appreciative in dealing with students. - The lecturer succeeded in making the event appealing.
Methodical aspects	- Methods and teaching/learning forms (individual, partner, group work, work in plenary) were appropriate. - The lecturer was able to present complex content in an understandable way. - The lecturer gave appropriate feedback or responded appropriately to the group.
Documents, course materials and media: design and use	- The quality of the media content (presentations, scripts, exercise sheets, e-lectures, etc.) was appropriate. - The media and (online) tools used were used sensibly.
Technical support for online events	- I was satisfied with the supervision and support during the digital course. - I was satisfied with the technical support. - The virtual classroom was suitable for the course.

2.2.2. Data Collection

For module 1, students were able to report their experiences via email or Microsoft Teams. As a result, the feedback providers were known, allowing specific queries for the further development of the program. For the evaluation, the responses were then aggregated and anonymized. In the further course, DIU program managers asked students to complete a systematic and anonymous evaluation at the course and module levels. For this purpose, DIU program managers used in-house, already established standardized questionnaires that are used for evaluation in all study programs at DIU [16]. For module 2, students answered an evaluation questionnaire with 23 questions in 5 categories (Table 2), which they could answer with values on a scale of 1 (strongly agree) to 6 (strongly disagree). In addition, students had the opportunity to indicate in free text fields what they particularly liked or disliked about the course, what they would recommend to improve the quality of the course and the lecturer's performance.

2.2.3. (Statistical) Analyses

Authors used the Gioia method [17] to evaluate the information from the feedbacks for module 1, some of which were very detailed. The Gioia method allows for qualitative evaluation with inductive and summary category building, allowing for creative influence with systematic accuracy. It assumes that the organizational world is socially constructed and its participants are knowledgeable individuals who can explain their intentions, thoughts and actions.

For module 2, authors calculated means and standard deviations to describe the student population and evaluation variables and used charts for illustration. In addition, they screened the free texts for concise statements, which are presented as examples in the results.

3. Results

3.1. Use Cases for Computer-Supported Collaborative Learning

The COVID-19 pandemic has quickly changed professional and private life, and a tremendous need emerged to hold meetings exclusively online, organize video conferences or create videos for lessons and further education. The lecture halls, meeting areas and learning spaces were empty (Figure 2). Teaching and learning shifted to virtual space under high time pressure, leading to a variety of innovative use cases, that were described and analyzed using the MSM Master's program.

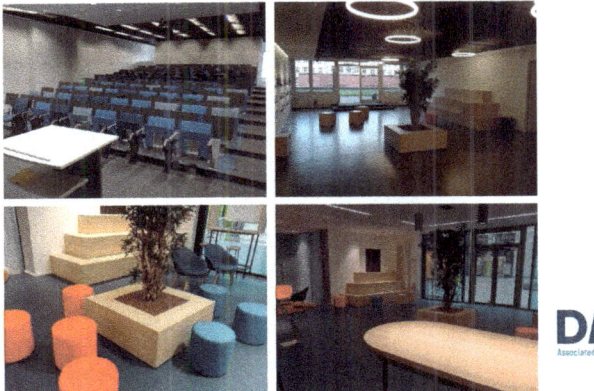
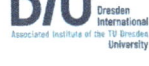

Figure 2. On-site teaching and learning spaces at Dresden International University.

3.1.1. Single Point of Truth for a Highly Effective Organization of the Master Program

All relevant information for the organizational management of the study program is available on one single data platform (example view in Figure 3). This includes, for example, all study documents, timetables, applications, forms, support information, step-by-step instructions, relevant literature, etc. The exchange with the program management and the lecturers is chat-based and transparent for all members. This dramatically reduces the effort required for bilateral communication and email.

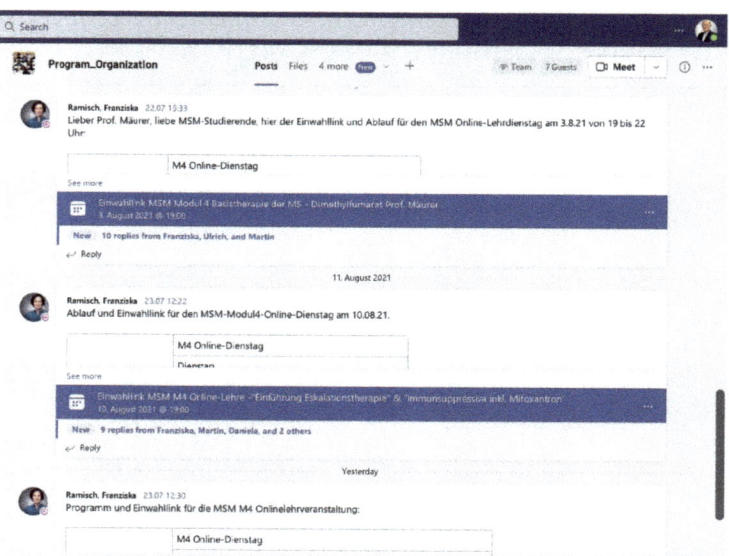

Figure 3. Communication of access information to online events as single point of truth.

3.1.2. Online Classroom in a Remote Learning Environment for Synchronous and Self-Directed Asynchronous Learning

Students have access to a wide range of tools and resources for remote learning via the digital hub (example view in Figure 4). Lecturers present their content as live lectures and can use functionalities for synchronous learning such as file sharing, various forms of participant feedback and real-time interaction or group workspaces. In addition, all documents for a course are available in chronological order. This gives students the flexibility to study the content at their own pace, at their own time and with their own device (asynchronous learning).

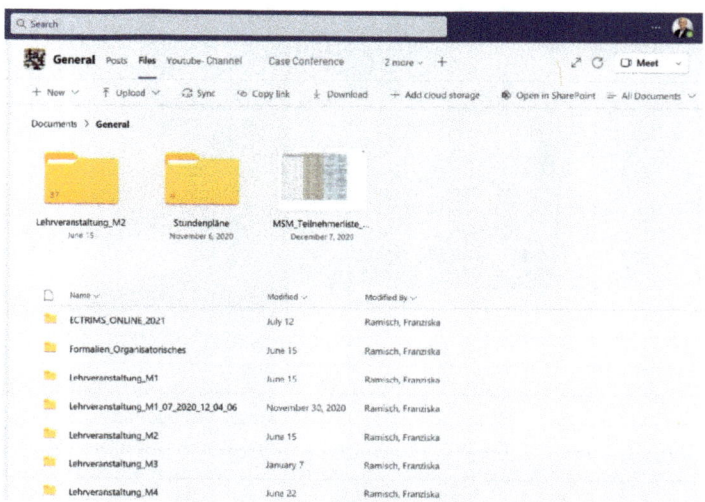

Figure 4. Learning modules that fit into vocational qualification.

3.1.3. Flexible Knowledge Transfer in the Learning Video Portal

The digital hub allows synchronous lessons, lectures and events to be held in special channels and to securely share and interact on video content from presentations. Microsoft Stream, the video service from Microsoft Teams [18], makes it possible to create live lectures, record them automatically and make them available regardless of location and time. The app simplifies uploading, organizing, and sharing video content across the Master's program. Students call up the recording of a missed learning session or recall session at a time of their choice in the video portal (Figure 5).

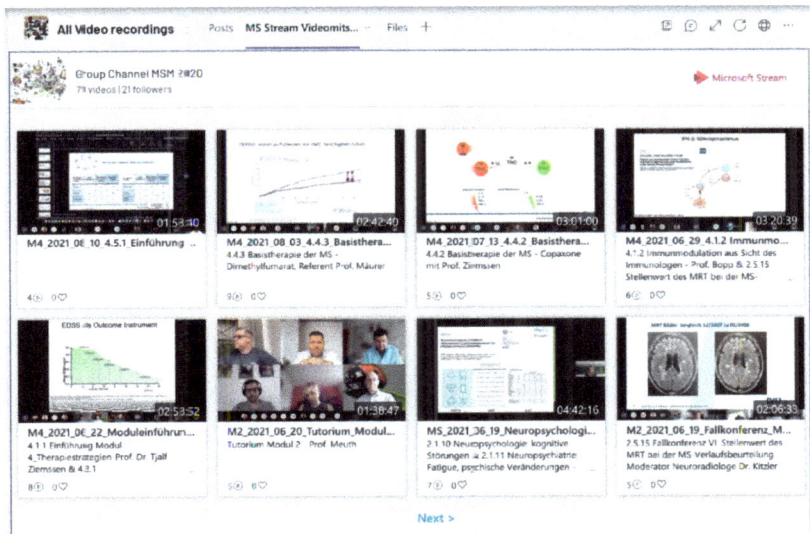

Figure 5. Live streaming and video on demand portal.

3.1.4. Set up of Special Learning Areas for Peer-to-Peer Learning

Joint activity learning areas are presented in an organized, structured, and consistent manner. In the MSM master's program, there are two light house examples of how specific learning areas can be established: case conferences and journal clubs. In the case conference students present their own case or—if they do not have patient contact—a published case to the lecturers and the other students (peer-to-peer-learning). In journal clubs, they discuss professional articles and several students can participate in analyzing a single article. In this process, participants discuss all articles according to fixed criteria: background, method, results, discussion and conclusion. The case conferences and journal clubs are organized using the wiki functionality in Microsoft Teams (Figure 6). Students autonomously enter their contributions into the given schedule grid and provide the information to be presented online. These approaches also allow lecturers to assess students' learning and experience more deeply regarding their areas of interest.

Since the start of the course, the platform has been used regularly by the students and the amount of learning content is continuously growing. In the future, exams will also take place on the digital hub and the lecturers will use the digital hub to supervise the preparation of master's theses.

3.2. Evaluation of Student's Feedback

3.2.1. Participants

Most of the 19 participants (89%) in the first matriculation of the Master's program are physicians with advanced training in neurology, but there are also biologists. Slightly more than half (53%) of the 19 students are women, which means that there is a balanced gender ratio. Students are on average 39.4 ± 8.9 years old, ranging from 28 to 60 years.

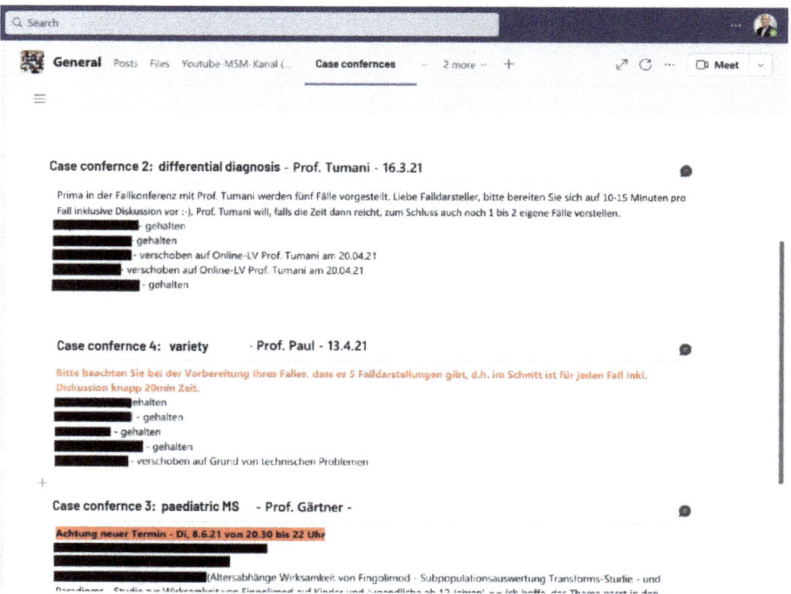

Figure 6. Students work and learn on a project basis.

Four students gave very detailed feedback on module 1. For module 2, the participants of the study program evaluated a total of 36 courses with regard to content, structure, and set-up of the course, with regard to the lecturer, methodological aspects, and quality and use of course materials. Response rates ranged from 16% to 84%, meaning that not all course participants always rated each single course. Since the master's program is currently still running and not all modules have been completed or started, not all modules could be evaluated yet.

3.2.2. Evaluation Survey

Four students gave detailed feedback on module 1 with 55 statements. There were 24 statements on the aggregated dimensions "Communicative and didactic quality of teaching" and 15 statements on the topic "Difficulties in studying". For example, students praised the "communicative and didactic quality of teaching": "In my opinion, everyone was a real asset in their own way and I found the often very different presentations and lectures very good throughout.", and the interactivity: "The highlight of module 1 for me was the opportunity for interaction". "Difficulties in studying" were addressed by two students and included, in particular, the large amount of time needed to rework the learning materials for certain groups of participants with non-medical backgrounds: "Especially for me as a non-neurologist, the module was also a good introduction; but also demanding and a lot of reworks was needed." Other statement dimensions related to the quality of teaching and the provision as well as the practical or research relevance of the content, the commitment of the university and the lecturers to the students, the organization of teaching and the examination system were rated positively overall.

In module 2, students evaluated 36 lectures (status: May 2021). They rated all evaluation categories with a mean of 1.2 or 1.3, indicating strong or certain agreement with the respective items, which the authors interpret as high satisfaction with the respective topic. Means and standard deviations for evaluation categories are presented in Table 3.

Table 3. Average score of satisfaction.

Category	Mean ± Standard Deviation
Content, structure and organization of the event	1.35 ± 0.80
Lecturer	1.28 ± 0.75
Methodical aspects	1.33 ± 0.79
Documents, course materials and media: design and use	1.29 ± 0.70
Technical support for online events	1.18 ± 0.44

In the category "content, structure and organization of the event", the students gave strong to certain agreement that the objectives of the event were clearly recognizable (1.26 ± 0.74) and that the content structure ("red thread") of the overall event was sensible (1.32 ± 0.77), as well as that the event time was used in a way that promoted learning (1.37 ± 0.81). For the students, the relevance of the content covered for practice became clear (1.31 ± 0.75) and they were able to contribute their personal competencies and previous experience appropriately (1.47 ± 1.01). In category "lecturer" the students gave strong to certain agreement that the lecturer has stimulated the discussion of the topics (1.27 ± 0.74), emphasized active participation of the students (1.37 ± 0.89), succeeded in making the event appealing (1.31 ± 0.76) and was appreciative in dealing with students (1.15 ± 0.56). The students also rated the "methodical aspects" very highly. They gave strong to certain agreement, that teaching/learning forms (individual, partner, group work, work in plenary) were appropriate (1.42 ± 0.86) that the lecturer was able to present complex content in an understandable way (1.27 ± 0.72) and gave appropriate feedback or responded appropriately to the group (1.32 ± 0.79). The quality of the media content (presentations, scripts, exercise sheets, e-lectures, etc.) was appropriate (1.32 ± 0.71) and the media and (online) tools used were used sensibly (1.27 ± 0.69)—students gave strong to certain agreement to these items in category "documents, course materials and media: design and use". Finally, students rated positively the aspects of "technical support of the online events"—they gave strong to certain agreement with the items satisfaction with technical support (1.09 ± 0.31) and supervision during the courses (1.21 ± 0.43), and the suitability of the virtual classroom for the course (1.26 ± 0.54).

Figure 7 shows the proportions of agreement in a stacked bar graph, clearly showing the large proportions of strong and certain agreement with the items. A percentage of 75% to 85% of students strongly agreed with each item, indicating a high level of student satisfaction with the implementation of module 2.

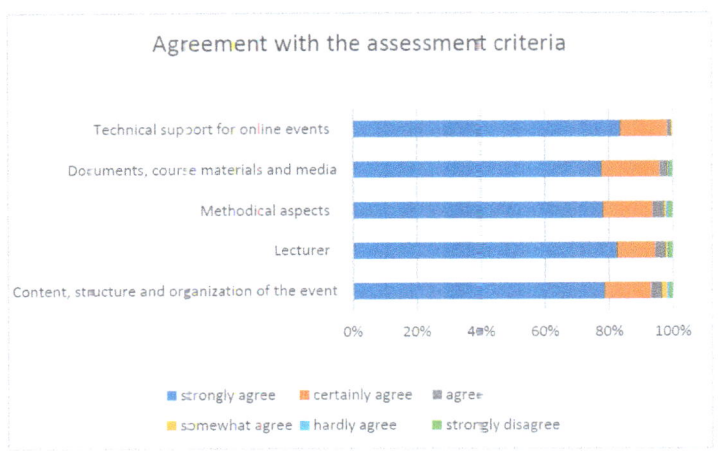

Figure 7. Proportions of satisfaction with the implementation of module 2.

In the free text ratings, the students gave a lot of praise regarding the content and the competence of the lecturers, e.g., "extremely exciting topic", "broad coverage of the subject", "very interesting, practice-oriented presentation of the clinical pictures" or "Prof. XY gave a very clear and comprehensible lecture with many good examples" and "Prof. XY managed to give an exciting and very informative lecture and at the same time to emphasize the relevance of this topic, which is rather neglected in the neurological study of MS". However, the students also criticized the speed of presentation and comprehensibility: "the topics of motor disorders and pain in MS came far too short", "very fast pace in the presentation of some studies", "unfortunately, the lecture was very technical and not very didactically prepared" or "The breakdown of the technical approach to the students' world of understanding is only partially successful". The students also made suggestions for improving the quality of the course as well as the performance of the lecturer, exemplified by the following: "the questions asked in between were good, could be made interactive and use the 'mentimeter' [app for real-time feedback] for example", "The material should be distributed over two lectures or another lecture [...] should be planned", and "It would be nice for future years of study (not possible this time due to Corona) to hold tutorials in a classroom context in order to further promote active engagement with the topic and especially the exchange in the group".

4. Discussion

This paper explored the innovative use of a cloud-based digital hub for computer-supported collaborative learning in the MSM master's program as well as student evaluation of the first semester of the master's program, considering the challenges of the COVID-19 pandemic.

Since the MSM master's program is aimed at professionals in neurology, it was planned from the beginning with a strong online component. Due to the start of the master's program in the midst of the COVID-19 pandemic, the organizers had to very quickly adjust the teaching formats towards even more online courses. In a short time, DIU succeeded in establishing Microsoft Teams as a cloud-based digital hub and technical basis as well as a central teaching, learning, communication and cooperation platform, which proved to be very effective. The centralized data platform served the highly efficient organization of the master's program. Thus, online classrooms were available in a distance learning environment for synchronous and self-paced asynchronous learning. The establishment of a learning video portal and special learning areas for peer-to-peer learning made flexible knowledge transfer possible. However, this master's program benefited from digitization not only in learning and teaching, but also through the opportunities for close coordination between the lecturers and the course management with the academic management and module coordinators, as well as among the students themselves.

For the first two modules of the program, the authors collected student feedback and analyzed it both qualitatively and quantitatively. The students rated the courses in the modules and the modules as a whole as good to very good. They were very satisfied with the content of the courses, with the knowledge transfer by the lecturers and with the interaction with each other, as well as with the lecturers. Some of the students wished for more time for certain topics, more interaction with lecturers and would have liked to have covered some specific topics such as magnetic resonance imaging (MRI) on-site in a face-to-face event. Such face-to-face events were also planned, but due to the circumstances of the COVID-19 pandemic, they could only be held as online events.

Nevertheless, authors indicate some limitations in the interpretation of the results. For example, there is a relatively small underlying response rate for individual courses, which is unfavorable for evaluation given the already small number of participants in the program. However, it is important to keep in mind that the evaluation of the courses and modules also took place under pandemic conditions, and students' ambitions to evaluate the courses online may not have been as high after a day full of online events. It should also be noted that the evaluation of the first two modules is only part of the evaluation of the program. The evaluation of the other modules and the entire master's program by the students is still pending. In addition, there is no comparative data on student satisfaction with the quality of the master's program under "normal conditions" because it was not implemented in the period before the COVID-19 pandemic. Therefore, whether this master's program will improve MS therapy and make a valuable contribution to the scientific advancement of the entire MS field remains to be seen.

The present work shows that, despite the aforementioned challenges, the MSM master's program is proving to be a great success, not least because of the fruitful interactions between lecturers and students. In addition, there are a few learnings that will promptly inform further implementation of the program.

Only the widespread use of digitization and digital tools made it possible to respond quickly to the imposed changes in the face of the COVID-19 pandemic and to effectively implement adjustments and necessary rescheduling. Above all, however, the "emergency mode" provided many insights and hints into the future "new normal". The pandemic showed the limitations of a traditional "bricks and mortar" university and highlighted the growing importance of using online tools. At the same time the value of a physical place for learning and teaching became very clear. On-site learning in presence will have in future a very special quality and will be of particularly high value. Certainly, the planned on-site portions of the program in specialized clinical settings or active participation in expert meetings will help open new perspectives for students [19]. By using digital tools a new format has gained more attention: the "flipped classroom", where the students actively work on the contents during the knowledge transfer stage before interacting with the lecturers and peers where they assimilate what they have read, watched or otherwise attempted [20–22].

The use cases for computer-based collaborative learning implemented in the first two modules of the master's program will be expanded and applied in the remaining modules. The digital implementation of the MSM master's program enables a "learning study program" using a rapid implementation of the PDCA (Plan–Do–Check–Act) cycle. Agility as one of the important current megatrends thus offers a high practical value for the MSM master's program.

As a further learning, lecturers are encouraged to use less of a pure presentation style to deliver content, and to interact and share even more with students at eye level. New competencies for the lecturers in developing attractive didactic formats are required as well as a new understanding of the role of module coordinators in the digital world are necessary: An important lesson learned is that when the MSM master's program is carried out digitally, there is a special requirement for the module to be accompanied by a person as a learning coordinator responsible for the module. As learning coordinators, they are tasked with guiding adults in their professional development.

5. Conclusions

Although the MSM master's program was launched under pandemic conditions and the associated challenges, it was and still is possible to design, implement and continuously adapt a completely new, disease-centered study program thanks to a flexible online platform. Student response and feedback to date demonstrate both the high quality of the program and the potential of the Master's program to make an important contribution to the MS field.

Based on this extremely positive experience, an internationalization of the program is planned to allow neurologists and other interested parties from other countries to access this high-quality Master's program. The program will then be offered in English. Another idea for the future is to build a video platform for the public for knowledge around the MS. In addition, new opportunities for content, technical and didactic improvement as well as new digital developments are to be constantly used to further develop the Master's program. This also includes the technology of the digital twin, which will find its way more and more into patient care in the coming years. For MS patients, the digital twin is an important step towards innovative and individual disease management. A digital twin for MS is a digital image of the MS patient—paired with the patient's characteristics, it allows health care professionals to process large amounts of patient data. This can contribute to more personalized and effective care by integrating data from different sources in a standardized way, implementing individualized clinical pathways, supporting doctor–patient communication and facilitating shared decision making [23].

Author Contributions: Conceptualization, I.V., T.Z., R.H.W.F. and J.N.; methodology, F.R. and R.H.W.F.; formal analysis, I.V. and J.N.; writing—original draft preparation, I.V., F.R., R.H.W.F., J.N. and T.Z.; writing—review and editing, I.V., C.S., S.G.M., F.R., R.H.W.F., J.N. and T.Z.; supervision, T.Z.; project administration, F.R. All authors have read and agreed to the published version of the manuscript.

Funding: This research received no external funding.

Institutional Review Board Statement: Ethical review and approval were waived for this study according to local legislation and national guidelines.

Informed Consent Statement: Patient consent was waived, as the data used in this paper originate from the standardized quality management system of the university and have been processed in accordance with data protection regulations.

Data Availability Statement: The data presented in this study are available on reasonable request from the corresponding author.

Acknowledgments: We thank all MSM lecturers and students as well as MSM supporters and the DIU team.

Conflicts of Interest: I.V. and C.S. declare no conflict of interest. S.M. received lecture fees and travel expenses for attending meetings from Almirall, Amicus Therapeutics Germany, Bayer Health Care, Biogen, Celgene, Diamed, Genzyme, MedDay Pharmaceuticals, Merck Serono, Novartis, Novo Nordisk, ONO Pharma, Roche, Sanofi- Aventis, Chugai Pharma, QuintilesIMS and Teva. He received research grants from: Bundesministerium für Bildung und Forschung (BMBF), Deutsche Forschungsgesellschaft (DFG), Else-Kröner-Fresenius-Stiftung, Deutscher Akademischer Austauschdienst, Hertie Stiftung, Interdisziplinäres Zentrum für Klinische Forschung (IZKF) Münster, Deutsche Stiftung Neurologie und Almirall, Amicus Therapeutics Germany, Biogen, Diamed, Fresenius Medical Care, Genzyme, Merck Serono, Novartis, ONO Pharma, Roche and Teva. R.H.W.F., F.R. and J.N. are members of the DIU, which hosts the program. T.Z. received personal compensation from Biogen, Bayer, Celgene, Novartis, Roche, Sanofi and Teva for consulting services and additional financial support for the research activities from Bayer, BAT, Biogen, Novartis, Teva and Sanofi.

References

1. Giovannoni, G. Disease-modifying treatments for early and advanced multiple sclerosis: A new treatment paradigm. *Curr. Opin. Neurol.* **2018**, *31*, 233–243. [CrossRef] [PubMed]
2. Multiple Sklerose Management (M.Sc.). Available online: https://www.di-uni.de/studium-weiterbildung/medizin/ms-management (accessed on 23 July 2021).
3. Postgraduate Study: Neuroscience and Neurodegeneration. Available online: https://www.sheffield.ac.uk/postgraduate/taught/courses/2021/neuroscience-and-neurodegeneration-msc?utm_source=findamasters&utm_campaign=courseid[56921]&utm_medium=featcourselisting&utm_content=button (accessed on 23 July 2021).
4. Master in Neuroimmunology 2021. Available online: https://www.cem-cat.org/en/corse/master-neuroimmunology (accessed on 23 July 2021).
5. MAS Neurophysiotherapie—Fachexperte/Fachexpertin in Multiple Sklerose, Morbus Parkinson und Stroke. Available online: https://advancedstudies.unibas.ch/studienangebot/kurs/mas-neurophysiotherapie--fachexpertefachexpertin-in-multiple-sklerose-morbus-parkinson-und-stroke-206474 (accessed on 23 July 2021).
6. MS-Schwester/MS-Therapiemanagement: DMSG Fachfortbildung für 'MS-Schwestern'. Available online: https://www.dmsg.de/service/fachfortbildungen/ms-schwester/ (accessed on 23 July 2021).
7. The British MS Healthcare Professionals Society. Available online: https://neurologyacademy.org/ms-academy (accessed on 23 July 2021).
8. Abrahamsson, S.; Dávila López, M. Comparison of online learning designs during the COVID-19 pandemic within bioinformatics courses in higher education. *Bioinformatics* **2021**, *37*, i9–i15. [CrossRef] [PubMed]

9. Brown, A.; Kassam, A.; Paget, M.; Blades, K.; Mercia, M.; Kachra, R. Exploring the global impact of the COVID-19 pandemic on medical education: An international cross-sectional study of medical learners. *Can. Med. Educ. J.* **2021**, *12*, 28–43. [CrossRef] [PubMed]
10. Gherheș, V.; Stoian, C.E.; Fărcașiu, M.A.; Stanici, M. E-Learning vs. Face-To-Face Learning: Analyzing Students' Preferences and Behaviors. *Sustainability* **2021**, *13*, 4381. [CrossRef]
11. Langegård, U.; Kiani, K.; Nielsen, S.J.; Svensson, P.-A. Nursing students' experiences of a pedagogical transition from campus learning to distance learning using digital tools. *BMC Nurs.* **2021**, *20*, 23. [CrossRef]
12. Paechter, M.; Maier, B. Online or face-to-face? Students' experiences and preferences in e-learning. *Internet High. Educ.* **2010**, *13*, 292–297. [CrossRef]
13. Simamora, R.M. The Challenges of Online Learning during the COVID-19 Pandemic: An Essay Analysis of Performing Arts Education Students. *Stud. Learn. Teach.* **2020**, *1*, 86–103. [CrossRef]
14. Martin, L.; Tapp, D. Teaching with Teams: An introduction to teaching an undergraduate law module using Microsoft Teams. *Innov. Pract. High. Educ.* **2019**, *3*, 58–66.
15. Poston, J.; Apostel, S.; Richardson, K. Using Microsoft Teams to Enhance Engagement and Learning with Any Class: It's Fun and Easy. *Pedagog. Conf. Proc.* **2020**, *6*, 1–7.
16. Dresden International University: Mission, Vision & Goals. Available online: https://www.di-uni.de/en/the-university/mission-vision-and-goals (accessed on 23 July 2021).
17. Gioia, D.A.; Corley, K.G.; Hamilton, A.L. Seeking Qualitative Rigor in Inductive Research: Notes on the Gioia Methodology. *Organ. Res. Methods* **2012**, *16*, 15–31. [CrossRef]
18. Microsoft. Set Up for Live Evetns in Microsoft Teams. Available online: https://docs.microsoft.com/en-us/microsoftteams/teams-live-events/set-up-for-teams-live-events (accessed on 16 August 2021).
19. Watson, J.F. *Blended Learning: The Convergence of Online and Face-to-Face Education. Promising Practices in Online Learning*; ERIC Number: ED509636; North American Council for Online Learning: Washington, DC, USA, 2008.
20. Al Mamun, M.A.; Azad, M.A.K.; Al Mamun, M.A.; Boyle, M. Review of flipped learning in engineering education: Scientific mapping and research horizon. *Educ. Inf. Technol* **2021**. [CrossRef] [PubMed]
21. Bingen, H.M.; Steindal, S.A.; Krumsvik, R.; Tveit. B. Nursing students studying physiology within a flipped classroom, self-regulation and off-campus activities. *Nurse Educ. Pract.* **2019**, *35*, 55–62. [CrossRef] [PubMed]
22. Khan, M.S.H.; Abdou, B.O. Flipped classroom: How higher education institutions (HEIs) of Bangladesh could move forward during COVID-19 pandemic. *Soc. Sci. Humanit. Open* **2021**, *4*, 100187. [CrossRef] [PubMed]
23. Voigt, I.; Inojosa, H.; Dillenseger, A.; Haase, R.; Akgün, K.; Ziemssen, T. Digital Twins for Multiple Sclerosis. *Front. Immunol.* **2021**, *12*, 669811. [CrossRef] [PubMed]

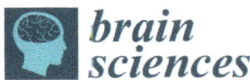

Review

A Mobile App for Measuring Real Time Fatigue in Patients with Multiple Sclerosis: Introducing the Fimo Health App

Jana Mäcken [1,*], Marie Wiegand [2], Mathias Müller [3], Alexander Krawinkel [3] and Michael Linnebank [4,5]

1. Department of Health Economics and Clinical Epidemiology, University Hospital Cologne, 50935 Cologne, Germany
2. Department of Psychology, University of Cologne, 50923 Cologne, Germany; marie.wiegand@outlook.ce
3. Fimo Health, 50827 Koln, Germany; mathias.muller@fimo.io (M.M.); Alexander.krawinkel@fimo.io (A.K.)
4. Evangelische Kliniken Gelsenkirchen, 45879 Gelsenkirchen, Germany; linnebank@evk-ge.de
5. Faculty of Health, University Witten/Herdecke, 58455 Witten, Germany
* Correspondence: maecken@wiso.uni-koeln.de

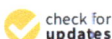

Citation: Mäcken, J.; Wiegand, M.; Müller, M.; Krawinkel, A.; Linnebank, M. A Mobile App for Measuring Real Time Fatigue in Patients with Multiple Sclerosis: Introducing the Fimo Health App. *Brain Sci.* **2021**, *11*, 1235. https://doi.org/10.3390/brainsci11091235

Academic Editors: Tjalf Ziemssen and Rocco Haase

Received: 30 July 2021
Accepted: 15 September 2021
Published: 18 September 2021

Publisher's Note: MDPI stays neutral with regard to jurisdictional claims in published maps and institutional affiliations.

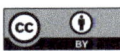

Copyright: © 2021 by the authors. Licensee MDPI, Basel, Switzerland. This article is an open access article distributed under the terms and conditions of the Creative Commons Attribution (CC BY) license (https://creativecommons.org/licenses/by/4.0/).

Abstract: Although fatigue is one of the most disabling symptoms of MS, its pathogenesis is not well understood yet. This study aims to introduce a new holistic approach to measure fatigue and its influencing factors via a mobile app. Fatigue is measured with different patient-reported outcome measures (Visual Analog Scale, Fatigue Severity Scale) and tests (Symbol Digit Modalities Test). The influencing vital and environmental factors are captured with a smartwatch and phone sensors. Patients can track these factors within the app. To individually counteract their fatigue, a fatigue course, based on the current treatment guidelines, was implemented. The course implies knowledge about fatigue and MS, exercises, energy-conservation management, and cognitive behavioral therapy. Based on the Transtheoretical Model of Behavior Change, the design of the Fimo health app follows the ten strategies of the process of change, which is a proven approach to designing health intervention programs. By monitoring fatigue and individual influencing factors, patients can better understand and manage their fatigue. They can share their data and insights about fatigue and its influencing factors with their doctors. Thus, they can receive individualized therapies and drug plans.

Keywords: fatigue; multiple sclerosis; mHealth; intervention; mobile application

1. Introduction

Worldwide, more than 2.3 million people suffer from multiple sclerosis (MS); thus, it is one of the world's most common neurological diseases [1]. MS is a neurodegenerative disorder of the central nervous system affecting young and middle-aged people and is known to cause a variety of clinical symptoms such as neurological impairments, pain, and fatigue [2]. Fatigue can be defined as "a subjective lack of physical and/or mental energy that is perceived by the individual or caregiver to interfere with usual or desired activity" [3]. People living with MS (pwMS) describe fatigue as one of the most disabling symptoms, as it impacts daily living, leisure activities, and work, and reduces the quality of life [4]. Moreover, it is the main reason for early retirement among pwMS and, consequently, a burden for social security systems [5].

The pathogenesis of MS-related fatigue is not well understood yet [6]. Nevertheless, two types of fatigue can be distinguished: Primary fatigue arises directly from the disease mechanisms of MS, such as demyelination, inflammation, or axonal loss. Secondary fatigue, on the other hand, is the consequence of sleep problems, pain, medication, or deconditioning [7]. The National Multiple Sclerosis Society (2021) identified ten secondary causes that contribute to the severity of fatigue: stress, mood disorders such as depression or anxiety, poor diet, comorbidities, sleep disorders, nocturia, pain and spasticity, decreased physical activity/muscle weakness and deconditioning, environmental factors, and side effects from medication [8]. Due to its multifaceted origins and complexity, fatigue is difficult to treat [7]. Treatment recommendations suggest addressing secondary contributing factors first [8]. Although in some cases, disease-modifying drugs can be an effective solution for special cases of fatigue, fatigue is not clearly understood yet [9]. However, fatigue is highly individual, as these factors vary between patients. Meta-analyses support the benefit of non-pharmacological interventions, whereas the evidence regarding pharmacological treatments is not conclusive [10,11]. Energy-conservation management, exercising, and cognitive behavioral therapy were especially able to significantly reduce fatigue—up to 30% [12,13]. However, these interventions could be even more effective after taking the individual influencing factors of pwMS into account.

This study aims to introduce a new holistic approach to measure fatigue and the influencing factors via a mobile app. The objective of the Fimo health app is to help pwMS treat their fatigue. In the first step, fatigue and the influencing factors are measured. This information helps pwMS and their physicians to better understand the occurrence of fatigue and enable more tailored interventions. To individually counteract their fatigue, pwMS also have the opportunity to engage in a fatigue course. The course provides knowledge about fatigue and MS, exercises, energy-conservation management, and cognitive behavioral therapy.

The approach of the Fimo health app is based on the transtheoretical model of behavior change, which will be broadly introduced. The design of the app follows the ten strategies of the process of change, which is a proven approach in the design of health intervention programs. Each step and its implementation in the Fimo health app is explained. The discussion summarizes the current state of the art and its advantages for physicians.

2. Measuring Fatigue

Fatigue is, due to its multifaceted origins and complexity, difficult to capture [7]. However, two types of measures for fatigue can be distinguished: patient-reported outcome measures and measures of changes in motor or cognitive functions. Patient-reported outcome measures capture fatigue as a subjective symptom by addressing patients to rate their fatigue or different aspects of it. Performance-based measures, on the other hand, measure fatigue more objectively, e.g., based on the decline of cognitive processing speed [14]. Both types of measures are used to detect fatigue within the Fimo health app.

2.1. Patient-Reported Outcome Measures

Different patient-reported outcome measures are used to measure fatigue. The visual analog scale (VAS) is used to detect fatigue three times, or every four hours, during waking hours (Figure 1). PwMS have the option to set a reminder to register their VAS. PwMS are asked to rate their current level of fatigue on a scale from 0 to 10, whereby higher levels indicate more fatigue. Previous research showed that a very high correlation between VAS measurements and a series of drawings of faces with expressions of increasing distress [6,15]. Answering the VAS takes only a couple of seconds and has been shown to be a valid tool to measure fatigue among pwMS [16].

Besides the VAS, the Fatigue Severity Scale (FSS) is also used to detect fatigue [17]. The FSS is a nine-item instrument designed to assess fatigue as a symptom of several chronic conditions, including MS. PwMS answer the FSS once a week to detect long-term changes. The FSS has demonstrated good internal consistency, reliability, and validity [18]. Moreover, the Chalder Fatigue Scale is implemented, as it has shown to be more sensitive to change compared to the FSS [19]. The Chalder Fatigue Scale consists of eleven items covering physical and mental fatigue, and pwMS are asked to answer the questionnaire once a week. The completion of the Chalder Fatigue Scale only takes 2–3 min and has been validated among pwMS [20,21].

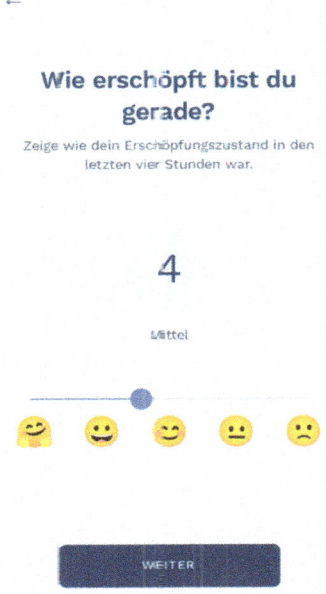

Figure 1. The VAS implemented in the Fimo health app

2.2. Performance-Based Measures for Fatigue

Fatigue correlates with declines in processing speed, reaction time, and/or accuracy over time, which are measured in different tests [22]. Performance-based tests capture the decline, thus measuring fatigue more objectively compared to self-reports. Among pwMS, the Symbol Digit Modalities Test (SDMT) is widely used to test cognitive declines in processing speed and has been proven to be valid and reliable [23]. During the 90 s assessment, pwMS are asked to sort nine numbers to different symbols according to the number. The score is the number of correct symbols. The SDMT was tested to be valid in a mobile and longitudinal setting with tests every three days [24]. Within the Fimo health app, pwMS are therefore asked to answer the test every three days.

2.3. Measuring Influencing Factors

Previous research identified several factors influencing fatigue, such as stress, mood disorders including depression or anxiety, poor diet, comorbidities, sleep disorders, nocturia, pain and spasticity, decreased physical activity or muscle weakness and deconditioning, environmental factors (temperature, humidity, light), and side effects from medication [8]. The vital parameters heart rate, stress level, steps, and sleep are measured with Garmin devices and are displayed within the Fimo health app.

The environmental factors temperature, humidity, light, and noise are captured by using the GPS location. Within the Fimo health app, users have the option to display the parameters and set them in relation to their individual fatigue level. All data are stored on German servers and anonymized in accordance with GDPR compliance.

3. Transtheoretical Model of Health Behavior Change

The transtheoretical model (TTM) of health behavior change is a dynamic model consisting of different stages of change and integrated processes and principles of inteventions depending on individuals' readiness to act on a new healthier behavior [25]. Six stages of health behavior change, based on people's motivation, can be distinguished:

1. Precontemplation: people are not ready and do not intend to take action;
2. Contemplation: people are beginning to realize that their behavior is problematic;
3. Preparation: people are ready to take action in the immediate future;
4. Action: people take action and modify their health behaviors;
5. Maintenance: people sustain their actions over a longer period;
6. Termination: people do not have the temptation to switch back to old behaviors.

While moving through these stages, people apply different strategies and techniques, depending on their motivation and goals. These processes result in strategies that help people make and maintain change. These strategies and techniques are summarized as the ten processes of change, with some processes being more relevant to a specific stage of change than others [26]. These ten processes can be divided into inner cognitive-affective processes on the one hand and behavioral processes on the other hand. They are based on several major theories of intervention describing key ways in which people change their behaviors [27]. The TTM has been applied successfully in energy conservation and exercise programs for pwMS in previous research [28,29].

Other Behavior Change Techniques

Alongside the TTM, we implemented various concrete health behavior change techniques extracted from the Taxonomy of Behavior Change Techniques by Abraham and Michie [30]. We combined the techniques to "provide information about behavior-health link", (i.e., general information about behavioral risk—for example, susceptibility to poor health outcomes or mortality risk in relation to the behavior) with "prompt intention formation" (i.e., encouraging the person to decide to act or set a general goal). This combination has been shown to be particularly effective in mHealth apps for mental and physical health [31]. For prompting intention formation, pwMS are asked to formulate SMART goals. The SMART technique is used to ensure that goals are specific, measurable, attainable, relevant, and timely. Additionally, basic gamification elements—for instance, collecting points based on the participation in the fatigue course, rewards for daily usage, a point system for activity within the app, and weekly reports—are implemented.

4. Overview of the Fatigue Course

The Fimo fatigue course consists of eight weekly modules, which consist of individual daily chapters based on the current treatment guidelines [32]. The topics of the chapters can be divided into four main topics: basic knowledge about MS and fatigue, dealing with difficult emotions, exercises and energy-conservation management (Figure 2). Several studies and meta-analyses showed that these measures were most effective in treating fatigue among pwMS [10,33–35]. The selection of the topics is based on a systematic literature review on exercise and behavioral interventions for pwMS suffering from fatigue. Covering studies between 2006 and 2021, 467 studies were identified. After removing duplicates and excluding studies based on the exclusion criteria (no RCT, wrong type of intervention, non-MS sample, or no self-reported fatigue measure), 31 articles were included. Moreover, the design of the course was discussed through expert interviews with four neurologists. Additionally, a patient board was introduced to measure and improve the user experience of pwMS.

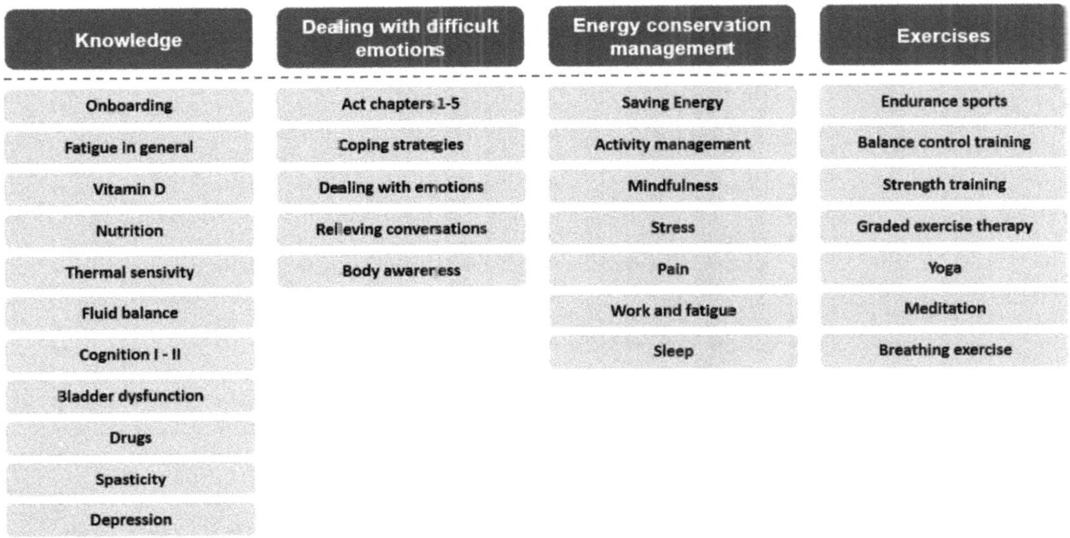

Knowledge	Dealing with difficult emotions	Energy conservation management	Exercises
Onboarding	Act chapters 1-5	Saving Energy	Endurance sports
Fatigue in general	Coping strategies	Activity management	Balance control training
Vitamin D	Dealing with emotions	Mindfulness	Strength training
Nutrition	Relieving conversations	Stress	Graded exercise therapy
Thermal sensitivity	Body awareness	Pain	Yoga
Fluid balance		Work and fatigue	Meditation
Cognition I - II		Sleep	Breathing exercise
Bladder dysfunction			
Drugs			
Spasticity			
Depression			

Figure 2. Overview of the Fimo fatigue course.

Different exercises are applied to treat fatigue and range from endurance sports, such as running, balance, strength, and aerobic exercises, to yoga. These exercises are explained in short videos, and pwMS can choose to complete the exercises that suit them most. The knowledge about MS and fatigue covers several relevant topics that are presented in an interactive way that includes dialogues, texts, graphics, and videos. The energy-conservation management section contains information and practical tips on how to structure daily routines to save energy. The content of the topic dealing with emotions and feelings is based on Acceptance and Commitment Therapy (ACT) [36], which is a psychotherapeutic approach that originated from Cognitive Behavioral Therapy (CBT). It combines classical behavior-therapy-oriented approaches with acceptance- and mindfulness-based techniques. Positive effects of ACT on fatigue among pwMS have been shown in previous research [37,38]. ACT techniques aim at psychological flexibility, which is described as being able to fully contact the present moment while acting in line with personal values [39]. The overarching goal is hence not a reduction of (physical) symptoms but an increase in the quality of life [40].

Specific ACT chapters were implemented in the fatigue course at several points. The four main topics concerning basic knowledge about MS and fatigue, how to deal with emotions and feelings, exercising with fatigue, and energy-conservation management are also to be found throughout the eight modules, repetitively.

Ten Processes of Change within the Fatigue Course

The content of the Fimo fatigue course addresses the ten steps of the TTM. Meta-analyses showed greater effects in programs that are tailored to the ten steps of the transtheoretical model [41]. Thus, the fatigue course within the Fimo health app is designed on the ten processes of change to help pwMS to counteract their fatigue efficiently.

- Step 1: Consciousness raising:

The first step aims at increasing awareness about the causes and consequences of fatigue. This can be accomplished by providing information, education, or personal feedback concerning health behaviors. The fatigue course contains information about fatigue in general, as well as on interventions that have been proven to reduce fatigue, such as aerobic exercises, energy-conservation management, or meditation [11]. Furthermore, the vital and environmental factors are constantly monitored, and pwMS receive feedback on which factors influence their personal fatigue.

- Step 2: Dramatic relief:

In the second step, the experience of increased negative emotions, e.g., fear, anxiety, or worry, that goes along with one's health problems, unhealthy behavior, and self-image, are at focus. It is followed by a reduced effect or anticipated relief if the appropriate action is taken [26]. However, the second step can also be positive if feelings such as inspiration or hope arise when hearing about a new solution or about how other people changed their health behaviors.

PwMS and fatigue particularly tend to struggle with catastrophizing and pressurizing thoughts [38], as well as worries about the future and negative feelings [42]. As these unpleasant inner experiences might be triggered in pwMS within the first chapter, they are provided with information on how to face these feelings in the chapter "dealing with emotions". Practical exercises directly targeting these negative feelings, thoughts, and worries are provided in separate ACT chapters. They enable pwMS to distance themselves from their detrimental thoughts, shift their attention back into the present moment, and cope with difficult emotions. Hence, ACT is perfectly suitable to address the second step of the TTM.

- Step 3: Self-reevaluation:

This step is about realizing that health behavior change is an important part of one's identity. It also involves appraising one's values with respect to problematic behavior and creating a new self-image. Being aware and accepting one's identity in all facets are core processes of ACT. Respective mindfulness exercises support the patients in letting go of their rigid self-image as MS patients and reevaluating their self-image. Moreover, pwMS learn about body-consciousness, how it might have changed due to their illness, and how to gain it back.

- Step 4: Environmental reevaluation:

Step four is about how the presence or absence of a personal behavior affects one's social environment. In the case of fatigue, social relationships might suffer as pwMS are less available. Several chapters of the course address this aspect. PwMS are encouraged to practice gratitude while focusing on their social network in one of the ACT exercises. Moreover, they learn how they can address their social networks and share their sorrows in the chapter "relieving conversations". Moreover, energy-conservation management methods and tips are taught to optimize time allocation and use times without fatigue more efficiently.

- Step 5: Self-liberation:

The self-liberation is both the belief that one can change and the commitment and re-commitment to act on that belief. It is about believing in one's ability to change and making commitments to act on that belief. To encourage pwMS to commit to and increase exercising, a SMART-goal setting is applied at the beginning of the chapters that include exercises. Furthermore, possible barriers which could hinder reaching a goal are identified, and possible solutions are suggested. All methods and interventions applied in the Fimo fatigue course are based on evidence and the clinical guidelines on treating fatigue among pwMS [29]. The effectiveness of the interventions is summarized and shared with the users to encourage changing their health behavior.

As pwMS especially suffer from a reduced quality of life [39], the exercises of the remaining ACT chapters encourage pwMS to identify their personal values and implement these into their daily lives. Thus, they aim to improve their quality of life despite the physical changes that pwMS might have to go through. By developing concrete action plans, these ACT chapters further contribute to the fifth step of self-liberation and commitment.

- Step 6: Social liberation:

    Step 6 is about noticing public support and realizing that society is supportive of healthy behaviors. PwMS learn how to address their networks as well as the workplace. More than 40% of pwMS reduce their numbers of working hours, and 25% retire earlier due to their fatigue [43]. By dealing openly with the illness at work, misunderstandings, such as complaints because of absenteeism, can be reduced, pwMS are likely to experience support from colleagues, and it is easier to accept the fact of a changed workability.

- Step 7: Counterconditioning:

    In step 7, pwMS learn how they can substitute problematic behaviors with healthier behaviors. Several chapters of the course address this step. Within the last ACT chapter, pwMS learn how to identify possible barriers along their way towards healthier behavior as well as how to develop a step-by-step action plan. In the chapters concerning fatigue and daily routines, pwMS learn how to structure their daily routines effectively and improve their sleep and nutrition. Another important factor that has yet to be shown to be effective is stress management [44]. PwMS learn to implement breaks in their daily routines and do breathing exercises. Furthermore, they have the option to track their stress level in the Fimo health app and to analyze and reflect on the situations in which they experience stress.

- Step 8: Stimulus control:

    This step is about removing cues for unhealthy habits and adding prompts for healthier alternatives. This step is addressed by providing the opportunity to track vital and environmental factors that influence fatigue. Thus, the possible causes of fatigue can be identified, and pwMS can modify their health behavior to tackle fatigue. PwMS can adjust their routines and implement, for example, mindfulness and/or exercises in their daily schedules, at whatever the best time is, based on their fatigue levels. Additionally, pwMS have the option to set reminders for exercising.

- Step 9: Contingency management:

    Step 9 involves providing consequences for taking steps in a particular direction by rewarding continued healthy behavior. PwMS have the option to self-monitor their behavior based on the vital parameters measured and displayed in the app. Based on the activity measure, they can check if they have reached their exercising goal or, for example, if their stress levels decreased after applying mindfulness exercises over some time. Furthermore, gamification elements are implemented within the Fimo fatigue course, and pwMS can collect points based on their participation within the course as an additional motivation.

- Step 10: Helping relationships:

    In this step, pwMS should find people that are supportive of their change and combine caring, trust, openness, and acceptance of the new behavior. Two modules in the Fimo fatigue course address this step: "relieving conversations" and "work and fatigue". In "relieving conversations", pwMS learn that they can and should accept help from friends and family. PwMS learn to handle feelings, such as being a burden to others because of their disease, and that they can better manage their disease with social support. The chapter "work and fatigue" further contributes to this step by encouraging PwMS to deal openly with the illness at work. Thus, hurdles and misunderstandings, such as complaints because of absenteeism, might be reduced. On the contrary, through open communication with their employer and colleagues, pwMS will probably even experience support in difficult situations.

5. Discussion

The aim of the Fimo health app was to offer a holistic approach for pwMS to tackle fatigue, which is described as one of the most disabling symptoms as it impacts daily living, leisure activities, work and reduces the overall quality of life [4]. Thus, fatigue and the influencing factors are measured within the Fimo health app. To individually counteract fatigue, an eight-week fatigue course based on the current treatment guidelines is implemented [32]. The fatigue course consists of four different pillars covering knowledge about MS and fatigue, dealing with difficult emotions, exercises, and energy-conservation management.

By doing so, the Fimo health app has several advantages for pwMS and physicians. Monitoring fatigue and the influencing factors helps pwMS to better understand and manage their fatigue as they know which factors matter. They can counteract by applying the learned methods according to their individual influencing factors. PwMS have the option to share their data and insights about fatigue and the influencing factors with their doctors, which we strongly advise. Thus, based on the new information, doctors can individualize therapies and drug plans, which would improve the treatment of pwMS substantially. Doctors would receive more objective information about the occurrence of fatigue and could measure the success of therapies. Compared to other solutions, the Fimo health app offers a more holistic approach by measuring fatigue and the influencing factors as well as offering a course.

However, the app also has some current limitations. At the moment, only Garmin devices can be connected. Integrating interfaces from other providers is intended for the future. Moreover, data can only be shared via a PDF export with doctors due to data protection reasons, which makes the implementation in the varied hospital information systems complex. Besides, we are working on a better interplay between our measured data and the fatigue course. In the long run, pwMS should receive recommendations about which exercise would help to reduce their fatigue based on their individual and current influencing factors. However, more data are needed to train the algorithm. The Fimo health app is not on the market yet, as we are in the process of applying for a Digitale Gesundheitsanwendung (DiGA).

Previous research showed that fatigue fluctuates over time and even throughout the day [45,46]. These fluctuations are difficult to capture. Mobile health solutions offer new possibilities, particularly for complex chronic diseases such as MS and fatigue. PwMS are especially suited to adopt mobile health solutions, as they usually show their first symptoms between the ages of 20 and 40 [47]. Hence, the Fimo health app is a useful tool to gain new insight into the occurrence and treatment of fatigue.

Author Contributions: Conceptualization, J.M. and M.W.; methodology, J.M.; writing—original draft preparation, J.M.; writing—review and editing, M.W. and A.K.; visualization, M.M.; supervision, M.L. All authors have read and agreed to the published version of the manuscript.

Funding: This research was funded by Start-up transfer.NRW, grant number FIMO MS App AZ: 2004su030.

Institutional Review Board Statement: Not applicable.

Informed Consent Statement: Not applicable.

Conflicts of Interest: The authors declare no conflict of interest.

References

1. National MS Society. What Is Multiple Sclerosis? 2021. Available online: https://www.nationalmssociety.org/What-is-MS/MS-FAQ-s (accessed on 28 July 2021).
2. Beckerman, H.; Blikman, L.J.; Heine, M.; Malekzadeh, A.; Teunissen, C.E.; Bussmann, J.B.; Kwakkel, G.; Van Meeteren, J.; de Groot, V. The effectiveness of aerobic training, cognitive behavioural therapy, and energy conservation management in treating MS-related fatigue: The design of the TREFAMS-ACE programme. *Trials* **2013**, *14*, 250. [CrossRef] [PubMed]
3. Multiple Sclerosis Council for Clinical Practice Guidelines, Fatigue Guidelines Development Panel of the Multiple Sclerosis Council for Clinical Practice Guidelines. Fatigue and Multiple Sclerosis. In *Evidence—Based Management Strategies for Fatigue in Multiple Sclerosis*; Paralyzed Veterans of America: Washington, DC, USA, 1998.
4. Van den Akker, L.E.; Beckerman, H.; Collette, E.H.; Twisk, J.W.; Bleijenberg, G.; Dekker, J.; Knoop, H.; de Groot, V. Cognitive behavioral therapy positively affects fatigue in patients with multiple sclerosis: Results of a randomized controlled trial. *Mult. Scler.* **2017**, *23*, 1542–1553. [CrossRef] [PubMed]
5. Smith, M.M.; Arnett, P.A. Factors related to employment status changes in individuals with multiple sclerosis. *Mult. Scler. J.* **2005**, *11*, 602–609. [CrossRef] [PubMed]

6. Palotai, M.; Wallack, M.; Kujbus, G.; Dalnoki, A.; Guttmann, C. Usability of a Mobile App for Real-Time Assessment of Fatigue and Related Symptoms in Patients With Multiple Sclerosis: Observational Study. *JMIR mHealth uHealth* **2021**, *9*, e19564. [CrossRef]
7. Langeskov-Christensen, M.; Bisson, E.J.; Finlayson, M.L.; Dalgas, U. Potential pathophysiological pathways that can explain the positive effects of exercise on fatigue in multiple sclerosis: A scoping review. *J. Neurol. Sci.* **2017**, *373*, 307–320. [CrossRef] [PubMed]
8. National MS Society. Fatigue. 2021. Available online: https://www.nationalmssociety.org/For-Professionals/Clinical-Care/Managing-MS/Symptom-Management/Fatigue (accessed on 27 July 2021).
9. Sverrningsson, A.; Falk, E.; Celius, E.G.; Fuchs, S.; Schreiber, K.; Berkö, S.; Sun, J.; Perner, I.K.; Tynergy Trial Investigators. Results from the TYNERGY Trial; A Study in the Real Life Setting. *PLoS ONE* **2013**, *8*, e58643. [CrossRef]
10. Asano, M.; Finlayson, M.L. Meta-Analysis of Three Different Types of Fatigue Management Interventions for People with Multiple Sclerosis: Exercise, Education, and Medication. *Mult. Scler. Int.* **2014**, *2014*, 798285. [CrossRef]
11. Rooney, S.; Moffat, F.; Wood, L.; Paul, L. Effectiveness of fatigue management interventions in reducing severity and impact of fatigue in people with progressive multiple sclerosis: A systematic review. *Int. J. MS Care* **2019**, *21*, 35–46. [CrossRef] [PubMed]
12. Ahmadi, A.; Arastoo, A.A.; Nikbakht, M.; Zahednejad, S.; Rajabpour, M. Comparison of the Effect of 8 weeks Aerobic and Yoga Training on Ambulatory Function, Fatigue and Mood Status in MS Patients. *Iran. Red. Crescent. Med. J.* **2013**, *15*, 449–454. [CrossRef]
13. Razazian, N.; Yavari, Z.; Farnia, V.; Azizi, A.; Kordavani, L.; Bahmani, D.S.; Holsboer-Trachsler, E.; Brand, S. Exercising Impacts on Fatigue, Depression, and Paresthesia in Female Patients with Multiple Sclerosis. *Med. Sci. Sports Exerc.* **2016**, *48*, 796–803. [CrossRef]
14. Krupp, L.B. Fatigue in multiple sclerosis. *CNS Drugs* **2003**, *17*, 225–234. [CrossRef] [PubMed]
15. Fadaeizadeh, L.; Emami, H.; Samiei, K. Comparison of visual analogue scale and faces rating scale in measuring acute postoperative pain. *Arch. Iran. Med.* **2009**, *12*, 73–75.
16. Kos, D.; Nagels, G.; D'Hooghe, M.B.; Duportail, M.; Kerckhofs, E. A rapid screening tool for fatigue impact in multiple sclerosis. *BMC Neurol.* **2006**, *6*, 27. [CrossRef] [PubMed]
17. Krupp, L.B.; LaRocca, N.G.; Muir-Nash, J.; Steinberg, A.D. The fatigue severity scale: Application to patients with multiple sclerosis and systemic lupus erythematosus. *Arch. Neurol.* **1989**, *46*, 1121–1123. [CrossRef] [PubMed]
18. Schwid, S.R.; Covington, M.; Segal, B.M.; Goodman, A.D. Fatigue in multiple sclerosis: Current understanding and future directions. *J. Rehabil. Res. Dev.* **2002**, *39*, 211–224.
19. Rietberg, M.; van Wegen, E.E.H.; Kwakkel, G. Measuring fatigue in patients with multiple sclerosis: Reproducibility, responsiveness and concurrent validity of three Dutch self-report questionnaires. *Disabil. Rehabil.* **2010**, *32*, 1870–1876. [CrossRef]
20. Chilcot, J.; Norton, S.; Kelly, M.E.; Moss-Morris, R. The Chalder Fatigue Questionnaire is a valid and reliable measure of perceived fatigue severity in multiple sclerosis. *Mult. Scler. J.* **2016**, *22*, 677–684. [CrossRef]
21. Braley, T.J.; Chervin, R.D. Fatigue in multiple sclerosis: Mechanisms, evaluation, and treatment. *Sleep* **2010**, *33*, 1061–1067. [CrossRef]
22. Andreasen, A.K.; Spliid, P.E.; Andersen, H.; Jakobsen, J. Fatigue and processing speed are related in multiple sclerosis. *Eur. J. Neurol.* **2010**, *17*, 212–218. [CrossRef]
23. Benedict, R.H.B.; DeLuca, J.; Phillips, G.; LaRocca, N.; Hudson, L.D.; Rudick, R. Validity of the Symbol Digit Modalities Test as a cognition performance outcome measure for multiple sclerosis. *Mult. Scler. J.* **2017**, *23*, 721–733. [CrossRef] [PubMed]
24. Van Oirschot, P.; Heerings, M.; Wendrich, K.; den Teuling, B.; Martens, M.B.; Jongen, P.J. Symbol digit modalities test variant in a smartphone app for persons with multiple sclerosis: Validation study. *JMIR mHealth uHealth* **2020**, *8*, e18160. [CrossRef]
25. Prochaska, J.O.; Velicer, W.F. The transtheoretical model of health behavior change. *Am. J. Health Promot.* **1997**, *12*, 38–43. [CrossRef]
26. Liu, K.T.; Kueh, Y.C.; Arifin, W.N.; Kim, Y.; Kuan, G. Application of Transtheoretical Model on Behavioral Changes, and Amount of Physical Activity Among University's Students. *Front. Psychol.* **2018**, *9*, 2402. [CrossRef]
27. Prochaska, J.O.; Redding, C.A.; Evers, K.E. The transtheoretical model and stages of change. In *Health Behavior: Theory, Research, and Practice*; John Wiley & Sons: Hoboken, NJ, USA, 2015; Volume 97.
28. Matuska, K.; Mathiowetz, V.; Finlayson, M. Use and perceived effectiveness of energy conservation strategies for managing multiple sclerosis fatigue. *Am. J. Occup. Ther.* **2007**, *61*, 62–69. [CrossRef]
29. Schüler, J.; Wolff, W.; Dettmers, C. Exercise in Multiple Sclerosis: Knowing is Not Enough—The Crucial Role of Intention Formation and Intention Realization. *Neurol. Ther.* **2019**, *8*, 5–11. [CrossRef] [PubMed]
30. Abraham, C.; Michie, S. A taxonomy of behavior change techniques used in interventions. *Heal. Psychol.* **2008**, *27*, 379. [CrossRef] [PubMed]
31. de Korte, E.; Wiezer, N.; Roozeboom, M.B.; Vink, P.; Kraaij, W. Behavior change techniques in mhealth apps for the mental and physical health of employees: Systematic assessment. *JMIR mHealth uHealth* **2018**, *6*, e167. [CrossRef] [PubMed]
32. Berthele, A.; Hemmer, B. S2k-Leitlinie: Diagnose und Therapie der Multiplen Sklerose, Neuromyelitis-optica-Spektrum-Erkrankungen und MOG-IgG-assoziierten Erkrankungen. *DGNeurologie* **2021**, *4*, 251–275. [CrossRef]
33. Grossman, P.; Kappos, L.; Gensicke, H.; D'Souza, M.; Mohr, D.; Penner, I.-K.; Steiner, C. MS quality of life, depression, and fatigue improve after mindfulness training: A randomized trial. *Neurology* **2010**, *75*, 1141–1149. [CrossRef]

34. Heine, M.; Verschuren, O.; Hoogervorst, E.L.; van Munster, E.; Hacking, H.G.; Visser-Meily, A.; Twisk, J.W.; Beckerman, H.; de Groot, V.; Kwakkel, G.; et al. Does aerobic training alleviate fatigue and improve societal participation in patients with multiple sclerosis? A randomized controlled trial. *Mult. Scler.* **2017**, *23*, 1517–1526. [CrossRef]
35. Mathiowetz, V.G.; Matuska, K.M.; Finlayson, M.L.; Luo, P.; Chen, H.Y. One-year follow-up to a randomized controlled trial of an energy conservation course for persons with multiple sclerosis. *Int. J. Rehabilit. Res.* **2007**, *30*, 305–313. [CrossRef]
36. Hayes, S.C.; Strosahl, K.; Wilson, K.G. *Acceptance and Commitment Therapy: An Experiential Approach to Behaviour Change*; Guilford Press: New York, NY, USA, 1999.
37. Sheppard, S.C.; Forsyth, J.P.; Hickling, E.J.; Bianchi, J. A Novel Application of Acceptance and Commitment Therapy for Psychosocial Problems Associated with Multiple Sclerosis. *Int. J. MS Care* **2010**, *12*, 200–206. [CrossRef]
38. Jacobsen, H.B.; Kallestad, H.; Landrø, N.I.; Borchgrevink, P.C.; Stiles, T.C. Processes in acceptance and commitment therapy and the rehabilitation of chronic fatigue. *Scand. J. Psychol.* **2017**, *58*, 211–220. [CrossRef] [PubMed]
39. Hayes, S.C.; Luoma, J.B.; Bond, F.W.; Masuda, A.; Lillis, J. Acceptance and Commitment Therapy: Model, processes and outcomes. *Behav. Res. Ther.* **2006**, *44*, 1–25. [CrossRef] [PubMed]
40. Hayes, S.C.; Levin, M.E.; Plumb-Vilardaga, J.; Villatte, J.L.; Pistorello, J. Acceptance and Commitment Therapy and Contextual Behavioral Science: Examining the Progress of a Distinctive Model of Behavioral and Cognitive Therapy. *Behav. Ther.* **2013**, *44*, 180–198. [CrossRef]
41. Noar, S.M.; Benac, C.N.; Harris, M.S. Does tailoring matter? Meta-analytic review of tailored print health behavior change interventions. *Psychol. Bull.* **2007**, *133*, 673. [CrossRef]
42. Rodriguez-Rincon, D.; Leach, B.; Pollard, J.; Parkinson, S.; Gkousis, E.; Lichten, C.; Sussex, J.; Manville, C. *Exploring the Societal Burden of Multiple Sclerosis: A Study into the Non-Clinical Impact of the Disease, Including Changes with Progression*; RAND Corporation: Santa Monica, CA, USA, 2019.
43. Heinonen, T.; Castrén, E.; Luukkaala, T.; Mäkinen, K.; Ruutiainen, J.; Kuusisto, H. The retirement rate due to multiple sclerosis has decreased since 1995–A retrospective study in a Finnish central hospital. *Mult. Scler. Relat. Disord.* **2020**, *45*, 102360. [CrossRef]
44. Nejati, S.; Esfahani, S.R.; Rahmani, S.; Afrookhteh, G.; Hoveida, S. The Effect of Group Mindfulness-based Stress Reduction and Consciousness Yoga Program on Quality of Life and Fatigue Severity in Patients with MS. *J. Caring Sci.* **2016**, *5*, 325–335. [CrossRef]
45. Johansson, S.; Ytterberg, C.; Hillert, J.; Holmqvist, L.W.; von Koch, L. A longitudinal study of variations in and predictors of fatigue in multiple sclerosis. *J. Neurol. Neurosurg. Psychiatry* **2008**, *79*, 454–457. [CrossRef]
46. Powell, D.J.H.; Liossi, C.; Schlotz, W.; Moss-Morris, R. Tracking daily fatigue fluctuations in multiple sclerosis: Ecological momentary assessment provides unique insights. *J. Behav. Med.* **2017**, *40*, 772–783. [CrossRef]
47. Scholz, M.; Haase, R.; Schriefer, D.; Voigt, I.; Ziemssen, T. Electronic health interventions in the case of multiple sclerosis: From theory to practice. *Brain Sci.* **2021**, *11*, 180. [CrossRef] [PubMed]

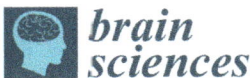

Review

Developing a Digital Solution for Remote Assessment in Multiple Sclerosis: From Concept to Software as a Medical Device

Anneke van der Walt [1,2,*], Helmut Butzkueven [1], Robert K. Shin [3], Luciana Midaglia [4], Luca Capezzuto [5], Michael Lindemann [5], Geraint Davies [5], Lesley M. Butler [5], Cristina Costantino [5] and Xavier Montalban [6]

1. Department of Neuroscience, Central Clinical School, Monash University, Melbourne, VIC 3004, Australia; helmut.butzkueven@monash.edu
2. The Alfred, Melbourne, VIC 3004, Australia
3. MedStar Georgetown University Hospital, Washington, DC 20007, USA; Robert.K.Shin@gunet.georgetown.edu
4. Servei de Neurologia-Neuroimmunologia, Centre d'Esclerosi Múltiple de Catalunya (Cemcat), Institut de Recerca Vall d'Hebron (VHIR), Hospital Universitari Vall d'Hebron, Universitat Autònoma de Barcelona, 08035 Barcelona, Spain; lmidaglia@cem-cat.org
5. F. Hoffmann-La Roche Ltd., 4070 Basel, Switzerland; luca.capezzuto@roche.com (L.C.); michael.lindemann@roche.com (M.L.); geraint.davies.gd1@roche.com (G.D.); lesley.butler@roche.com (L.M.B.); costantino.cristina@gene.com (C.C.)
6. Multiple Sclerosis Centre of Catalonia (Cemcat), Department of Neurology/Neuroimmunology, Hospital Universitari Vall d'Hebron, Universitat Autònoma de Barcelona, 08035 Barcelona, Spain; xavier.montalban@cem-cat.org
* Correspondence: anneke.vanderwalt@monash.edu; Tel.: +61-3-99030555

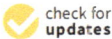

Citation: van der Walt, A.; Butzkueven, H.; Shin, R.K.; Midaglia, L.; Capezzuto, L.; Lindemann, M.; Davies, G.; Butler, L.M.; Costantino, C.; Montalban, X. Developing a Digital Solution for Remote Assessment in Multiple Sclerosis: From Concept to Software as a Medical Device. *Brain Sci.* **2021**, *11*, 1247. https://doi.org/10.3390/brainsci11091247

Academic Editors: Michelle Ploughman and Stephen D. Meriney

Received: 13 August 2021
Accepted: 16 September 2021
Published: 21 September 2021

Publisher's Note: MDPI stays neutral with regard to jurisdictional claims in published maps and institutional affiliations.

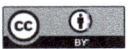

Copyright: © 2021 by the authors. Licensee MDPI, Basel, Switzerland. This article is an open access article distributed under the terms and conditions of the Creative Commons Attribution (CC BY) license (https://creativecommons.org/licenses/by/4.0/).

Abstract: There is increasing interest in the development and deployment of digital solutions to improve patient care and facilitate monitoring in medical practice, e.g., by remote observation of disease symptoms in the patients' home environment. Digital health solutions today range from non-regulated wellness applications and research-grade exploratory instruments to regulated software as a medical device (SaMD). This paper discusses the considerations and complexities in developing innovative, effective, and validated SaMD for multiple sclerosis (MS). The development of SaMD requires a formalised approach (design control), inclusive of technical verification and analytical validation to ensure reliability. SaMD must be clinically evaluated, characterised for benefit and risk, and must conform to regulatory requirements associated with device classification. Cybersecurity and data privacy are also critical. Careful consideration of patient and provider needs throughout the design and testing process help developers overcome challenges of adoption in medical practice. Here, we explore the development pathway for SaMD in MS, leveraging experiences from the development of Floodlight™ MS, a continually evolving bundled solution of SaMD for remote functional assessment of MS. The development process will be charted while reflecting on common challenges in the digital space, with a view to providing insights for future developers.

Keywords: multiple sclerosis; software as a medical device; digital health; participatory health; monitoring; smartphone-based assessments; clinical validation; technical validation; MS apps; digital health solution development

1. Introduction

Multiple sclerosis (MS) is an inflammatory demyelinating and degenerative disease [1] characterised by a wide clinical variability in disease trajectory between individuals [2]. Clinical monitoring is intermittently, and often inconsistently [3,4], applied via in-clinic measures, such as the Expanded Disability Status Scale (EDSS) [5] and magnetic resonance imaging; detecting early disease progression is thus challenging [3,4]. Progressive worsening in specific domains (e.g., cognition [6]) can be subtle or subclinical, especially in the early stages of the disease, but tends to increase in frequency and severity over time. The worsening of disability is a multidimensional process and difficult to detect [7,8]. At present, the diagnosis of progression in MS is typically retrospective with a heavy reliance on clinical history, requiring progressive worsening for more than 6 months based on EDSS score, without evidence of relapses [3,4]. Monitoring in MS relies on infrequent outpatient assessments (typically occurring once or twice annually) with a lack of objective assessments of progression available to healthcare professionals (HCPs). New clinical and research tools are therefore needed to address the unmet need of early detection and ongoing assessment of progressive worsening, rendering this an inviting area for innovation in the digital health space.

Remote digital solutions such as smartphone-based apps, wearables, and decision support algorithms are increasingly utilised in research and clinical trial settings [9] and are beginning to emerge in routine medical care. This paper will focus on smartphone technology, which is ubiquitous and broadly accessible [10,11], making it a viable approach for facilitating remote assessment [12–14]. Smartphones can be used in a patients' home environment as frequently as required and their use is increasingly familiar and unobtrusive. Further, most off-the-shelf smartphones contain sensors with the capacity to gather objective data unaffected by inter- and intra-rater variability. Measurements and patient-reported information captured with smartphone technology have the potential to enable more frequent, decentralised, and home-based care to supplement the infrequent in-clinic assessments typically offered to patients. Mutually sharing this information with patients can help focus the clinical conversation or empower shared decision making. Smartphone-based digital solutions are thus ideally placed to contribute to improving clinical care management for people living with MS (PLwMS) [15,16] and providing personalised healthcare [17].

Today, smartphone applications, performing a variety of functions, are available to support PLwMS. Many of these tools are non-regulated wellness applications designed to support day-to-day disease management, for example through symptom or medication intake tracking, visit-scheduling, provision of disease education, and connectivity to supportive care facilities or patient social media networks [18–23]. Other smartphone-based solutions enable assessment of functional parameters affected by the disease, such as mobility and cognition, or therapeutic benefit, such as for fatigue or depression [24]. Data and digital biomarkers collected by patient-facing apps may provide clinical value by generating new insights into the MS disease course, ultimately improving the understanding of individual disease trajectories and response to intervention. Despite their promise, however, smartphone-based solutions have not yet been fully integrated into routine medical practice.

The development journey of a smartphone-based solution for remote assessment of PLwMS will be presented here as a case study to illustrate the design and development process, validation, regulatory and clinical requirements, as well as deployment in the emergent digital health landscape. The process will be discussed from the perspective of industry developers and academic collaborators, from ideation through to technical solution development and version iteration, certification, and deployment. The Floodlight programme is a Roche-led initiative that aims to create digital solutions to facilitate functional assessment in MS. The first Floodlight app was an assessment suite for clinical research that required provisioned smartphones. More recent versions have been developed under design control to ensure that they meet the regulatory standards of reliability and meaningfulness associated with software as a medical device (SaMD)—standalone software that can perform medical functions without being part of a specific medical device hardware [25]—and to enable access for use on personal smartphones in a variety of integrated MS care settings.

2. Concept, Proof of Concept, and Assessment of Unmet Needs

The MS digital health space is still largely uncharted. Close partnerships between developers, researchers, HCPs, and PLwMS, from inception and throughout the design process, is essential to ensure that technical solutions, such as smartphone apps, are grounded in science and adequately address unmet patient and/or healthcare needs. Technical development typically begins with the identification and prioritisation of user needs, then the ideation of possible solutions, followed by a "design, test, and iterate" build cycle to ensure those needs are fulfilled. For SaMD development, this creative cycle must also be balanced with clinical, technical, and regulatory processes to ensure the required rigour is achieved. In parallel, it must be established that the solution provides output that is meaningful to both PLwMS and HCPs and that can be readily embedded in the relevant healthcare system.

Technical development for SaMD may begin after proof of concept (PoC) has already been established in a research setting. In the Floodlight PoC study, sensor-based measurement was shown to effectively capture reliable and clinically relevant measures of functional impairment in three domains: cognition, gait, and balance, and hand motor function [26,27]. The Floodlight PoC study constituted sufficient evidence to allow for the use of these assessments in a research setting, but further development under design control was required for deployment in a clinical setting as SaMD. Implementing a secondary, more rigorous technical design step also provided evidence to support face validity and inform features that would facilitate the user experience.

The Double Diamond (DD) model (Figure 1), an iterative approach commonly used in software development, was utilised to guide the process of gaining user insights for the design of the new Floodlight solution. DD is a non-linear model based on divergent–convergent thinking, where a topic is first explored more widely or deeply (divergent) before a focused approach is taken with a singular design solution (convergent) [28]. The iterative aspect of development is then retained through the ongoing acquisition and utilisation of new real-world user insights, experiences, and behaviours to inform subsequent refinement of the solution.

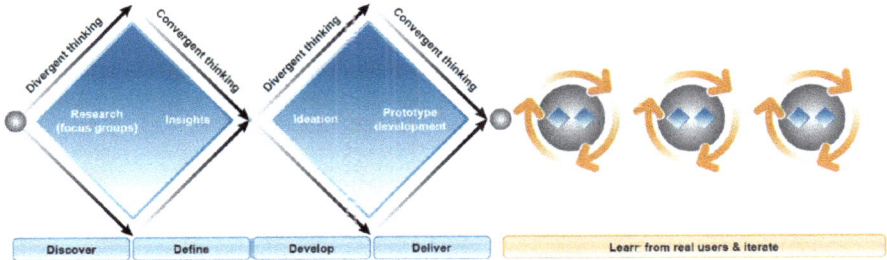

Figure 1. Double Diamond model, an iterative approach with rapid prototyping.

In the initial divergent phase, focus groups with MS experts and PLwMS were conducted to identify the signs and symptoms that might best represent the emergence of progression and to define the current in-clinic standards used to assess functional loss. This process then fed into the convergent phase, which prioritised the assessment of hand motor function, gait, and cognition, all domains frequently affected in PLwMS with worsening disease [29–37]. These findings served to substantiate the selection of domain assessments tested in the Floodlight PoC study. During the second divergent phase, exploration of how to technically design the solution and implement the assessments took place, followed by the prioritisation and consolidation of a singular, defined approach for technical development. In order to inform iterative updates and advancements to the solution in the future, mechanisms, such as an analytics platform, were then incorporated to collect insights from real-world users.

This design effort yielded a preliminary structure for the new Floodlight solution, named Floodlight™ MS (currently v1.2). Floodlight MS would provide five assessments for measurement of function across three domains, as well as a Patient Journal (Figure 2). A "bundling approach", wherein the five assessments would be verified, validated, and independently registered as SaMD, was taken to enable flexibility to change, update, and add new features or assessments without compromising the solution as a whole.

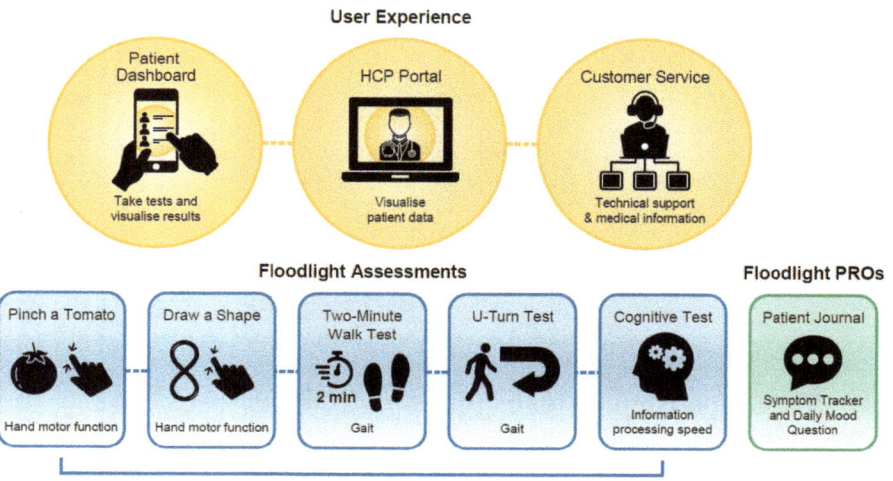

Figure 2. Illustration of current version of Floodlight™ MS v1.2 app and assessments. HCP, healthcare professional; PRO, patient-reported outcome.

3. Desirability: Challenges in Developing a Digital Solution That PLwMS and HCPs Need and Use

Identifying and balancing the needs and desires of different users when creating a digital solution can be challenging. Prior to initiating design control, the Jobs-to-be-Done (JTBD) framework [38] was used to define concrete user need statements for Floodlight MS. JTBD is an outcome-driven innovation strategy used to provide an in-depth understanding of user goals in a structured manner. Core functional desired outcomes (e.g., "Minimize the time it takes to determine how the patient's past symptoms have changed since their last consultation"), as well as emotional and related jobs that might impact the ability to achieve an outcome (e.g., "Avoid feeling guilty for not spending enough time with a patient"), were collected for each user type. For Floodlight MS solution design, users were defined as (1) individuals with MS who are trying to live their lives while managing their MS, and (2) neurologists who are maintaining MS patients' quality of life.

JTBD outcome statements reframed the needs related to management of MS into user needs that can be addressed through a technical solution and that can be used to establish parameters for device quality system requirements. To determine which of the needs was most underserved, the desired outcome statements were quantitatively ranked by 202 PLwMS and 211 HCPs in terms of importance of the outcome and current satisfaction in performing the job. For PLwMS, the most underserved needs concerned gaining a better understanding of their health status and treatment management. For HCPs the most underserved needs included monitoring changes in the health status of PLwMS, assessing the impact of MS on daily life, and driving patient compliance. For Floodlight MS, facilitation of improved conversations between PLwMS and their neurologists emerged as a defining priority.

JTBD analysis also clarified factors that might limit the ability of PLwMS to interact with an app, such as comorbidities and disability status. The findings indicated that assessments within the solution must be convenient, with a reasonable duration and frequency. Different levels of user ability in terms of digital skills, as well as aspects such as dexterity and cognitive and visual impairments, would be likely to impact engagement. For many commercial applications, engagement is a key performance indicator and revenue driver. In digital health, however, solutions should only strive for sufficient engagement to support successful outcomes, in order to strike the balance between benefit and burden to the users

To ensure safety and effectiveness during use, human factors that may affect an individual user's performance need to be identified and addressed. Errors are frequently caused by the design of the user interface with which users interact. Formative testing with an additional cohort of users is a step in the design control process that serves to identify potential hazardous situations, assess overall usability, and ensure that the interface can be clearly understood and operated per intended use In formative testing for Floodlight MS, PLwMS expressed satisfaction with an MS-specific solution, which they identified would be a key part of the conversation with their neurologist. PLwMS also indicated that they were more likely to utilise the solution if it were prescribed by an HCP. Formative testing with neurologists was used to assess HCP willingness to adopt the solution and potential barriers to adoption. Neurologists reported that they saw the solution as complementary to their current processes, as long as the data were readily interpretable and easily accessible.

Formative testing informed a significant decision in the developmental journey for the Floodlight programme: the adoption of a prescription-based model for Floodlight MS. This model prioritised partnering with HCPs in a coordinated care setting to identify appropriate patient users, support onboarding and oversee generation and interpretation of patient data. These findings were substantiated by Floodlight Open, a global open-access study, entirely operated via digital interfaces, that was designed to assess adherence to using the app and the feasibility of a "bring your own device" research version of the Floodlight assessment suite provided directly to PLwMS. In line with the adherence issues reported in similar fully digital studies conducted in real-world settings [39], overall adherence in Floodlight Open was low. This contrasts with the controlled environment of the Floodlight PoC study, where good adherence and patient satisfaction were observed [26]. Moreover, in Floodlight Open, adherence rates were positively impacted by concomitant studies that provided clinical coordination. Together, these findings suggested that a supportive clinical care environment would be required to maintain long-term use of the Floodlight MS solution.

Insufficient adherence to remote digital health solutions often presents a challenge to long-term engagement [39]. This is a significant obstacle for developers of apps intended for users with MS, where engagement may be required throughout the user's lifetime. Adherence to the use of a digital health solution over time may be regarded as a behaviour, determined by factors such as the user's motivation, ability, and other aspects such as forgetfulness. Behavioural design is based on insights from behavioural science, which can be implemented to aid in evoking desired user behaviour, and is recognised as a key element for development of digital health solutions to increase the likelihood of achieving the desired outcomes [40–42]. For example, the concept of the "neurological loop" has been used to explain how habits are formed via a three-step loop composed of cue, routine, and reward; solutions can thus be designed to provide users with strategic rewards to elicit repeated behaviour, based on specific cues [43]. A behavioural design approach was adopted to identify features that might enable users of Floodlight MS to achieve the outcome of improving clinical conversations. Fogg's behaviour model (Behaviour = Motivation × Ability × Prompt [44]) was used as a framework to audit the design to identify facilitators and barriers to engagement in terms of motivation, ability, and prompts [44,45]. Feedback architecture was then designed to ensure appropriate communication with users and rewards (motivational prompts) for short-, medium-, and long-term outcomes. For example, the PLwMS interface home screen was designed to incorporate prompts for action, a progress indicator, and an appointment calendar to orient use of Floodlight MS around the care conversation. Further, notification and content architecture were also devised to sustain motivation across different use cases.

As there is great variability in symptomology and disease course between individuals living with MS, solutions designed for these users need to accommodate diverse characteristics and varied needs, preferences, and behaviours when utilising smartphones. The complexity of addressing individual preferences and needs in a "one-size-fits-all" approach is typified in the end-user reaction to app gamification. The utility of gamification (the use of game design elements in other contexts) is widely discussed in relation to digital health solution development, as it may aid in increasing motivation and sustaining usage (i.e., increasing adherence [46]); however, any elements need to be applied cautiously in the context of healthcare and must support the desired outcome, which, for Floodlight MS, is the use of data for a care conversation. The topic of gamification—where, in the context of the Floodlight programme experience, some users considered it an inappropriate approach to disease assessment—may represent an example of possible divergent perspectives from different users and user types, which further illustrates the importance of behavioural strategies in studying use patterns. Even after final solution design, regular testing of the applied concepts should be conducted to ensure the usability of the features for all users, aligning with the specific needs of PLwMS. Moreover, careful consideration must be given to how the solution is implemented to ensure effective use. The application of behavioural science, for example through built-in analytics, whilst continuing to develop, test, and iterate on a periodic release cycle, will be important to enable iterative development throughout the solution lifecycle.

4. Regulatory Standards: Data Security, Verification and Validation

Challenges and compromises are involved in creating a digital solution that is not only meaningful to end users, but also technically and scientifically robust and aligned with regulatory standards. Digital solutions producing measures adoptable in medical care must meet the standards of device regulatory agencies on design control, cybersecurity and data privacy, risk analysis, and clinical evaluation—all elements considered in the certification of SaMD [25].

To satisfy regulatory requirements, each of the assessments provided by Floodlight MS were subject to technical verification, as well as clinical and analytical validation (Figure 3). Individual assessments and data features were selected for SaMD certification based upon evidence obtained from the Floodlight PoC study and insights from DD.

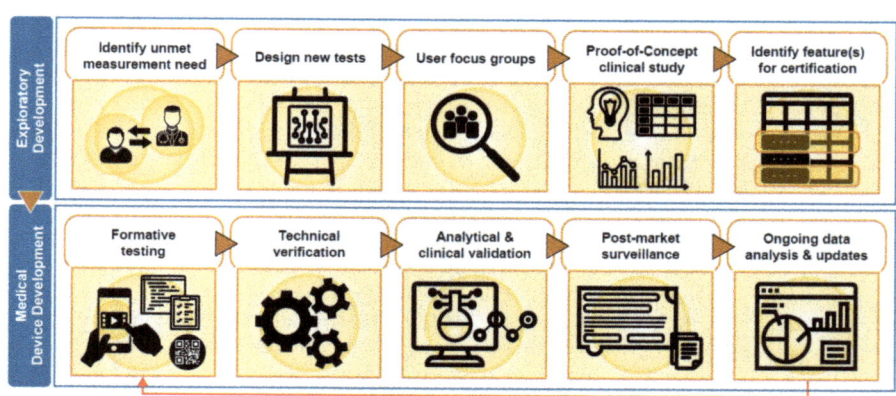

Figure 3. Development of Floodlight™ MS software as a medical device.

Technical verification requires assurance that the software is built to the specified requirements. These include elements such as: software unit testing to ensure the functionality of each component, software system testing of new features or components to expose defects in interfaces and interactions between integrated components, and software verification testing to check that the software meets the specified requirements. In modern software development, an agile process is typically implemented to embed quality testing into development, including efforts such as in-sprint level manual testing (in which incremental development and testing occur in tandem) and automation tests to support regression efforts (a software testing practice that ensures an application still functions as expected after any change).

Analytical validation is needed to ensure SaMD output is reliable, accurate, and precise: it demonstrates how well SaMD fulfil their intended use by accurately measuring the desired parameters and generating the correct outputs [47,48]. Analytical validation includes testing the user experience of the solution. This does not require patient or disease-specific assessment, so testing can be conducted in healthy individuals and/or via simulations. For each of the Floodlight MS assessments, robot testing was conducted across 26 mobile devices, representing over 70% of the global smartphone market. Acceptance criteria consisted of three components: observed variability when the same test is repeated on the same smartphone multiple times (within device error), observed variability when the same test is repeated on different smartphones (between device error), and distance between mean measurement of all smartphones to a theoretical ground truth (systemic bias). All smartphones tested passed acceptance criteria with the exception of the Alcatel 7 phone which failed due to a device chipset issue where screen sizes are not properly reported by the device, rendering the tomatoes in the Floodlight MS "Pinch A Tomato Test" larger than the acceptable range defined in SaMD specifications. All operating systems were also validated. Testing demonstrated that the operating system of the mobile device did not influence data captured. Finally, a series of security tests were conducted, ranging from threat modelling to penetration testing, to ensure data security in the final product.

Whereas analytical validation establishes reliability, a process of clinical evaluation establishes clinical association and validation and is used to determine the sufficiency of evidence and the requirement for further clinical investigation. Clinical evaluation is a systematic and methodologically sound process used to continuously generate, collect, analyse, and assess the clinical data pertaining to a device in order to verify and validate the safety and performance of the device, including any clinical benefits, in the target user population and when used as intended [49]. Each assessment in the Floodlight MS solution was subject to evaluation, supported by multiple evidence sources, including the Floodlight PoC study and an observational study with PLwMS that provided an assessment by clinical content area experts that the process of, and results from, the Floodlight MS assessments achieved their intended purpose.

Post-marketing surveillance of SaMD is also required to provide ongoing monitoring of any defects and/or safety concerns, in order to ensure that solutions are safe and effective during real-world use. The post-market clinical follow-up plan, which is part of the clinical evaluation, specifies methods and procedures for collection and evaluation of clinical data from on-market use to confirm safety and performance. In addition to implementing subsequent clinical trials and real-world evidence generation initiatives, customer support should be present to capture reportable SaMD events for investigation, such as technical defects and safety issues, in order to fully comply with regulatory requirements. For Floodlight MS, customer support was tailored to respond to users' needs (HCPs and PLwMS) in a specific geography, for example by offering local language support, in addition to addressing technical and medical questions.

Significant effort from the developer is required to achieve robust, regulatory-grade clinical validation. Given the rapidly evolving nature of digital technology, it is also critical for developers to find effective approaches to continuously advance solution design. Likewise, continual technological advancement presents a challenge to regulators, who must concurrently advance policy in order to foster growth of digital innovation for better disease management [17]. To this end, regulatory agencies are actively facilitating collaborative initiatives within the digital community to advance digital health innovation [50].

Two key aspects of this dialogue are data safety and cybersecurity, as it is crucial to not only establish and maintain robust data privacy and security, but also to adapt them to comply with local requirements across geographies (e.g., General Data Protection Regulation in the EU, the Health Insurance Portability and Accountability Act in the USA, etc.). Data security can be divided into technical (obtaining and storage of data), methodological (the software application and infrastructure used to deliver it), and procedural aspects (data usage, data access, and security breaches), and each of these must be carefully considered at each stage of design and development [51]. Demonstrating a robust approach to personal data security is also a means to build users' trust: 45% of users worry about the unwanted use of their data when using mobile devices for health-related activities [52,53], and there are legitimate concerns over user identification, data sharing with third parties, or accidental data leakage [52]. As data privacy and security provisions must be placed at the fore from the start of a user's interaction with a digital solution, Floodlight MS users are presented with a data privacy notice during the sign-up process. This contains detailed information on the treatment of their personal information, which is in line with the applicable regulatory frameworks. Different types of security measures are in place for Floodlight MS, including password-protected access with automatic logout after a period of inactivity, and data encryption in transit and at rest. Moreover, the legal manufacturer of the device ensures that appropriate training and processes for data management operators are set up and that action plans are ready in case of any incidents.

After regulatory clearance has been achieved, the hurdles of adoption into medical practice, making the solution accessible, and providing ongoing monitoring and managing the system need to be overcome. All these aspects will involve the collaborative efforts of multiple healthcare stakeholders such as PLwMS, HCPs, and payers, as these hurdles cannot be overcome without participation from all relevant parties [17].

5. Taking an Adaptive Approach

Agility is key when developing digital solutions, requiring a fluid approach to facilitate an iterative developmental process that aligns with the design control and requisite regulatory requirements. The rapidly changing technological environment contrasts markedly with classical drug development with its careful, largely linear and standardised processes [54,55]. Once a new solution is developed and deployed, post-market data can serve to further validate clinical effectiveness, evolve technical capabilities, and refine the user experience, and may even support subsequent regulatory engagement and reassessment.

Real-world evidence generation and non-interventional studies are often more efficient than, and can be complementary to, interventional trials. For the Floodlight programme, non-interventional studies and real-world evidence generated with Floodlight MS serves to complement assessment of Floodlight test technology in more formal clinical trial settings. Research is also being conducted to improve the clinical utility of the test suite, support clinical analysis, develop quality control features, and advance the understanding of sensor data [56–59].

The development path outlined here culminated in the release of Floodlight MS, which contains the five assessments registered as SaMD. Additional features, such as the Patient Journal, designed to help users reach the outcome of improved care conversations, are grouped separately and are thus able to be more frequently and flexibly iterated and improved upon based on user feedback, without necessitating resubmission to regulatory authorities. This continual iteration is enabled by recurring development cycles, which allow improvements to be implemented frequently, generating updated versions several times throughout the year. Floodlight MS is set to continue evolving, and thus certain topics covered in this paper may be revisited as knowledge advances.

The use of different technical deployment models, tailoring the means by which the solution is provided, may also provide the flexibility needed to meet local regulatory requirements and enable interoperability and integration in a complex and fragmented electronic health records landscape [60,61]. Three deployment models were designed for Floodlight MS: (i) a standalone solution with an HCP-facing web-based portal for data access, (ii) a standalone solution that can be integrated with electronic health records, and (iii) a software development kit (SDK). The SDK enables rapid, tailored integration of the Floodlight MS assessments into a third-party solution, for example into the DreaMS digital research tool advanced by the Research Center for Clinical Neuroimmunology and Neuroscience, Basel (RC2NB) [62]. The SDK approach also allows for integration into solutions developed in-house. Tailoring the deployment model for a digital solution may enable greater interoperability and the capability to address diverse and local needs on a greater scale.

6. Future Horizons

The provision and adoption of technological solutions and the sharing of information globally has the potential to drive knowledge acquisition and positively affect healthcare worldwide [63]. Digital solutions offer great promise in delivering increasingly individualised, easily accessible, and effective healthcare, with the capacity to evolve with time and adapt to the changing needs of PLwMS and HCPs The impact of the COVID-19 pandemic has given additional proof of such versatility and usefulness, highlighting how barriers can be overcome through the adoption of digital tools [64], where capturing digital data remotely may mean that symptom tracking can be maintained even when clinic visits are not possible. Ultimately, digital solutions must contribute to the long-term resolution of broader health system challenges, such as lack of access to care, lack of frequent monitoring, costly and ineffective treatment, and delayed diagnosis of MS disease progression.

Fundamentally, digital solutions such as Floodlight MS aim to improve outcomes for PLwMS To reach this objective, continued collaboration and partnership with the entire MS community is needed, not only to continually refine individual solutions but also to create robust standards for implementation, interpretation, and interoperability. Ongoing investment into the clinical development of a digital solution will also enable continuous improvement, enhancing the clinical utility and sustained actionability of a given solution. This is especially relevant for solutions such as Floodlight MS, which generate data that may be used to improve our understanding of the disease or create digital biomarkers. The use of such data could serve to bridge the gap between clinical trials and medical care, for example, by enabling the creation of a baseline dataset in routine care prior to clinical trial enrolment; or by enabling a more immediate comparison of population outcomes to individual performance using the same reliable, objective outcome measures.

The sharing and secondary use of the data collected using digital solutions will be important for shaping the future of research, regulation, and policymaking in the digital healthcare sphere. Platforms such as the European Health Data Space are being developed to facilitate data sharing across sectors [65]. Key areas centre around health data exchange, access to health data for research and policymaking, and a single market for digital health products and services. Structuring projects to generate data for secondary use in collaboration with the scientific community will help to shape the digital space by furthering research, as well as from a regulatory perspective in terms of enabling better fit-for-purpose and evidence-based policymaking.

The Floodlight programme has undertaken a path of SaMD design and development to support safe and effective use of Floodlight MS, a bundled digital assessment solution for PLwMS. The incorporation of design strategies commonly used in software development informed features to support user adherence, clinical utility, and readiness for integration into today's fragmented global healthcare landscape. This effort is underpinned by an iterative and collaborative clinical validation, technical refinement, and deployment approach intended to drive continual evolution of the technology. Ultimately, the emergence of robust digital solutions may help to change the way that disease progression is measured in MS, enabling optimisation of care, and helping to bridge clinical trial and medical practice data.

Author Contributions: Writing—Review and Editing, A.v.d.W., H.B., R.K.S., L.M., L.C., M.L., G.D., L.M.B., C.C. and X.M. All authors have read and agreed to the published version of the manuscript.

Funding: The author(s) disclosed receipt of the following financial support for the research, authorship and/or publication of this article: F. Hoffmann-La Roche Ltd., Basel, Switzerland provided financial support for the publication of this manuscript.

Acknowledgments: We would like to thank all the Floodlight partnering institutions and scientific collaborators. We would also like to thank the F. Hoffmann-La Roche Ltd. Floodlight team members, particularly Mike Baker, Camille André, JP Guyon, Seya Colloud, Jorge Cancela, Licinio Craveiro, Alexandre Breton, Susanne Clinch, Jens Schjodt-Eriksen, Catherine Wu, Shibir Desai, Teri Kanerva, Christian Gossens, Timothy Kilchenmann, and Christine Eighteen. Writing and editorial assistance for this manuscript was provided by Terri Desmonds of Articulate Science, UK, and funded by F. Hoffmann-La Roche Ltd.

Conflicts of Interest: The authors declared the following potential conflicts of interest with respect to the research, authorship and/or publication of this article: A.v.d.W. received travel support, speaker honoraria and served on advisory boards for Biogen, Merck, Genzyme, Novartis and Teva. H.B. has received institutional (Monash University) funding from Biogen, F. Hoffmann-La Roche Ltd., Merck and Novartis; has carried out contracted research for Novartis, Merck, F. Hoffmann-La Roche Ltd. and Biogen; has taken part in speakers' bureaus for Biogen, Genzyme, F. Hoffmann-La Roche Ltd. and Merck; has received personal grants from Oxford PharmaGenesis and Biogen (prior to 30 June 2018). R.K.S. has received consulting fees and speaker honoraria from Biogen, Bristol Myers Squibb, EMD Serono, Genentech, Novartis and Sanofi Genzyme. L.M. has nothing to disclose. L.C. is an employee of F. Hoffmann-La Roche Ltd. M.L. is a consultant for F. Hoffmann-La Roche Ltd. via Inovigate. G.D. is an employee of F. Hoffmann-La Roche Ltd. L.M.B. is an employee of F. Hoffmann-La Roche Ltd. C.C. is an employee and shareholder of F. Hoffmann-La Roche Ltd. X.M. has received speaking honoraria and/or travel expenses for participation in scientific meetings, and/or has been a steering committee member of clinical trials, and/or participated in advisory boards of clinical trials in the past years with Actelion, Alexion, Bayer, Biogen, Bristol Myers Squibb/Celgene, EMD Serono, Genzyme, F. Hoffmann-La Roche Ltd., Immunic Therapeutics, Janssen Pharmaceuticals, MedDay, Merck, Mylan, NervGen Pharma Corp., Novartis, Sanofi Genzyme, Teva Pharmaceuticals, TG Therapeutics, EXCEMED, Multiple Sclerosis International Federation and National Multiple Sclerosis Society.

References

1. Filippi, M.; Bar-Or, A.; Piehl, F.; Preziosa, P.; Solari, A.; Vukusic, S.; Rocca, M.A. Multiple sclerosis. *Nat. Rev. Dis. Primers* **2018**, *4*, 43. [CrossRef]
2. Lorscheider, J.; Buzzard, K.; Jokubaitis, V.; Spelman, T.; Havrdova, E.; Horakova, D.; Trojano, M.; Izquierdo, G.; Girard, M.; Duquette, P. Defining secondary progressive multiple sclerosis. *Brain* **2016**, *139*, 2395–2405. [CrossRef]
3. Allen-Philbey, K.; Middleton, R.; Tuite-Dalton, K.; Baker, E.; Stennett, A.; Albor, C.; Schmierer, K. Can we improve the monitoring of people with multiple sclerosis using simple tools, data sharing, and patient engagement? *Front. Neurol.* **2020**, *11*, 464. [CrossRef] [PubMed]
4. Lublin, F.D.; Reingold, S.C.; Cohen, J.A.; Cutter, G.R.; Sørensen, P.S.; Thompson, A.J.; Wolinsky, J.S.; Balcer, L.J.; Banwell, B.; Barkhof, F. Defining the clinical course of multiple sclerosis: The 2013 revisions. *Neurology* **2014**, *83*, 278–286. [CrossRef]
5. Kurtzke, J.F. Rating neurologic impairment in multiple sclerosis: An expanded disability status scale (EDSS). *Neurology* **1983**, *33*, 1444. [CrossRef]
6. Amato, M.P.; Portaccio, E.; Goretti, B.; Zipoli, V.; Hakiki, B.; Giannini, M.; Pastò, L.; Razzolini, L. Cognitive impairment in early stages of multiple sclerosis. *Neurol. Sci.* **2010**, *31*, 211–214. [CrossRef] [PubMed]
7. Inojosa, H.; Proschmann, U.; Akgün, K.; Ziemssen, T. Should we use clinical tools to identify disease progression? *Front. Neurol.* **2021**, *11*, 1890. [CrossRef] [PubMed]
8. Manouchehrinia, A.; Zhu, F.; Piani-Meier, D.; Lange, M.; Silva, D.G.; Carruthers, R.; Glaser, A.; Kingwell, E.; Tremlett, H.; Hillert, J. Predicting risk of secondary progression in multiple sclerosis: A nomogram. *Mult. Scler.* **2019**, *25*, 1102–1112. [CrossRef]
9. Inan, O.; Tenaerts, P.; Prindiville, S.; Reynolds, H.; Dizon, D.; Cooper-Arnold, K.; Turakhia, M.; Pletcher, M.; Preston, K.; Krumholz, H. Digitizing clinical trials. *Jpn. Digit. Med.* **2020**, *3*, 1–7. [CrossRef]

10. Haase, R.; Schultheiss, T.; Kempcke, R.; Thomas, K.; Ziemssen, T. Modern communication technology skills of patients with multiple sclerosis. *Mult. Scler.* **2013**, *19*, 1240. [CrossRef]
11. Center, P.R. Cell Phone and Smartphone Ownership Demographics. Available online: www.pewinternet.org/data-trend/mobile/cell-phone-and-smartphone-ownership-demographics/ (accessed on 15 June 2021).
12. Prasad, S.; Ramachandran, R.; Jennings, C. Development of Smartphone Technology to Monitor Disease Progression in Multiple Sclerosis (P01. 144). *Neurology* **2012**, *78*. [CrossRef]
13. Bove, R.; White, C.C.; Giovannoni, G.; Glanz, B.; Golubchikov, V.; Hujol, J.; Jennings, C.; Langdon, D.; Lee, M.; Legedza, A. Evaluating more naturalistic outcome measures: A 1-year smartphone study in multiple sclerosis. *Neurol. Neuroimmun. Neuroinflamm.* **2015**, *2*, e162. [CrossRef] [PubMed]
14. Boukhvalova, A.K.; Kowalczyk, E.; Harris, T.; Kosa, P.; Wichman, A.; Sandford, M.A.; Memon, A.; Bielekova, B. Identifying and quantifying neurological disability via smartphone. *Front. Neurol.* **2018**, *9*, 740. [CrossRef] [PubMed]
15. Feys, P.; Giovannoni, G.; Dijsselbloem, N.; Centonze, D.; Eelen, P.; Lykke Andersen, S. The importance of a multi-disciplinary perspective and patient activation programmes in MS management. *Mult. Scler.* **2016**, *22*, 34–46. [CrossRef] [PubMed]
16. Marziniak, M.; Brichetto, G.; Feys, P.; Meyding-Lamadé, U.; Vernon, K.; Meuth, S.G. The use of digital and remote communication technologies as a tool for multiple sclerosis management: Narrative review. *JMIR Rehabil. Assist. Technol.* **2018**, *5*, e7805. [CrossRef] [PubMed]
17. Cancela, J.; Charlafti, I.; Colloud, S.; Wu, C. Digital health in the era of personalized healthcare: Opportunities and challenges for bringing research and patient care to a new level. *Digit. Health* **2021**, 7–31. [CrossRef]
18. Scholz, M.; Haase, R.; Schriefer, D.; Voigt, I.; Ziemssen, T. Electronic health interventions in the case of multiple sclerosis: From theory to practice. *Brain Sci.* **2021**, *11*, 180. [CrossRef]
19. Lavorgna, L.; Russo, A.; De Stefano, M.; Lanzillo, R.; Esposito, S.; Moshtari, F.; Rullani, F.; Piscopo, K.; Buonanno, D.; Morra, V.B. Health-related coping and social interaction in people with multiple sclerosis supported by a social network: Pilot study with a new methodological approach. *Interact. J. Med. Res.* **2017**, *6*, e7402. [CrossRef]
20. Allam, A.; Kostova, Z.; Nakamoto, K.; Schulz, P.J. The effect of social support features and gamification on a Web-based intervention for rheumatoid arthritis patients: Randomized controlled trial. *J. Med. Internet Res.* **2015**, *17*, e3510. [CrossRef]
21. Fernandez-Luque, L.; Elahi, N.; Grajales, F., 3rd. An analysis of personal medical information disclosed in YouTube videos created by patients with multiple sclerosis. *Stud. Health Technol. Inform.* **2009**, *150*, 292–296.
22. Biogen. Aby App—By above MS. Available online: https://www.abovems.com/en_us/home/ms-support-events/aby-app.html (accessed on 22 July 2021).
23. Settle, J.R.; Maloni, H.W.; Bedra, M.; Finkelstein, J.; Zhan, M.; Wallin, M.T. Monitoring medication adherence in multiple sclerosis using a novel web-based tool: A pilot study. *J. Telemed. Telecare* **2016**, *22*, 225–233. [CrossRef]
24. De Angelis, M.; Lavorgna, L.; Carotenuto, A.; Petruzzo, M.; Lanzillo, R.; Brescia Morra, V.; Moccia, M. Digital Technology in Clinical Trials for Multiple Sclerosis: Systematic Review. *J. Clin. Med.* **2021**, *10*, 2328. [CrossRef] [PubMed]
25. International Medical Device Regulators Forum. Available online: http://www.imdrf.org/docs/imdrf/final/technical/imdrf-tech-140918-samd-framework-risk-categorization-141013.pdf (accessed on 12 July 2021).
26. Midaglia, L.; Mulero, P.; Montalban, X.; Graves, J.; Hauser, S.L.; Julian, L.; Baker, M.; Schadrack, J.; Gossens, C.; Scotland, A. Adherence and satisfaction of smartphone-and smartwatch-based remote active testing and passive monitoring in people with multiple sclerosis: Nonrandomized interventional feasibility study. *J. Med. Internet Res.* **2019**, *21*, e14863. [CrossRef]
27. Montalban, X.; Graves, J.; Midaglia, L.; Mulero, P.; Julian, L.; Baker, M.; Schadrack, J.; Gossens, C.; Ganzetti, M.; Scotland, A. A smartphone sensor-based digital outcome assessment of multiple sclerosis. *Mult. Scler.* **2021**, 13524585211028561. [CrossRef] [PubMed]
28. British Design Council. What Is the Framework for Innovation? Design Council's Evolved Double Diamond. Available online: https://www.designcouncil.org.uk/news-opinion/what-framework-innovation-design-councils-evolved-double-diamond (accessed on 12 July 2021).
29. Heesen, C.; Böhm, J.; Reich, C.; Kasper, J.; Goebel, M.; Gold, S. Patient perception of bodily functions in multiple sclerosis: Gait and visual function are the most valuable. *Mult. Scler.* **2008**, *14*, 988–991. [CrossRef] [PubMed]
30. Bethoux, F.; Bennett, S. Evaluating walking in patients with multiple sclerosis: Which assessment tools are useful in clinical practice? *Int. J. MS Care* **2011**, *13*, 4–14 [CrossRef] [PubMed]
31. Dubuisson, N.; Baker, D.; Thomson, A.; Marta, M.; Gnanapavan, S.; Turner, B.; Giovannoni, G.; Schmierer, K. Disease modification in advanced MS: Focus on upper limb function. *Mult. Scler.* **2017**, *23*, 1956–1957. [CrossRef]
32. Ortiz-Rubio, A.; Cabrera-Martos, I.; Rodríguez-Torres, J.; Fajardo-Contreras, W.; Díaz-Pelegrina, A.; Valenza, M.C. Effects of a home-based upper limb training program in patients with multiple sclerosis: A randomized controlled trial. *Arch. Phys. Med. Rehabilit.* **2016**, *97*, 2027–2033. [CrossRef]
33. Kister, I.; Bacon, T.E.; Chamot, E.; Salter, A.R.; Cutter, G.R.; Kalina, J.T.; Herbert, J. Natural history of multiple sclerosis symptoms. *Int. J. MS Care* **2013**, *15*, 146–156. [CrossRef] [PubMed]
34. Costa, S.L.; Genova, H.M.; DeLuca, J.; Chiaravalloti, N.D. Information processing speed in multiple sclerosis: Past, present, and future. *Mult. Scler.* **2017**, *23*, 772–789. [CrossRef]
35. Oreja-Guevara, C.; Ayuso Blanco, T.; Brieva Ruiz, L.; Hernández Pérez, M.Á.; Meca-Lallana, V.; Ramió-Torrentà, L. Cognitive dysfunctions and assessments in multiple sclerosis. *Front. Neurol.* **2019**, *10*, 581. [CrossRef]

36. Patti, F.; Amato, M.; Trojano, M.; Bastianello, S.; Tola, M.; Goretti, B.; Caniatti, L.; Di Monte, E.; Ferrazza, P.; Brescia Morra, V. Cognitive impairment and its relation with disease measures in mildly disabled patients with relapsing—Remitting multiple sclerosis: Baseline results from the Cognitive Impairment in Multiple Sclerosis (COGIMUS) study. *Mult. Scler.* **2009**, *15*, 779–788. [CrossRef] [PubMed]
37. Krishnan, V.; Jaric, S. Hand function in multiple sclerosis: Force coordination in manipulation tasks. *Clin. Neurophysiol.* **2008**, *119*, 2274–2281. [CrossRef] [PubMed]
38. Ulwick, T. What Is Jobs-to-be-Done? Available online: https://jobs-to-be-done.com/what-is-jobs-to-be-done-fea59c8e39eb (accessed on 12 July 2021).
39. Pratap, A.; Neto, E.C.; Snyder, P.; Stepnowsky, C.; Elhadad, N.; Grant, D.; Mohebbi, M.H.; Mooney, S.; Suver, C.; Wilbanks, J. Indicators of retention in remote digital health studies: A cross-study evaluation of 100,000 participants. *Jpn. Digit. Med.* **2020**, *3*, 1–10. [CrossRef] [PubMed]
40. Burrus, O.; Gupta, C.; Ortiz, A.; Zulkiewicz, B.; Furberg, R.; Uhrig, J.; Harshbarger, C.; Lewis, M.A. Principles for developing innovative HIV digital health interventions: The case of Positive Health Check. *Med. Care* **2018**, *56*, 756–760. [CrossRef]
41. Pagoto, S.; Bennett, G.G. How behavioral science can advance digital health. *Transl. Behav. Med.* **2013**, *3*, 271–276. [CrossRef]
42. Klonoff, D.C. Behavioral theory: The missing ingredient for digital health tools to change behavior and increase adherence. *J. Diabetes Sci. Technol.* **2019**, *13*, 276–281. [CrossRef] [PubMed]
43. Duhigg, C. *The Power of Habit: Why We Do What We Do and How to Change*; Random House: New York, NY, USA, 2013; pp. 1–371.
44. Fogg, B.J. *Tiny Habits: The Small Changes That Change Everything*; Eamon Dolan Books: Boston, MA, USA, 2019. [CrossRef]
45. Fogg, B.J. A behavior model for persuasive design. In Proceedings of the 4th International Conference on Persuasive Technology, Claremont, CA, USA, 26–29 April 2009; pp. 1–7. [CrossRef]
46. Cugelman, B. Gamification: What it is and why it matters to digital health behavior change developers. *JMIR Serious Games* **2013**, *1*, e3139. [CrossRef]
47. Mathews, S.C.; McShea, M.J.; Hanley, C.L.; Ravitz, A.; Labrique, A.B.; Cohen, A.B. Digital health: A path to validation. *Jpn. Digit. Med.* **2019**, *2*, 1–9. [CrossRef]
48. Food and Drug Administration. Software as a Medical Device (SAMD). Clinical Evaluation-Guidance for Industry and Food and Drug Administration Staff. Retrieved June; 2017; Volume 29, p. 2020. Available online: https://www.fda.gov/files/medical%20devices/published/Software-as-a-Medical-Device-%28SAMD%29--Clinical-Evaluation---Guidance-for-Industry-and-Food-and-Drug-Administration-Staff.pdf (accessed on 15 September 2021).
49. Article 2 of Regulation (EU) 2017/745-MDR. *Off. J. Eur. Union* **2017**, L 117/1–L 117/175. Available online: https://eur-lex.europa.eu/legal-content/EN/TXT/?uri=OJ%3AL%3A2017%3A117%3ATOC (accessed on 15 September 2021).
50. FDA. FDA Digital Devices: Digital Health Center of Excellence Services. Available online: https://www.fda.gov/medical-devices/digital-health-center-excellence/digital-health-center-excellence-services (accessed on 12 July 2021).
51. Bennett, K.; Bennett, A.J.; Griffiths, K.M. Security considerations for e-mental health interventions. *J. Med. Internet Res.* **2010**, *12*, e61. [CrossRef] [PubMed]
52. Commission, E. *Green Paper on Mobile Health ("mHealth")*. 2014, pp. 1–20. Available online: https://digital-strategy.ec.europa.eu/en/library/green-paper-mobile-health-mhealth (accessed on 12 July 2021).
53. Recruitment, B.C.P. *Leveraging Mobile Health Technology for Patient Recruitment*. 2012, pp. 1–16. Available online: https://docplayer.net/10235751-Leveraging-mobile-health-technology-for-patient-recruitment-an-emerging-opportunity.html (accessed on 12 July 2021).
54. Leclerc, O.; Smith, J. How New Biomolecular Platforms and Digital Technologies Are Changing R&D. Available online: https://www.mckinsey.com/industries/pharmaceuticals-and-medical-products/our-insights/how-new-biomolecular-platforms-and-digital-technologies-are-changing-r-and-d (accessed on 12 July 2021).
55. Izmailova, E.S.; Wagner, J.A.; Ammour, N.; Amondikar, N.; Bell-Vlasov, A.; Berman, S.; Bloomfield, D.; Brady, L.S.; Cai, X.; Calle, R.A. Remote digital monitoring for medical product development. *Clin. Transl. Sci.* **2021**, *14*, 94–101. [CrossRef]
56. Cheng, W.-Y.; Bourke, A.K.; Lipsmeier, F.; Bernasconi, C.; Belachew, S.; Gossens, C.; Graves, J.S.; Montalban, X.; Lindemann, M. U-turn speed is a valid and reliable smartphone-based measure of multiple sclerosis-related gait and balance impairment. *Gait Posture* **2021**, *84*, 120–126. [CrossRef] [PubMed]
57. Creagh, A.; Simillion, C.; Scotland, A.; Lipsmeier, F.; Bernasconi, C.; Belachew, S.; van Beek, J.; Baker, M.; Gossens, C.; Lindemann, M. Smartphone-based remote assessment of upper extremity function for multiple sclerosis using the Draw a Shape Test. *Physiol. Meas.* **2020**, *41*, 054002. [CrossRef]
58. Creagh, A.P.; Simillion, C.; Bourke, A.K.; Scotland, A.; Lipsmeier, F.; Bernasconi, C.; van Beek, J.; Baker, M.; Gossens, C.; Lindemann, M. Smartphone-and smartwatch-based remote characterisation of ambulation in multiple sclerosis during the two-minute walk test. *IEEE J. Biomed. Health Inform.* **2020**, *25*, 838–849. [CrossRef]
59. Bourke, A.K.; Scotland, A.; Lipsmeier, F.; Gossens, C.; Lindemann, M. Gait characteristics harvested during a smartphone-based self-administered 2-minute walk test in people with multiple sclerosis: Test-retest reliability and minimum detectable change. *Sensors* **2020**, *20*, 5906. [CrossRef]
60. Bernat, J.L. Ethical and quality pitfalls in electronic health records. *Neurology* **2013**, *80*, 1057–1061. [CrossRef]
61. Romero, M.R.; Staub, A. Specialty Task Force: A Strategic Component to Electronic Health Record (EHR) Optimization. *Stud. Health Technol. Inform.* **2016**, *225*, 1051–1052.

62. D'Souza, M.; Papadopoulou, A.; Girardey, C.; Kappos, L. Standardization and digitization of clinical data in multiple sclerosis. *Nat. Rev. Neurol.* **2021**, *17*, 119–125. [CrossRef]
63. Organisation, W.H. *Digital Implementation Investment Guide (DIIG): Integrating Digital Interventions into Health Programmes.* 2020, pp. 1–182. Available online: https://www.who.int/publications/i/item/9789240010567 (accessed on 12 July 2021).
64. Breuer, R.; Zurkiya, D.N.; Samorezov, J.; Patangay, A.; Zerbi, C.; Company, F.M. Omnichannel Engagement in Medtech: The Time Is Now. Available online: https://www.mckinsey.com/industries/pharmaceuticals-and-medical-products/our-insights/omnichannel-engagement-in-medtech-the-time-is-now (accessed on 12 July 2021).
65. Iacob, N.; Simonelli, F. Towards a European Health Data Ecosystem. *Eur. J. Risk Regul.* **2020**, *11*, 884–893. [CrossRef]

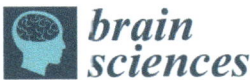

Article

Automated Analysis of the Two-Minute Walk Test in Clinical Practice Using Accelerometer Data

Katrin Trentzsch [1], Benjamin Melzer [1,2], Heidi Stölzer-Hutsch [1], Rocco Haase [1], Paul Bartscht [1], Paul Meyer [1,2] and Tjalf Ziemssen [1,*]

1. Center of Clinical Neuroscience, Neurological Clinic, University Hospital Carl Gustav Carus, TU Dresden, Fetscherstr. 74, 01307 Dresden, Germany; katrin.trentzsch@uniklinikum-dresden.de (K.T.); benjamin.n.melzer@outlook.com (B.M.); Heidi.Stoelzer-Hutsch@uniklinikum-dresden.de (H.S.-H.); Rocco.Haase@uniklinikum-dresden.de (R.H.); paul@bartscht.name (P.B.); paul.meyer.15@web.de (P.M.)
2. Institute of Biomedical Engineering, TU Dresden, Fetscherstr. 29, 01307 Dresden, Germany
* Correspondence: Tjalf.Ziemssen@uniklinikum-dresden.de Tel.: +49-351-458-4465; Fax: +49-351-458-5717

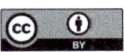

Citation: Trentzsch, K.; Melzer, B.; Stölzer-Hutsch, H.; Haase, R.; Bartscht, P.; Meyer, P.; Ziemssen, T. Automated Analysis of the Two-Minute Walk Test in Clinical Practice Using Accelerometer Data. *Brain Sci.* **2021**, *11*, 1507. https://doi.org/10.3390/brainsci11111507

Academic Editors: Maryam Zoghi and Marco Luigetti

Received: 19 October 2021
Accepted: 11 November 2021
Published: 13 November 2021

Publisher's Note: MDPI stays neutral with regard to jurisdictional claims in published maps and institutional affiliations.

Copyright: © 2021 by the authors. Licensee MDPI, Basel, Switzerland. This article is an open access article distributed under the terms and conditions of the Creative Commons Attribution (CC BY) license (https://creativecommons.org/licenses/by/4.0/).

Abstract: One of the core problems for people with multiple sclerosis (pwMS) is the impairment of their ability to walk, which can be severely restrictive in everyday life. Therefore, monitoring of ambulatory function is of great importance to be able to effectively counteract disease progression. An extensive gait analysis, such as the Dresden protocol for multidimensional walking assessment, covers several facets of walking impairment including a 2-min walk test, in which the distance taken by the patient in two minutes is measured by an odometer. Using this approach, it is questionable how precise the measuring methods are at recording the distance traveled. In this project, we investigate whether the current measurement can be replaced by a digital measurement method based on accelerometers (six Opal sensors from the Mobility Lab system) that are attached to the patient's body. We developed two algorithms using these data and compared the validity of these approaches using the results from 2-min walk tests from 562 pwMS that were collected with a gold-standard odometer. In 48.4% of pwMS, we detected an average relative measurement error of less than 5%, while results from 25.8% of the pwMS showed a relative measurement error of up to 10%. The algorithm had difficulties correctly calculating the walking distances in another 25.8% of pwMS; these results showed a measurement error of more than 20%. A main reason for this moderate performance was the variety of pathologically altered gait patterns in pwMS that may complicate the step detection. Overall, both algorithms achieved favorable levels of agreement (r = 0.884 and r = 0.980) with the odometer. Finally, we present suggestions for improvement of the measurement system to be implemented in the future.

Keywords: multiple sclerosis; gait analysis; mobility; digital tools and applications

1. Introduction

Multiple sclerosis (MS) is a chronic inflammatory, progressive disease of the central nervous system. Based on its multifocal, inflammatory lesions in the central nervous system, MS is characterized by deficits in different neurological functional systems, which leads to a wide range of symptoms and a highly individualized course of the disease [1,2]. It is important to phenotype the different symptoms of MS to adapt the management of the disease [3,4]. For many people with MS (pwMS) the limitation on the ability to walk is a clinical hallmark of their disease. Walking problems have a major impact on important areas of life and contribute significantly to the patient's quality of life. Up to 85% of pwMS report impairments in their ability to walk [5]. Kister et al. stated that 5 years after disease onset, 45% of pwMS reported mild gait deficits, and after 30 years of disease, only 18% of pwMS were able to walk without problems or with minimal limitations [6]. Different pathophysiological components such as spasticity, paresis, or sensitivity and balance disorders contribute to the development of patient-specific gait disorders [7,8].

In pwMS, walking impairments are characterized by a decreased gait speed, walking endurance, step rate, and cadence in addition to an increased variability of gait [9–11]. All these gait impairments increase with the progression of the disease. In routine clinical practice, limitations in mobility are primarily assessed with the Expanded Disability Status Scale (EDSS). Less frequently, various time-based walking tests are applied, which are often subject to intraindividual and interindividual variation [12–14]. For a better detection of mobility impairments and a high-quality, clinically relevant characterization of pwMS, an objective multimodal assessment of gait changes, such as the Dresden protocol for multidimensional walking assessment (DMWA), is important [15–17]. Different walking domains, such as gait quality, maximal walking speed, patient-reported outcomes, and also gait endurance should be assessed, with the aim to provide a more objective and standardized measurement of walking ability in addition to the EDSS [16].

Specifically, testing of walking endurance is used as an important marker in various medical settings. The Cooper 12-min walk test was originally developed for physical fitness [18]. As time progressed, shorter versions of this endurance walk test, such as the six- and two-minute walk test (6MWT, 2MWT) were developed [19]. In medicine, the gold standard of endurance testing is considered to be the 6MWT [7]. However, some patients are unable to walk for longer than two minutes. So, the 6MWT is often too strenuous and time consuming for cardiac patients and also for pwMS, so the 2MWT became a practical alternative in this case [19–21]. This is a popular and well-established walking test to obtain a detailed impression of walking ability [22] that can be well compared to the 6MWT [20,22,23].

For subtle changes in gait and the detection of an early deterioration in endurance, an accurate measurement of the distance covered is required. Estimating the total distance by multiplying the number of gaits covered does not meet the requirement for accuracy. Unlike an estimate of the total distance travelled, an odometer objectively measures the distance travelled. An odometer is clinically approved and considered the gold standard. Odometers are in principle well suited for measuring longer distances with quite high measuring accuracy [24]. For this reason, they are widely used for the measurement of walking distance in clinical environments [16,25–28]. An odometer is a measuring wheel with an integrated counter, a handpiece, and a digital display. It is designed for distance measurements on flat ground. For this purpose, the odometer is pushed over the floor in such a way that the wheel rolls permanently without slip. Although an odometer objectively measures the distance travelled, it does not measure the exact distance travelled by the patient within the given time. Using a stopwatch, the tester must measure exactly two minutes so that the odometer can be stopped afterwards, which creates a delay effect of the distance measurement. Patients can show different evasive movements when walking the distance. This is due, among other things, to the pathological gait pattern and obstacles in the course. Furthermore, the turn at the end of the gait is displayed inaccurately because the reversal angle with the odometer is different. In addition, there is the possibility of a speed influence that is subconsciously transferred from the tester with the odometer to the person being tested. To prevent a lower inter-rater reliability by changing the respective examiner, the person to be tested should walk the 2MWT completely alone.

The aim of the study is to address exactly this problem by improving the existing monitoring of multidimensional gait analysis in its complexity and efficiency and increasing its objectivity. A digitalization in this field, through the integration of appropriate algorithms can optimize the efficiency and quality of patient management [29]. The use of inertial measurement units (IMUs) is becoming increasingly popular for determining gait deficits, such as with the 6MWT [30]. In particular, the distance traveled is often calculated from IMU data [31–33]. Retory et al. compared the distance traveled, which was classically calculated from the product of the number of steps (from video recordings) with the median step length, with IMU data from an accelerometer and a correlation of $r = 0.99$ [32] was shown. When calculating the distance traveled using IMUs no other measurement instruments were needed, thus resulting in less bias in the measuring method.

Furthermore, the use of IMUs facilitated the application of the 2MWT in a setting outside the clinic. The development of such a digital measurement method is relevant to the structural shift towards home-based assistive devices for which simple digital measurement methods are needed, as well as to simplify the clinical measurement process while improving measurement accuracy.

For this purpose, we developed two algorithms using accelerometer data. These two approaches were compared and their basic functionality was evaluated in a monocentric study with the gold standard of odometers.

2. Materials and Methods

This work investigates whether the 2MWT with an odometer can be replaced by a 2MWT with accelerometers. From the sensor data of the body-worn sensors, the total distance can be determined using two developed algorithms. The first approach provides an overall evaluation of the total acceleration (Digiwalk algorithm, DWA) signals. The second approach calculates the total distance based on an average stride length (Mobility Lab algorithm, MLA). The primary focus of this study is to compare the accuracy of the DWA and MLA with the gold-standard odometer.

2.1. Population

Data from 562 patients were used for the analysis, which were recorded between July 2018 and February 2020 at the MS Center Dresden of University Hospital Carl Gustav Carus, Dresden. All pwMS completed a multidimensional gait analysis according to the DMWA protocol as part of their clinical outpatient visit. We included patients with a reliable diagnosis of MS, which were able to walk with or without assistive devices. Each participant was examined according to good clinical practice guidelines. The study was approved by the local ethics committee (BO-EK-320062021).

2.2. Procedure of the 2-Min Walk Test (2MWT)

For the 2MWT, the pwMS wore six Mobility Lab Opal sensors (APDM, Portland, OR, USA) and were asked to walk along a hospital corridor approximately 25 m long for two minutes. Walkers could be used during the test, but the patient had to be able to walk independently. Short breaks could also be taken, but these were recorded during the two minutes. To allow accurate distance measurement, the examiner walked behind the patient to match the patient's speed and not dictate his or her own walking pace. The distance traveled was recorded with an odometer, and the respective time needed was checked with a stopwatch. For each patient, the covered distance of the 2MWT was measured with the odometer and the file with the acceleration values was archived.

2.3. Distance Measurement with Acceleration Sensors

An accelerometer is a sensor that determines the acceleration it experiences by measuring the inertial force acting on a test mass. In the accelerometer-based measurement method, we used Mobility Lab Opal sensors (APDM, Portland, OR, USA) to measure spatiotemporal gait parameters of patients during walking trials. There were six individual sensor units that were attached to the patient's wrists, ankles, sternum, and lower back (Figure 1) [34].

Location of the motion sensors on specific body parts was used to obtain valid gait and balance parameters. Being consistent with other motion sensors worn on the body, the sensor to measure upper sway was placed in front of the sternum 2 cm below the jugular fossa [35]. Another sensor was placed on the lumbar spine at L5 to measure lower trunk balance [35–37]. To measure the arm swing, two sensors were placed at the left and right wrist, 4 cm from the dorsum of the hand [38]. The last two sensors for spatiotemporal gait parameters were attached to the forefoot [39,40]. Each sensor unit contained a three-axis accelerometer, three-axis gyroscope, and a magnetometer. Measurement data were collected after each walking test by plugging the sensors into the access point, which automatically generated a single file containing the raw kinematic measurements [41]. We used the acceleration data contained in these files to estimate the distance walked by the patient.

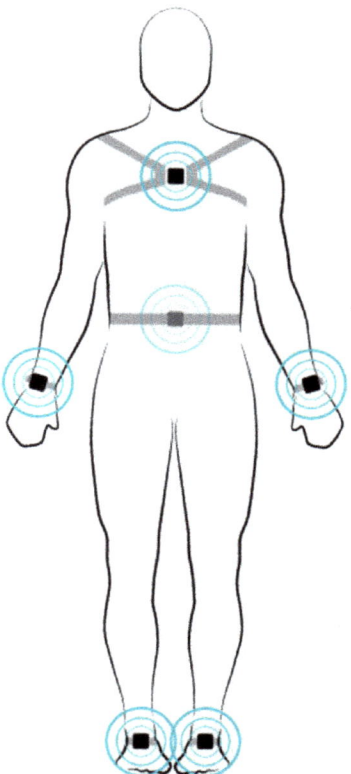

Figure 1. Demonstration of the six Mobility Lab sensors (APDM, Portland, OR, United States), both sensors applied to the forefoot serve as the basis for the calculation.

While accelerometers are a well-established method for gait analysis in the clinical environment, they are currently not commonly used for measuring walking distances [42]. However, acceleration measurements of any sensor unit carry a measurement error caused by tiny drift rates of the gyroscopes that must be compensated for by the algorithms employed [43]. In fact, extracting precise distance values from acceleration data requires exceptionally sophisticated algorithms that employ methods from the field of inertial navigation [43].

There are essentially two different algorithmic approaches to extract distance information from acceleration data.

2.3.1. Digiwalk Algorithm (DWA)

The underlying idea of the DWA is to calculate velocity from acceleration (a(t)) by integration over time. Repeating this procedure to integrate velocity over time results in the distance traveled (s(t)) at the following rate:

$$s(t) = \iint a(t) d^2 t$$

Foxlin and Bebek et al. demonstrated that two sensors that were each attached to an ankle provided sufficient information about the distance walked [43,44]. The reason being that the ankles experienced the greatest acceleration during walking which led to a high signal to noise ratio and a highly detectable movement signal. Furthermore, we leveraged the fact that each foot stands completely still for a brief moment during each walking cycle. Velocity and distance can be calculated from acceleration data by integration over time. Due to the drift of the acceleration sensors and the resulting double integration of a possible error, the calculated values deviated more from the real values over longer distances. To compensate for these errors, the periodical standstills of the feet allowed us to continuously set the velocity to zero whenever a resting foot was detected, which eliminated the drift of the calculated values. We followed the approach of Foxlin who proposed to apply these zero velocity updates (ZVU) to solve the problem of drifting values for velocity and distance [43]. To the extent that this method builds on the raw acceleration data from the Mobility Lab system, we called this approach the Digiwalk algorithm. The following section describes the DWA that we implemented to determine the distance traveled from the raw acceleration data. Figure 2 illustrates the process.

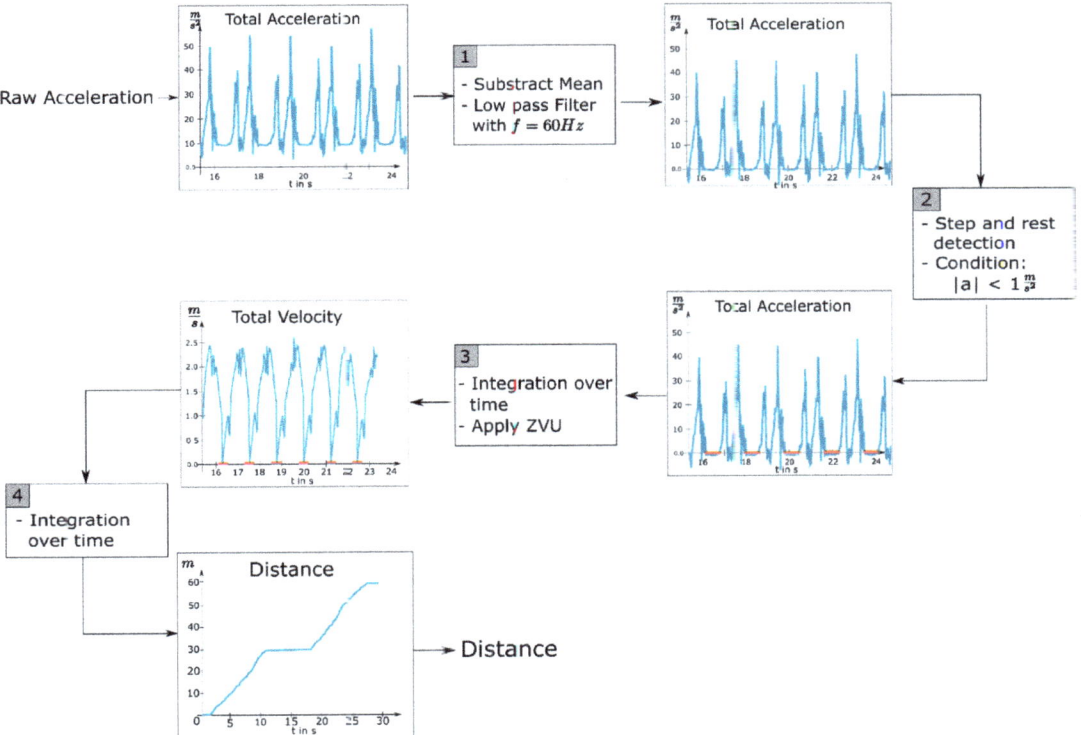

Figure 2. Flowchart for determining the distance walked; ZVU = zero velocity updates.

The first step was to preprocess and clean the acceleration data from the influence of gravity. Therefore, from each acceleration component a_x, a_y, and a_z, we subtracted its mean. Subsequently, we reduced unwanted frequency components in the signals (which were sampled at 128 Hz) by applying a low pass filter with a cut-off frequency of 60 Hz. Next, we detected the time periods during which each foot was resting. Since a resting foot should only experience the acceleration of gravity, which we removed from the signal, we searched for sections with a total acceleration of zero plus a threshold for measurement inaccuracy. We determined the optimal threshold in preliminary experiments to be 1 $\frac{m}{s^2}$ by varying the threshold value until each step of a test subject was detected for an appropriate duration (stance duration). The results of our step detection are illustrated in Figure 3, which shows the raw acceleration data of one foot as well as the time intervals in which the algorithm declared the foot was resting.

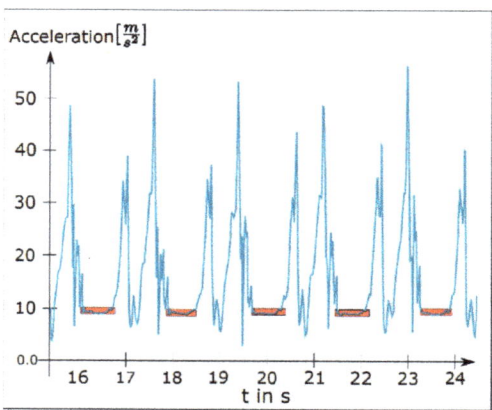

Figure 3. Total acceleration of one foot with detected resting periods (red).

In addition to the detection of a single resting foot, we also identified time periods during which the patient completely stopped walking. This occurred frequently during the walking tests since some patients were severely restricted in their ability to walk for longer periods of time. The patient was declared to be resting as soon as both feet were found to be resting simultaneously for more than one second. The integration process was paused for both feet as soon as the standstill of the patient was detected. To calculate the distance walked, we separately integrated each component of the acceleration signal twice over time. Integration was suspended for the time interval in which either one or both feet were detected to be resting and continued afterwards starting with an initial value of zero. The difference between the calculated velocity curves of one foot with and without ZVU can be seen in Figure 4.

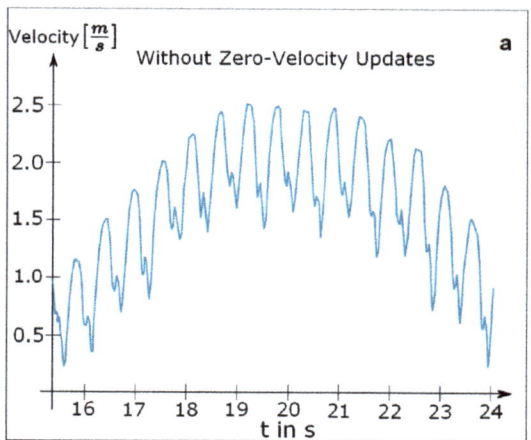 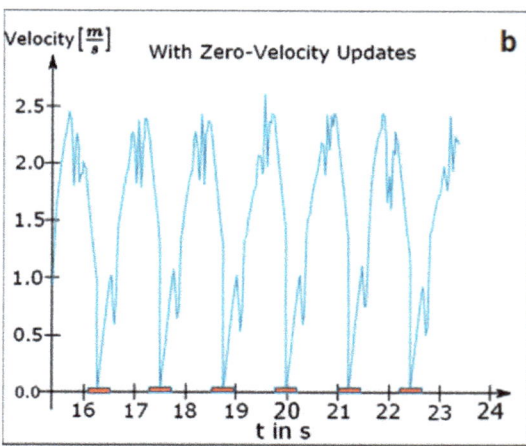

Figure 4. (a) Velocity curve of a single foot without zero velocity updates; (b) velocity curve of a single foot with zero velocity updates.

Even though each step was clearly visible in the velocity diagram without ZVU in Figure 4a, the curve contradictorily suggests that the foot never reached a velocity of zero. By contrast, the velocity curve with applied ZVU in Figure 4b depicts each step realistically with short periods of zero velocity while the foot is resting.

Finally, the difference between the calculated distances with and without stop detection is shown in Figure 5, which depicts an experiment in which a test subject walked to stop at t = 10 s for approximately 6 s. While the distance calculated without stop detection continued growing even though the test subject was standing still, the curve with stop detection stopped growing properly at this point.

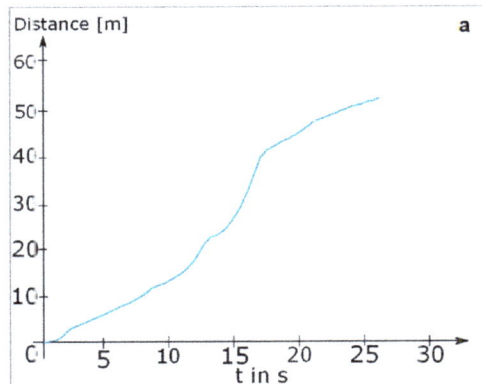
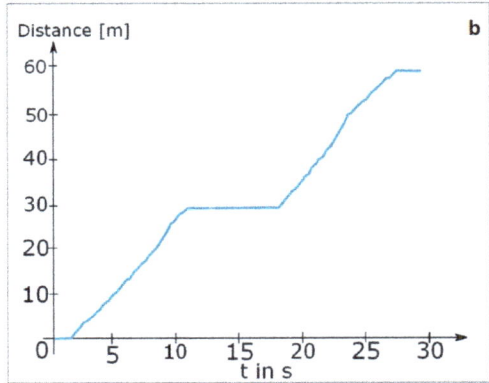

Figure 5. Acceleration of one foot with (a) calculated distance without rest detection; (b) calculated distance with rest detection.

2.3.2. Mobility Lab Algorithm (MLA)

Capela et al. presented a possible approach for inertial navigation [45]. They used raw accelerometer data processing for the 6MWT in a clinical setting and employed an activity detection to distinguish walking from standing times. By multiplying the average stride lengths by the number of steps taken, the walked distance was determined [45]. The number of steps could be recorded using a pedometer or peak identification of the acceleration data. In our work, we used the same approach as just described. The distance traveled in two minutes were estimated by multiplying the stride length by the number of steps per minute. As the calculation was based on the stride length output by the Mobility Lab System, we refer to it as the Mobility Lab algorithm.

2.4. Statistical Methods

Continuous variables were presented as mean ± standard deviation (SD) or median with interquartile range (IQR), where appropriate. Categorical variables were described in absolute numbers and percentages. We calculated the mean of the differences between the DWA, MLA, and odometer measurement series, the SD, and the 95% limits of agreement (=mean ± 1.96 × SD) to describe the agreement between the MLA and the DWA to the standardized odometer measurement method. Bland–Altman plots, Pearson's r, and intraclass correlation coefficients (ICC) were calculated to compare the three estimates of distance (odometer, DWA, MLA). ICC levels were interpreted according to the guidelines of Koo and Li (below 0.50: poor, between 0.50 and 0.75: moderate, between 0.75 and 0.90 good, above 0.90: excellent) [46]. Mean values were tested for significance using a t-test for systematic differentiation between the distance traveled by the different measurement methods and the use of assistive devices. In order to assess important variables influencing the measurement series and their measurement errors, Kendall's tau-b correlation analyses were performed. Kendall's tau-b (τb) has been defined for level 0.1 to 0.3 as weak, for level 0.3 to 0.5 as moderate, and above 0.5 as strong correlation. Linear model analyses were performed to determine variables influencing DWA and MLA. An identity linkage function linear model were used for normally distributed data with the factors of age, sex, degree of disability (via EDSS), the use of assistive devices, and subtype of MS (relapsing–remitting, primary progressive, and secondary progressive). The level of statistical significance was set at α = 5%. All statistical analyses were performed using IBM SPSS Statistics 27 (SPSS, Chicago, IL, USA).

3. Results

The analysis used data from 562 pwMS performing the 2MWT. There was an age distribution of 16 to 79 years among the patients, with a mean age of 43.15 (SD ± 12.31) years. A figure of 69.8% of the pwMS were female and the disease duration of patients averaged 8.57 (SD ± 7.51) years. An overview of patient characteristics is shown in Table 1.

Table 1. Characterization of people with multiple sclerosis (MS) presented as mean [mean] with standard deviation [SD] or median with interquartile range (IQR); MS = multiple sclerosis; RRMS = relapsing–remitting MS; PPMS = primary progressive MS; SPMS = secondary progressive MS; EDSS = Expanded Disability Status Scale; 2-min walk = 2MWT.

	pwMS (n = 562)
Mean age (years; mean ± SD)	43.15 ± 12.31
Females (N, %)	392 (69.8%)
Disease duration (years; mean ± SD)	8.57 ± 7.51
MS Subtype	
RRMS (N, %)	490 (87.2%)
PPMS (N, %)	55 (9.8%)
SPMS (N, %)	13 (3.0%)
EDSS (median, IQR)	2.5 (1.5–3.5)
Aids	
with	35 (6.2%)
without	527 (93.8%)
2MWT	
2MWT with odometer in m (mean, SD)	143.52 ± 32.57
2MWT with Digiwalk in m (mean, SD)	149.20 ± 32.33
2MWT with MobiLab in m (mean, SD)	140.61 ± 32.58

With the comparison of the respective mean values of the two measuring methods to the odometer it was shown that the DWA overestimated the values (149.20 ± 32.33) whereas the MLA, calculated using cadence and average step length, underestimated the covered distance (140.6 ± 32.58) compared with the distance measured by the odometer (143.52 ± 32.57) (Table 1, Figure 6).

Bland–Altman plots revealed upper and lower limits of agreement of 24.10 and −36.40 for the DWA and upper and lower limits of agreement of 15.68 and −9.84 for the MLA (Figure 6). The two algorithms showed good to excellent correlations with the odometer (DWA: r = 0.884, ICC = 0.871; MLA: r = 0.980, ICC = 0.976).

The relative measurement error was calculated for both algorithms, and the distribution is visualized in Figure 7. Most of the recordings showed a relatively small measurement error of 10% or less. The mean measurement error was 9.21 ± 14.7% for the DWA and 4.06 ± 4.61% for the MLA, respectively.

Comparing the covered distance between the DWA and the odometer, 272 data sets had a relative measurement error of less than 5%, which was 48.4% of the total number of data sets. However, 145 (25.8%) data sets remained with a measurement error of up to 10% and 25.8% had a measurement error of more than 20% error.

In the second approach, comparing the MLA and the odometer, a relative measurement error of less than 5% was present in 436 (77.6%) data sets. Another 85 data sets (15.1%) showed a measurement error of less than 10% and the remaining 7.3% had over 20% error.

The relative measurement errors were analyzed in relation to influencing variables such as age, degree of disability, and the use of assistive devices and are shown in Figure 8.

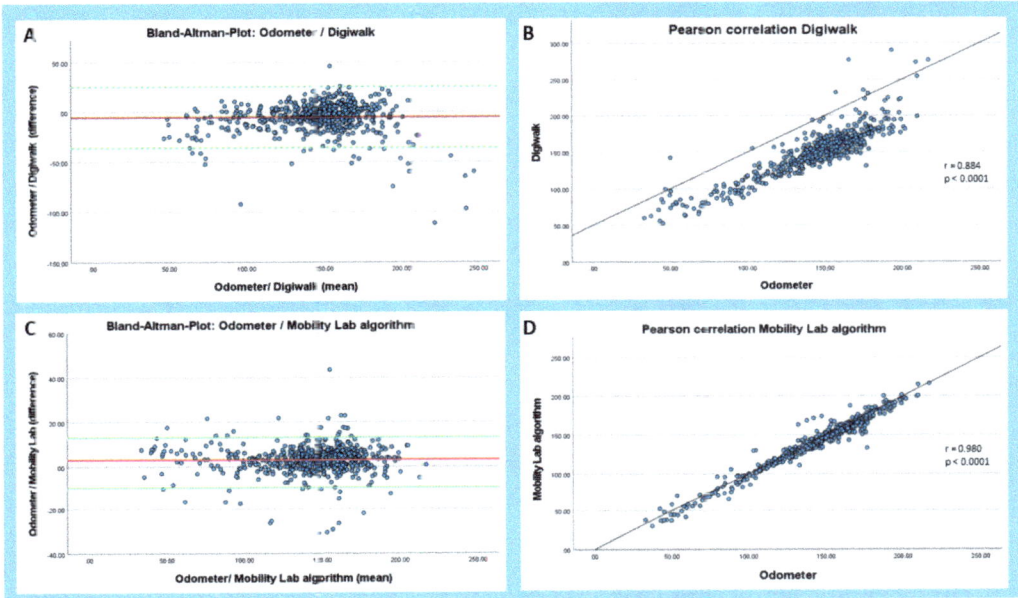

Figure 6. Bland–Altman and Pearson's correlation plots. (**A**) Bland–Altman plot of the Digiwalk measurement; (**B**) Pearson correlation of the Digiwalk measurement; (**C**) Bland–Altman plot of the Mobility Lab algorithm; (**D**) Pearson correlation of the Mobility Lab algorithm. The red line shows the mean of the differences between the two respective methods, and the dashed green horizontal lines show the upper and lower 95% limits of agreement (=mean ± 1.96 × SD). R = correlation coefficient.

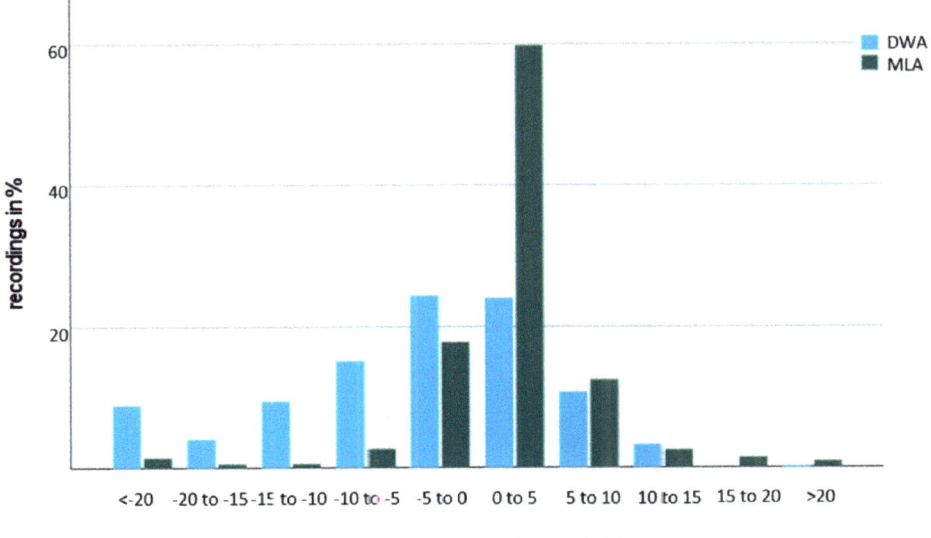

Figure 7. Histogram of the relative frequencies of relative measurement errors for the Digiwalk algorithm (DWA) and the Mobility Lab algorithm (MLA) compared to the current gold-standard odometer.

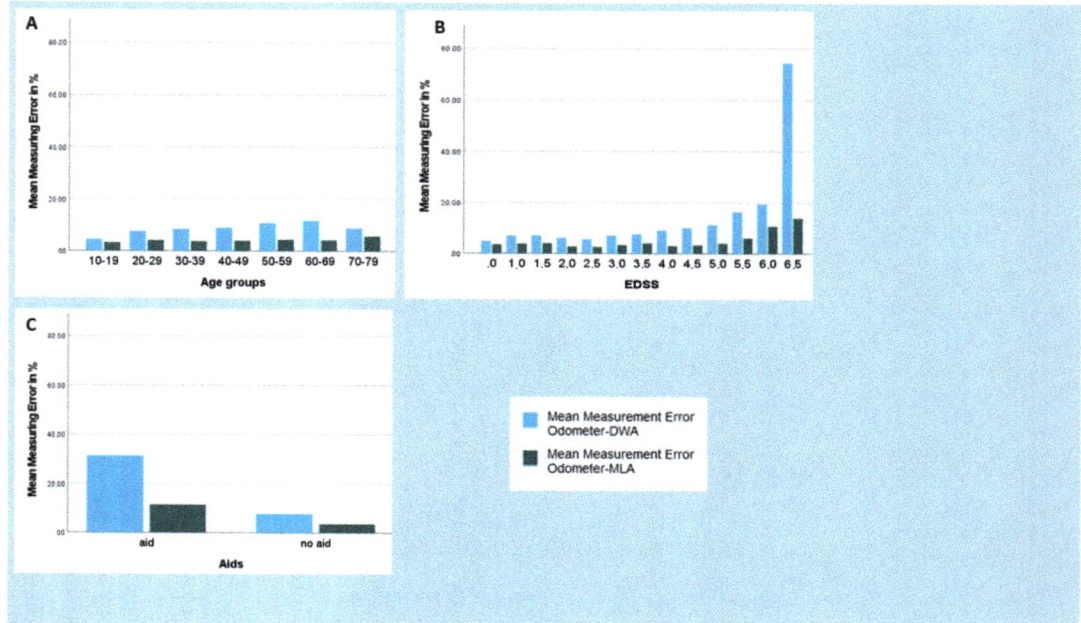

Figure 8. Representation of the relative measurement errors of the Digiwalk algorithm (DWA) and the Mobility Lab algorithm (MLA) in relation to the influence variables of age (**A**), Expanded Disability Status Scale (**B**), and use of aids (**C**).

When age (Figure 8A) of the pwMS was considered, the MLA measurement errors appeared to be independent of age. For the DWA, there was a peak in measurement error at the age of 60 to 69.

Measurement errors tended to increase with increasing disability slightly earlier with the DWA (EDSS 4.0) than with the MLA (EDSS 5.5) (Figure 8B).

The relative measurement errors also increased with the use of assistive devices, especially with DWA. The highest relative measurement error that occurred was 31.27% when measuring with the DWA with aids. In contrast, the lowest relative measurement error of 3.57% occurred when measuring with the MLA without aids (Figure 8C). The mean difference between the odometer and the DWA using assistive devices was -14.44 ± 16.39 m, compared to without assistive devices -5.10 ± 15.44 m ($p = 0.001$). Compared to the DWA, the mean difference between the odometer and the MLA was lower with aids 4.82 ± 7.28 m and without aids 2.79 ± 6.45 m ($p = 0.074$) (Table 2).

Table 2. Comparison of the measurement series with the aids (mean ± SD) by t-tests; 2MWT = two-minute walk test; OM = odometer; DWA = Digiwalk algorithm; MLA = Mobility Lab algorithm.

	With Aids	Without Aids	p
2MWT OM	70.98 ± 22.89	148.34 ± 29.91	<0.001
2MWT DWA	85.42 ± 16.55	153.44 ± 28.44	<0.001
2MWT ML	66.16 ± 23.19	145.55 ± 26.53	<0.001
Difference OM-DWA	−14.44 ± 16.39	−5.10 ± 15.44	0.001
Difference OM-MLA	4.82 ± 7.28	2.79 ± 6.45	0.074

The measurement error of the DWA showed a weak correlation with age ($\tau b = 0.0173$), the use of aids (-0.159), and disease disability (Table 3), as well as a moderate correlation with double support ($\tau b = 0.0359$). There were no such correlations for the MLA.

Table 3. Kendall's tau-b correlation between demographic data, clinical outcomes, and parameter of gait (n = 552); EDSS = Expanded Disability Status Scale; DWA = Digiwalk algorithm; MLA= Mobility Lab algorithm.

		Measurement Error DWA	Measurement Error MLA
Age	τ	0.173 **	0.091 **
Sex	τ	0.041	−0.007
Aids	τ	−0.159 **	0.147
Disease Duration	τ	0.073 *	0.001
Disease Disability (EDSS)	τ	0.241 **	−0.029
Parameter of gait			
Cadence	τ	−0.116 **	0.155 **
Stride Length	τ	−0.191 **	0.119 **
Double Support	τ	0.359 **	−0.010
Gait speed	τ	−0.184 **	0.143 **
Lateral Step variability	τ	0.177 **	0.075 **
Number of turns	τ	−0.164 **	0.051

* $p < 0.05$, ** $p < 0.01$. EDSS = Expanded Disability Status Scale, DWA = Digiwalk algorithm; MLA = Mobility Lab algorithm.

In a multifactorial linear model approach, level of disease disability was solely associated with the measurement error of the DWA (T = 6.395; $p < 0.001$; CI 95% 0.184 to 0.348), whereas disease disability (T = −3.464; $p = 0.001$; CI 95% −0.086 to −0.024) and age (T = 2.329; $p = 0.02$; CI 95% 0.003 to 0.039) where associated with the measurement errors of the MLA. Sex, the use of walking aids, and the subtype of MS were not associated with any algorithm in the respective linear model.

4. Discussion

Walk endurance tests are important to quantify walking parameters accurately [47,48]. Therefore, we applied two novel algorithm–based approaches using accelerator sensors in comparison to the current standard measurement using the odometer in the walking assessment of pwMS. Our results demonstrated that the DWA achieved a good performance (measurement error < 5%) in about half of the pwMS tested (48.4%) and the MLA in considerably more pwMS (77.6%). Overall, both algorithms achieved favorable levels of agreement (DWA: ICC = 0.871; MLA: ICC = 0.976) with the odometer. These results are comparable to other calculations based on accelerometers for measuring distance traveled [49].

Sensor data for the assessment of mobility in MS have gained interest over recent years. Creagh et al. demonstrated how signal-based features related to movement can be extracted from sensors in smartphones and smartwatches and showed good correlations with clinical outcomes [47]. Karle et al. performed initial approaches of a 2MWT outside a clinical environment for pwMS. For this, the average cadences were processed from the raw acceleration data of an activity monitor. An average cadence between a clinical environment and an outside environment was compared [48]. Unfortunately, both studies did not include a gold standard of measurement to verify the respective measurement system. Our approach including two algorithms aimed for the digitalization of walking assessment in the neurological practice through the integration of appropriate algorithms that could optimize patient management. While we demonstrated overall performances of good to excellent in the two algorithms in comparison to the gold standard, measurement errors in some subgroups of pwMS increased. It was reasonable to assume that the measurement error of a distance measurement with accelerometers was highly dependent on the gait pattern of the person. We investigated how accurately an irregular gait pattern affected accelerometer measurements. Thus, we found a robust association between disease disability of the pwMS and measurement error for both algorithms (MLA and DWA). Furthermore, there may have been an inherent error in the calculated relative measurement error because the measurement accuracy of the odometer was unknown.

For the DWA, there was a moderate correlation ($\tau = 0.359$) between double support and the measurement error. It should be taken into account that only six gait parameters (cadence, stride length, double support, gait speed, lateral step variability, and number of turns) were considered in our analyses. Nevertheless, there are many more spatiotemporal gait parameters that can be tested with respect to measurement error. For example, the number of breaks taken was not considered in our work. It should be noted that some pwMS, especially in older age or with increased degree of disability, were not able to perform the 2MWT continuously but needed short standing breaks in between.

Other measurement inaccuracies can also result from the rotation of the subjects at the turning point of the measurement course. An algorithm modification should be implemented for this. There must be an intelligent threshold for detecting the rotation. El-Gohary et al. proposed a threshold of $\pm 5°/s$ as the beginning and end of each rotation [50]. For general testing with differently impaired subjects, these thresholds need to be evaluated. Cheng et al. have already provided reliable algorithms for detecting rotations and rotation speeds. Similar processing algorithms can be implemented in the DWA in the future. More accurate detection of rotations will increase the accuracy of the total distance [51].

The DWA measurement error was more often positive than negative, whereas this seemed to be the other way round for the MLA. Positive error values mean that a distance value derived from the accelerometers was higher than the reference value. This in turn suggests that the DWA more often failed to detect steps, rather than misclassifying a signal segment as a step when there was none. In particular, the DWA was found to have difficulties to some degree in accurately detecting steps once the gait pattern deviated heavily from the norm. For this reason, the DWA tended to miss steps frequently in some pwMS, resulting in the acceleration not resetting correctly to zero. As a result, acceleration, velocity, and distance increased incorrectly. Additionally, the accurate detection of resting phases, as well as the differentiation between resting phases, slow walking, and turning, proved to be difficult. Any misjudgment of the person's current state led to acceleration errors, which in turn led to a rapidly growing error in the calculated distance.

In conclusion, the quality of the measurement was highly dependent on successful step detection, which in turn depended on the gait pattern being as regular as possible. Possible solutions to these problems are discussed in the next section.

5. Future

In the future, we will improve our analytical algorithm described here by adopting the approach of Foxlin, who implemented a measurement system to track the position of a walking person [43]. Since the distance walked can be calculated from the difference in position between two points in time, this approach would also be suitable for our approach. Foxlin tracks the position using calculations based on a complex sensor fusion of accelerometers and gyroscopes. The calculation errors of velocity, distance, and attitude originating from sensor drifts are compensated by only navigating in an open loop manner during the strides phase of each foot. Zero velocity updates are not directly applied to the velocity measurements by resetting it to zero but are fed into an extended Kalman filter (EKF) as pseudo measurements. The EKF corrects the state components acceleration, velocity, distance, attitude, and angular velocity after each measurement, reducing the position error that previously grew cubically in time to an error growing linearly with the number of steps taken. In this manner, the position drift that occurs during each stride phase is corrected by monitoring the correlation between velocity and position error. The performance of this measurement system was evaluated by indoor experiments in which a person walked for 322 s, covering 118.5 m, resulting in a position error of only 0.3%. It is however unclear, exactly how well this algorithm will perform on pathologically altered gait patterns, especially since the calculations also rely on detecting the stance of the phases of the feet.

A completely different approach would be the use of Bluetooth beacons which could eliminate the problem of accurately detecting the stance phases of the feet that has proven to be the main problem. Therefore, this approach could be tested in the future. Since the main weakness of this method is the position accuracy, further tests have to show how a position error of about 1 to 2 m affects the calculated distance.

Applying artificial intelligence is another possibility and is a promising approach. As we have shown, machine learning algorithms enable the integration and visualization of a wide variety of gait parameters in routine clinical practice [52]. Thus, model calculations could be performed based on the available spatiotemporal gait data to predict the distance traveled. For this, further studies are needed to determine the necessary input data and the most useful (combination of) sensor systems.

Author Contributions: Conceptualization, K.T. and B.M.; methodology, K.T., B.M. and R.H.; software, B.M. and P.M.; validation, R.H. and H.S.-H.; formal analysis, B.M., K.T., R.H. and H.S.-H.; investigation, B.M. and P.B.; resources, P.B. and H.S.-H.; data curation, B.M., P.B. and H.S.-H.; writing—original draft preparation, K.T. and B.M.; writing—review and editing, R.H., P.B., H.S.-H. and T.Z.; visualization, K.T., B.M. and H.S.-H.; supervision, T.Z.; project administration, K.T. All authors have read and agreed to the published version of the manuscript.

Funding: This research received no external funding.

Institutional Review Board Statement: The study was conducted according to the guidelines of the Declaration of Helsinki and approved by Ethics Committee at the Technical University Dresden. Approval number: EK-320062021. The patients/participants provided their written informed consent to participate in this study.

Informed Consent Statement: Informed consent was obtained from all subjects involved in the study.

Data Availability Statement: The data presented in this study are available on request from the corresponding author. The data are not publicly available due to patient confidentiality.

Conflicts of Interest: The authors declare no conflict of interest.

References

1. Goldenberg, M.M. Multiple Sclerosis Review. *Pharm. Ther.* **2012**, *37*, 175–184.
2. Lindner, M.; Klotz, L.; Wiendl, H. Mechanisms underlying lesion development and lesion distribution in CNS autoimmunity. *J. Neurochem.* **2018**, *146*, 122–132. [CrossRef]
3. Voigt, I.; Inojosa, H.; Dillenseger, A.; Haase, R.; Akgün, K.; Ziemssen, T. Digital Twins for Multiple Sclerosis. *Front. Immunol.* **2021**, *12*, 669811. [CrossRef] [PubMed]
4. Ziemssen, T.; Kern, R.; Thomas, K. Multiple sclerosis: Clinical profiling and data collection as prerequisite for personalized medicine approach. *BMC Neurol.* **2016**, *16*, 124. [CrossRef] [PubMed]
5. Comber, L.; Sosnoff, J.J.; Galvin, R.; Coote, S. Postural control deficits in people with Multiple Sclerosis: A systematic review and meta-analysis. *Gait Posture* **2018**, *61*, 445–452. [CrossRef]
6. Kister, I.; Chamot, E.; Salter, A.R.; Cutter, G.R.; Bacon, T.E.; Herbert, J. Disability in multiple sclerosis: A reference for patients and clinicians. *Neurology* **2013**, *80*, 1018–1024. [CrossRef]
7. Goldman, M.D.; Marrie, R.A.; Cohen, J. Evaluation of the six-minute walk in multiple sclerosis subjects and healthy controls. *Mult. Scler. J.* **2008**, *14*, 383–390. [CrossRef] [PubMed]
8. Shanahan, C.J.; Boonstra, F.M.C.; Lizama, L.E.C.; Strik, M.; Moffat, B.A.; Khan, F.; Kilpatrick, T.J.; Van Der Walt, A.; Galea, M.P.; Kolbe, S.C. Technologies for Advanced Gait and Balance Assessments in People with Multiple Sclerosis. *Front. Neurol.* **2018**, *8*, 708. [CrossRef]
9. Cameron, M.H.; Wagner, J.M. Gait Abnormalities in Multiple Sclerosis: Pathogenesis, Evaluation, and Advances in Treatment. *Curr. Neurol. Neurosci. Rep.* **2011**, *11*, 507–515. [CrossRef]
10. Sosnoff, J.J.; Sandroff, B.; Motl, R.W. Quantifying gait abnormalities in persons with multiple sclerosis with minimal disability. *Gait Posture* **2012**, *36*, 154–156. [CrossRef]
11. Dujmovic, I.; Radovanovic, S.; Martinovic, V.; Dackovic, J.; Maric, G.; Mesaros, S.; Pekmezovic, T.; Kostic, V.; Drulovic, J. Gait pattern in patients with different multiple sclerosis phenotypes. *Mult. Scler. Relat. Disord.* **2017**, *13*, 13–20. [CrossRef]
12. Meyer-Moock, S.; Feng, Y.-S.; Maeurer, M.; Dippel, F.-W.; Kohlmann, T. Systematic literature review and validity evaluation of the Expanded Disability Status Scale (EDSS) and the Multiple Sclerosis Functional Composite (MSFC) in patients with multiple sclerosis. *BMC Neurol.* **2014**, *14*, 58. [CrossRef] [PubMed]

13. Goodkin, D.E.; Cookfair, D.; Wende, K.; Bourdette, D.; Pullicino, P.; Scherokman, B.; Whitham, R. Inter- and intrarater scoring agreement using grades 1.0 to 3.5 of the Kurtzke Expanded Disability Status Scale (EDSS). *Neurology* **1992**, *42*, 859–863. [CrossRef] [PubMed]
14. Hobart, J.; Freeman, J.; Thompson, A. Kurtzke scales revisited: The application of psychometric methods to clinical intuition. *Brain* **2000**, *123*, 1027–1040. [CrossRef] [PubMed]
15. Decavel, P.; Sagawa, Y. Gait quantification in multiple sclerosis: A single-centre experience of systematic evaluation. *Neurophysiol. Clin. Neurophysiol.* **2019**, *49*, 165–171. [CrossRef]
16. Trentzsch, K.; Weidemann, M.L.; Torp, C.; Inojosa, H.; Scholz, M.; Haase, R.; Schriefer, D.; Akgün, K.; Ziemssen, T. The Dresden Protocol for Multidimensional Walking Assessment (DMWA) in Clinical Practice. *Front. Neurosci.* **2020**, *14*, 582046. [CrossRef] [PubMed]
17. Scholz, M.; Haase, R.; Trentzsch, K.; Stölzer-Hutsch, H.; Ziemssen, T. Improving Digital Patient Care: Lessons Learned from Patient-Reported and Expert-Reported Experience Measures for the Clinical Practice of Multidimensional Walking Assessment. *Brain Sci.* **2021**, *11*, 786. [CrossRef] [PubMed]
18. Cooper, K.H. A Means of Assessing Maximal Oxygen Intake. *JAMA* **1968**, *203*, 201–204. [CrossRef]
19. Butland, R.; Pang, J.; Gross, E.; Woodcock, A.; Geddes, D. Two-, six-, and 12-minute walking tests in respiratory disease. *Br. Med. J.* **1982**, *284*, 1607–1608. [CrossRef]
20. Gijbels, D.; Eijnde, B.; Feys, P. Comparison of the 2- and 6-minute walk test in multiple sclerosis. *Mult. Scler. J.* **2011**, *17*, 1269–1272. [CrossRef]
21. Brooks, D.; Parsons, J.; Tran, D.; Jeng, B.; Gorczyca, B.; Newton, J.; Lo, V.; Dear, C.; Silaj, E.; Hawn, T. The two-minute walk test as a measure of functional capacity in cardiac surgery patients. *Arch. Phys. Med. Rehabil.* **2004**, *85*, 1525–1530. [CrossRef]
22. Rossier, P.; Wade, D. Validity and reliability comparison of 4 mobility measures in patients presenting with neurologic impairment. *Arch. Phys. Med. Rehabil.* **2001**, *82*, 9–13. [CrossRef] [PubMed]
23. Scalzitti, D.; Harwood, K.J.; Maring, J.R.; Leach, S.J.; Ruckert, E.A.; Costello, E. Validation of the 2-Minute Walk Test with the 6-Minute Walk Test and Other Functional Measures in Persons with Multiple Sclerosis. *Int. J. MS Care* **2018**, *20*, 158–163. [CrossRef] [PubMed]
24. Von Messrädern, P. Merkblatt. 2015, pp. 1–9. Available online: https://www.ptb.de/cms/fileadmin/internet/fachabteilungen/abteilung_5/5.4_interferometrie_an_masverkoerperungen/5.45/merkblatt/Merkblatt_Messrad_a2.pdf (accessed on 20 May 2021).
25. Créange, A.; Serre, I.; Levasseur, M.; Audry, D.; Nineb, A.; Boerio, D.; Moreau, T.; Maison, P.; Sindefi-Sep, R. Walking capacities in multiple sclerosis measured by global positioning system odometer. *Mult. Scler. J.* **2007**, *13*, 220–223. [CrossRef]
26. Donovan, K.; Lord, S.; McNaughton, H.K.; Weatherall, M. Mobility beyond the clinic: The effect of environment on gait and its measurement in community-ambulant stroke survivors. *Clin. Rehabil.* **2008**, *22*, 556–563. [CrossRef] [PubMed]
27. Stockman, J. Six-Minute Walk Test in Children and Adolescents. *Yearb. Pediatr.* **2007**, *150*, 395–399. [CrossRef]
28. Peralta-Brenes, M.; Briceño-Torres, J.M.; Chacón-Araya, Y.; Moncada-Jiménez, J.; Villanea, M.S.; Johnson, D.K.; Campos-Salazar, C. Prediction of Peak Aerobic Power among Costa Rican Older Adults. *J. Clin. Diagn. Res.* **2018**, *12*, CC01–CC04. [CrossRef]
29. Scholz, M.; Haase, R.; Schriefer, D.; Voigt, I.; Ziemssen, T. Electronic Health Interventions in the Case of Multiple Sclerosis: From Theory to Practice. *Brain Sci.* **2021**, *11*, 180. [CrossRef]
30. Storm, F.A.; Cesareo, A.; Reni, G.; Biffi, E. Wearable Inertial Sensors to Assess Gait during the 6-Minute Walk Test: A Systematic Review. *Sensors* **2020**, *20*, 2660. [CrossRef]
31. Brooks, G.C.; Vittinghoff, E.; Iyer, S.; Tandon, D.; Kuhar, P.; Madsen, K.A.; Marcus, G.M.; Pletcher, M.J.; Olgin, J.E. Accuracy and Usability of a Self-Administered 6-Minute Walk Test Smartphone Application. *Circ. Heart Fail.* **2015**, *8*, 905–913. [CrossRef]
32. Retory, Y.; David, P.; Niedzialkowski, P.; De Picciotto, C.; Bonay, M.; Petitjean, M. Gait Monitoring and Walk Distance Estimation with an Accelerometer During 6-Minute Walk Test. *Respir. Care* **2019**, *64*, 923–930. [CrossRef] [PubMed]
33. Vienne-Jumeau, A.; Oudre, L.; Moreau, A.; Quijoux, F.; Edmond, S.; Dandrieux, M.; Legendre, E.; Vidal, P.P.; Ricard, D. Personalized Template-Based Step Detection from Inertial Measurement Units Signals in Multiple Sclerosis. *Front. Neurol.* **2020**, *11*, 261. [CrossRef] [PubMed]
34. Wearable Sensors—APDM Wearable Technologies. Available online: https://apdm.com/mobility/ (accessed on 31 May 2020).
35. Spain, R.; George, R.S.; Salarian, A.; Mancini, M.; Wagner, J.; Horak, F.; Bourdette, D. Body-worn motion sensors detect balance and gait deficits in people with multiple sclerosis who have normal walking speed. *Gait Posture* **2012**, *35*, 573–578. [CrossRef]
36. Mancini, M.; Horak, F.B. Potential of APDM mobility lab for the monitoring of the progression of Parkinson's disease. *Expert Rev. Med. Devices* **2016**, *13*, 455–462. [CrossRef] [PubMed]
37. Mancini, M.; Salarian, A.; Carlson-Kuhta, P.; Zampieri, C.; King, L.; Chiari, L.; Horak, F.B. ISway: A sensitive, valid and reliable measure of postural control. *J. Neuroeng. Rehabil.* **2012**, *9*, 59. [CrossRef] [PubMed]
38. Killeen, T.; Elshehabi, M.; Filli, L.; Hobert, M.A.; Hansen, C.; Rieger, D.; Brockmann, K.; Nussbaum, S.; Zörner, B.; Bolliger, M.; et al. Arm swing asymmetry in overground walking. *Sci. Rep.* **2018**, *8*, 12803. [CrossRef] [PubMed]
39. Washabaugh, E.P.; Kalyanaraman, T.; Adamczyk, P.; Claflin, E.S.; Krishnan, C. Validity and repeatability of inertial measurement units for measuring gait parameters. *Gait Posture* **2017**, *55*, 87–93. [CrossRef]
40. Werner, C.; Heldmann, P.; Hummel, S.; Bauknecht, L.; Bauer, J.M.; Hauer, K. Concurrent Validity, Test-Retest Reliability, and Sensitivity to Change of a Single Body-Fixed Sensor for Gait Analysis during Rollator-Assisted Walking in Acute Geriatric Patients. *Sensors* **2020**, *20*, 4866. [CrossRef] [PubMed]

41. APDM Wearable Technologies Inc. *User Guide Mobility Lab*; APDM Wearable Technologies Inc.: Portland, OR, USA, 2020.
42. Weidemann, M.L.; Trentzsch, K.; Torp, C.; Ziemssen, T. Remote-Sensoring—Neue Optionen des Progressionsmonitorings bei Multipler Sklerose. *Nervenarzt* **2019**, *90*, 1239–1244. [CrossRef] [PubMed]
43. Foxlin, E.; Intersense, A. Pedestrian tracking with shoe-mounted inertial sensors. *IEEE Comput. Graph. Appl.* **2005**, *25*, 38–46. [CrossRef] [PubMed]
44. Bebek, O.; Suster, M.A.; Rajgopal, S. Fu, M.J.; Huang, X.; Cavusoglu, M.C.; Young, D.J.; Mehregany, M.; Bogert, A.J.V.D.; Mastrangelo, C.H. Personal navigation via shoe mounted inertial measurement units. *ISEEE Trans. Instrum. Meas.* **2010**, *59*, 3018–3027. [CrossRef]
45. Capela, N.; Lemaire, E.D.; Baddour, N. Novel algorithm for a smartphone-based 6-minute walk test application: Algorithm, application development, and evaluation. *J. Neuroeng. Rehabil.* **2015**, *12*, 19. [CrossRef] [PubMed]
46. Koo, T.K.; Li, M.Y. A Guideline of Selecting and Reporting Intraclass Correlation Coefficients for Reliability Research. *J. Chiroprac. Med.* **2016**, *15*, 155–163. [CrossRef] [PubMed]
47. Creagh, A.P.; Simillion, C.; Bourke, A.K.; Scotland, A.; Lipsmeier, F.; Bernasconi, C.; van Beek, J.; Baker, M.; Gossens, C.; Lindemann, M.; et al. Smartphone- and Smartwatch-Based Remote Characterisation of Ambulation in Multiple Sclerosis During the Two-Minute Walk Test. *IEEE J. Biomed. Health Inform.* **2020**, *25*, 838–849. [CrossRef]
48. Karle, V.; Hartung, V.; Ivanovska, K.; Mäurer, M.; Flachenecker, P.; Pfeifer, K.; Tallner, A. The Two-Minute Walk Test in Persons with Multiple Sclerosis: Correlations of Cadence with Free-Living Walking Do Not Support Ecological Validity. *Int. J. Environ. Res. Public Health* **2020**, *17*, 9044. [CrossRef]
49. Truong, P.H.; Lee, J.; Kwon, A.-R.; Jeong, G.-M. Stride Counting in Human Walking and Walking Distance Estimation Using Insole Sensors. *Sensors* **2016**, *16*, 823. [CrossRef]
50. El-Gohary, M.; Pearson, S.; McNames, J.; Mancini, M.; Horak, F.; Mellone, S.; Chiari, L. Continuous Monitoring of Turning in Patients with Movement Disability. *Sensors* **2013**, *14*, 356–369. [CrossRef]
51. Cheng, W.-Y.; Bourke, A.K.; Lipsmeier, F.; Bernasconi, C.; Belachew, S.; Gossens, C.; Graves, J.S.; Montalban, X.; Lindemann, M. U-turn speed is a valid and reliable smartphone-based measure of multiple sclerosis-related gait and balance impairment. *Gait Posture* **2021**, *84*, 120–126. [CrossRef]
52. Trentzsch, K.; Schumann, P.; Śliwiński, G.; Bartscht, P.; Haase, R.; Schriefer, D.; Zink, A.; Heinke, A.; Jochim, T.; Malberg, H.; et al. Using Machine Learning Algorithms for Identifying Gait Parameters Suitable to Evaluate Subtle Changes in Gait in People with Multiple Sclerosis. *Brain Sci.* **2021**, *11*, 1049. [CrossRef]

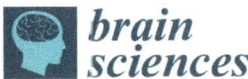

Review

Digital Biomarkers in Multiple Sclerosis

Anja Dillenseger [†], Marie Luise Weidemann [†], Katrin Trentzsch, Hernan Inojosa, Rocco Haase, Dirk Schriefer, Isabel Voigt, Maria Scholz, Katja Akgün and Tjalf Ziemssen *

Multiple Sclerosis Center Dresden, Center of Clinical Neuroscience, Department of Neurology, University Clinic Carl-Gustav Carus, Dresden University of Technology, Fetscherstrasse 74, 01307 Dresden, Germany; Anja.Dillenseger@uniklinikum-dresden.de (A.D.); MarieLuise.Weidemann@uniklinikum-dresden.de (M.L.W.); katrin.trentzsch@uniklinikum-dresden.de (K.T.); hernan.inojosa@uniklinikum-dresden.de (H.I.); Rocco.Haase@uniklinikum-dresden.de (R.H.); dirk.schriefer@uniklinikum-dresden.de (D.S.); Isabel.Voigt@uniklinikum-dresden.de (I.V.); maria.scholz@uniklinikum-dresden.de (M.S.); Katja.Akguen@uniklinikum-dresden.de (K.A.)
* Correspondence: Tjalf.Ziemssen@uniklinikum-dresden.de; Tel.: +49-351-458-5934; Fax: +49-351-458-5717
† These Authors have contributed equally to this work.

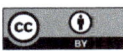

Citation: Dillenseger, A.; Weidemann, M.L.; Trentzsch, K.; Inojosa, H.; Haase, R.; Schriefer, D.; Voigt, I.; Scholz, M.; Akgün, K.; Ziemssen, T. Digital Biomarkers in Multiple Sclerosis. *Brain Sci.* **2021**, *11*, 1519. https://doi.org/10.3390/brainsci11111519

Academic Editor: Emilio Portaccio

Received: 20 October 2021
Accepted: 11 November 2021
Published: 16 November 2021

Publisher's Note: MDPI stays neutral with regard to jurisdictional claims in published maps and institutional affiliations.

Copyright: © 2021 by the authors. Licensee MDPI, Basel, Switzerland. This article is an open access article distributed under the terms and conditions of the Creative Commons Attribution (CC BY) license (https://creativecommons.org/licenses/by/4.0/).

Abstract: For incurable diseases, such as multiple sclerosis (MS), the prevention of progression and the preservation of quality of life play a crucial role over the entire therapy period. In MS, patients tend to become ill at a younger age and are so variable in terms of their disease course that there is no standard therapy. Therefore, it is necessary to enable a therapy that is as personalized as possible and to respond promptly to any changes, whether with noticeable symptoms or symptomless. Here, measurable parameters of biological processes can be used, which provide good information with regard to prognostic and diagnostic aspects, disease activity and response to therapy, so-called biomarkers Increasing digitalization and the availability of easy-to-use devices and technology also enable healthcare professionals to use a new class of digital biomarkers—digital health technologies—to explain, influence and/or predict health-related outcomes. The technology and devices from which these digital biomarkers stem are quite broad, and range from wearables that collect patients' activity during digitalized functional tests (e.g., the Multiple Sclerosis Performance Test, dual-tasking performance and speech) to digitalized diagnostic procedures (e.g., optical coherence tomography) and software-supported magnetic resonance imaging evaluation. These technologies offer a timesaving way to collect valuable data on a regular basis over a long period of time, not only once or twice a year during patients' routine visit at the clinic. Therefore, they lead to real-life data acquisition, closer patient monitoring and thus a patient dataset useful for precision medicine. Despite the great benefit of such increasing digitalization, for now, the path to implementing digital biomarkers is widely unknown or inconsistent. Challenges around validation, infrastructure, evidence generation, consistent data collection and analysis still persist. In this narrative review, we explore existing and future opportunities to capture clinical digital biomarkers in the care of people with MS, which may lead to a digital twin of the patient. To do this, we searched published papers for existing opportunities to capture clinical digital biomarkers for different functional systems in the context of MS, and also gathered perspectives on digital biomarkers under development or already existing as a research approach.

Keywords: multiple sclerosis; digital biomarkers; digital health technology; eHealth; precision medicine; personalized therapy; big data; digital twin

1. Introduction

Multiple sclerosis (MS) is a complex and chronic neurological disease of the central nervous system (CNS) that is characterized by a pathophysiological combination of neuroinflammation and neurodegeneration. As the inflammatory and neurodegenerative process can involve a variety of different neuroanatomical locations in the CNS, many functional neurological systems can be affected, ranging from visual, motor, cerebellar and sensory problems to complex cognitive symptoms. Since MS already occurs early in adulthood, accompanied by only a mildly reduced life expectancy, the highly heterogeneous disease, lasting over several decades, offers numerous inter-individually and intra-individually differences as well as different disease phenotypes evident in different disease stages [1]. Each of these individual differences and disease phenotypes must be addressed when it comes to treating MS as well as MS-related symptoms (e.g., spasticity, pain and gait problems). Additionally, as MS and its symptoms can change over time, it is crucial to detect these changes early in their development by using regular neurologic evaluation, questionnaires, functional tests, magnetic resonance imaging (MRI), laboratory checks and other assessments. Therefore, during this lifelong, chronic disease, a large amount of medical data accumulates, with important information pertaining to medical conditions and symptoms as well as diagnostic and therapeutic measures. In particular, the assessment of responders and non-responders to immunomodulatory therapies requires the long-term monitoring of different MS-related parameters, such as, for example, imaging, clinical assessments and biomarkers. If one adds the characterization of all different MS symptoms (e.g., depression and fatigue), the necessity for the complex and comprehensive collection of additional data becomes clear [1,2]. Since the collection of these data requires a lot of time, personnel and funds, using digital technology devices can facilitate this process and lead to the collection of so-called digital biomarkers. In this narrative review, we provide an overview of emerging digital biomarkers in the field of MS, their integration into regular monitoring and interesting approaches already in the testing phase, highlighting the need and benefits for the care of people with MS (pwMS). Searching for relevant literature in PubMed, specifying "digital biomarkers AND multiple sclerosis", showed to be inefficient. Therefore, we decided to search for different functional systems with better results, although results in connection with multiple sclerosis are limited. Much more research has been done with digital biomarkers in other diseases, e.g., Alzheimer's disease or depression [3–5]. Some of these digital biomarkers are now being investigated for their potential use in MS.

2. Digital Biomarkers
2.1. Definition of Digital Biomarkers

According to the National Institutes of Health (NIH, USA), biomarkers are objectively measured indicators of physiologic processes, pathologic processes or pharmacologic responses to a therapeutic intervention [6,7]. In MS, they can be subdivided into diagnostic (help to differentiate between different diseases, e.g., anti-aquaporin-4 antibodies, oligoclonal bands, etc.), prognostic (enable physicians to estimate how a disease might develop once it has been diagnosed, e.g., neurofilaments, oligoclonal bands, etc.), predictive (predict the treatment response and thus help to decide which patient is most likely to benefit from a certain treatment), disease activity (measure the inflammatory/neurodegenerative components of the disease, e.g., MRI, clinical parameters, etc.) and treatment response (responders versus non-responders of a certain treatment) biomarkers [6]. Especially with the focus on personalized medicine in pwMS, treatment response biomarkers can enable neurologists to differentiate patients regarding efficacy (e.g., neurofilament light chains, neutralizing antibodies against interferon-ß or natalizumab) or potential side effects (e.g., anti-varicella zoster virus antibodies, anti-John Cunningham virus antibodies) of a certain treatment [6]. The collection of such data is crucial to adapt the treatment of each patient individually to his/her results. However, it is also time-consuming if these data have to be gathered by physicians or other healthcare staff. With the increasing digitalization of healthcare, medicine now gains access to a new type of biomarker. So-called digital biomarkers enable the translation of up-to-date new data sources into informative, actionable knowledge. They can be used by healthcare professionals (HCPs) by implementing digital devices in their assessment (e.g., MRI, optical coherence tomography (OCT) and tablet-based neurostatus); they also enable data collection directly from the patient. They can collect such data directly as part of disease management on a regular basis, and thus ensure good monitoring and a prompt reaction to the progression of MS and the worsening of symptoms. Digital biomarkers mean objective, quantifiable physiological and behavioral data that are measured and collected by digital devices. The data collected by, e.g., portables, wearables, implantables or digestibles are typically used to generate, influence and/or predict health-related outcomes, and thus represent deep digital phenotyping, collecting clinically meaningful and objective digital data [8]. As digital technologies are usually less expensive than the process of collecting these data face to face, and as some of these data can be collected even without patients being actively involved (passive monitoring, e.g., by the use of wearables) data can also be collected more frequently and longitudinally. Health-related outcomes can vary, from explaining health and disease states, predicting drug responses or influencing health behaviors. In addition to this rather strict definition of digital biomarkers, digitalization in medicine also includes patient-reported measures (e.g., survey data), genetic information and other data that now can be collected by digital infrastructure. These data can complement the mentioned digital biomarkers, creating a digital multidimensional dataset.

Due to the technological transformation of healthcare, new technologies are leveraged to generate, track and collect new data. With the wealth of novel data, the responsibility is on the system to turn them into promising information that helps clinicians, researchers, patients and entrepreneurs to better understand states of disease and health [9].

2.2. Challenges of Digital Biomarkers

The path to implementing digital biomarkers in the clinic is complex, because the benefits that can be achieved by the use of digital biomarkers come with significant challenges (Table 1).

Table 1. Challenges in implementing digital biomarkers in the clinic.

Benefits	Challenges
Continuous real-time data	Privacy
Better real-world evidence	Adherence/retention
Greater power	High variability
Novel, sensitive endpoints	Validation required
Faster decisions	Complex analysis
Big data	Data storage

Digital biomarkers will, at least, face the same regulatory requirements as traditional biomarkers, and need to be tested for feasibility and reliability. The knowledge on how to establish and validate digital biomarkers is still limited. It can be challenging to identify relevant data and analyze them, and especially difficult in terms of how to use accurate baselines to relate this data for evaluation [10]. On the other hand, collecting continuous real-time data out of the patient's everyday life closes the data gap between visits, and thus can reveal changes in the disease course as soon as they occur. A continuous dataflow from patients to their treating physician could generate a big dataset that shows real-world evidence, therefore being more meaningful and enabling faster decision making. This is only possible with patients who are carefully educated about the need for such sensitive data and demonstrate appropriate adherence. To avoid patients getting obsessed with even minor, non-significant changes, as to decrease the potential of over-reactions and increased anxiety, networking between physician and patient is crucial to evaluate and discuss the significance of these biomarkers. Besides necessary reflections on data security and the possibility to store these data over a long period of time, a huge dataset arises through the use of digital devices, which requires complex analyses.

Digital biomarkers have great potential for medical domains that are not well-understood, especially if digital biomarkers lead the way to phenotypic signatures. Challenges around infrastructure, evidence generation, consistent data collection and workflow remain.

To be seen less as a challenge than as an aspect to be considered is the distribution and availability of digital devices for data collection. Not every patient can afford to buy wearables or a smartphone to collect their data during their everyday life. In addition, some patients will have difficulties with their usage, due to age-related reasons or impairments that prevent the handling of digital devices.

2.3. Classification of Digital Biomarkers

Digital biomarkers are basically collected by digital tools. A way to classify these measures focuses on what has been measured, and the added clinical value derived from that data. At this, measurements can be familiar, such as the measurement of blood pressure, or innovative, such as the continuous measurement of blood pressure. A known clinical value is one that is well-understood and has previously been validated., e.g., blood pressure can be used as an indicator of cardiovascular risk. Alternatively, the known measurement can additionally be used to detect a new finding, linking blood pressure to, e.g., major depression. These different digital biomarker categories will influence the level of evidence required for regulatory approval, validation and clinical implementation [7,9].

2.4. Clinical Digital Biomarkers in Multiple Sclerosis

Due to the increasing digitalization of health, a growing amount of patient data can be collected digitally in the care of pwMS (Figure 1). This not only refers to digital assessment results during clinical visits, but also daily patient-driven data collection, e.g., via the usage of smart devices, such as motion sensors, that arouse great interest in characterizing lifelong MS disease in a more granular way.

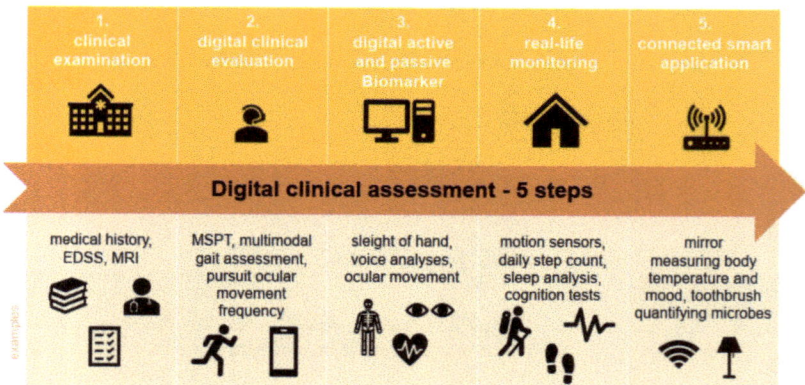

Figure 1. Developing a digital clinical assessment. (EDSS: Expanded Disability Status Scale; MRI: magnetic resonance imaging; and MSPT: Multiple Sclerosis Performance Test). © Multiple Sclerosis Center Dresden.

Figure 1 shows the five steps in digital clinical assessment from where we are now to where the future of digital clinical assessments could be. The typical clinical examination is still for the most part paper-based (except MRI, which is already digital), with, at best, subsequent digital storage of scanned documents in the hospital information system (step one). Digital clinical evaluations of, e.g., gait, patients' perception regarding symptoms (patient-reported outcomes) or the digital version of the Multiple Sclerosis Functional Composite (MSPT; Section 3.4) are not available for every neurologic practice or hospital for use in clinical routine, but are available mostly as part of clinical trials (step two). Digital biomarkers cannot only be collected actively. Additionally, passive monitoring and data collection are possible using, e.g., voice analysis during calls with patients (step three). As step two relates to digital data collection at given points in time during patients' visits, step three is already the transition towards data collection outside the clinical setting (e.g., passive collection of mobility via smartphones). Symptoms can vary over time, and disease progression may therefore be detected too late. For this reason, real-life monitoring is crucial (step four). Future devices could be smart applications, such as mirrors that automatically recognize body temperature and mood (step five).

Increasing evidence supports a forward-thinking chance of treatment decisions due to inter-individual highly variable clinical presentation, the extent of disease progression and a growing amount of defining biomarkers and surrogate endpoints, which personalize each disease presentation and favor our objective of a tailored treatment approach [1,11–13].

In the subsequent chapters, we will focus on digital biomarkers collected to investigate the involved functional systems or subdomains that are affected by different topographic lesions that occur during the course of MS. As MS is such a multidimensional disease, affecting different functional systems, collecting digital biomarkers capturing changes in those systems can offer insights into a comprehensively personalized disease.

3. Clinical Digital Biomarker by Functional Systems

3.1. Vision

Vision is one of the most affected functional systems in pwMS and often manifests itself in form of optic neuritis. Clinical signs can range from changes in color vision, reduced visual acuity or even complete loss of vision [14]. As atrophy of the retinal nerve fiber layer and ganglion cell layer was detected in 79% of pwMS and was 17 times higher in comparison to other neurological diseases, the measurement of the retinal nerve fiber layer can be used as a digital biomarker [15]. Using OCT, peripapillary retinal nerve fiber layer (pRNFL) thickness and macular volume can be measured to search for retinal atrophy [16]. Therefore, Martinez-Lapiscina et al. (2016) used models designed to determine the association of OCT-based metrics with the degree of disability, and included continuous variables such as pRNFL thickness as well as macular volume to quantify the effect (increase or decrease) on the risk of disability worsening associated with each unit of change (1 μm for pRNFL thickness and 1 mm^3 for macular volume). Th results suggested that regular monitoring of the peripapillary retinal fiber layer could be a useful digital biomarker to monitor the worsening of disability in MS, especially as it correlated with clinical and paraclinical parameters of vision, disability and MRI [16,17].

Another digital biomarker that can be used to monitor vision impairment is contrast vision. Testing visual acuity at low contrast ratios is significant, because in pwMS the threshold at which a letter can still be distinguished from the background is significantly higher than in healthy persons [18]. Sloan low-contrast letter acuity (LCLA) has been shown to correlate with MRI parameters and with OCT-detected retinal nerve fiber layer thickness [19]. The benefit of such contrast vision screenings is that they can also be used on mobile devices such as tablets or mobile phones, and can be easily done at home by patients themselves on a regular basis. How such a test can be put into practice is described in Section 4.1 in more detail.

Furthermore, virtual reality (VR)-based visual field testing may offer options for in-clinic and self-testing at home in the future. To date, VR vision testing is not ready to be counted as a digital biomarker because a "standard of care" test is missing. However, after completing VR training, MS patients presented promising improvements in cognitive and motor function [20].

3.2. Brainstem

Regarding brainstem functions for neurologists treating MS, oculomotor function and dysarthria are particularly suitable to be used as digital biomarkers.

Oculomotor function evaluation: Among the clinical signs of brainstem involvement, oculomotor disturbances are a common symptom, and often present early in the course of MS (such as in relapsing–remitting MS (RRMS)) [21]. The most frequently observed eye movement disorders are saccadic dysmetria (91%), internuclear ophthalmoplegia (68%), vestibulo-ocular reflex abnormalities and gaze-evoked nystagmus (36%) [22,23].

The development of eye-tracking technologies became more popular because these technologies offer the chance to obtain in-depth information about how people explore the world, indirectly provide insights into higher-order cognitive processes, e.g., preference, and investigate attentional deficits. Additionally, these technologies enable oculomotor insights from a medical point of view (e.g., kinematic of eye movement, frequency and metrics of saccades in addition to response latency) [24,25].

One option to analyze eye motor function is to measure the saccadic initiation time (SI time), which describes the time until an appropriate saccade appears, beginning with a central visual cue [26,27]. Because of its close connection with ocular nerve impairment, saccadic tests are popular and most frequently used to assess oculomotor function in MS [28,29]. To measure SI time, participants fixate a central cross, and after replacing the cross through an arrow they make saccadic eye movements towards periphery stars in the corner of a screen [27]. Nygaard et al. (2015) found that the SI time of RRMS patients was significantly longer compared to age- and gender-matched controls. The presence or absence of white matter or brainstem lesions between patients had no influence on the SI time. However, eye motor disturbances might be an early indicator for a disseminated MS [27]. Another study by Finke et al. (2012) found a significantly larger decrease in saccade peak velocity and amplitude in pwMS suffering from fatigue in comparison to non-fatigued pwMS as well as to healthy controls when performing a saccade fatigue task that lasted 10 min [30].

Further, the pursuit ocular movement (POM) frequency has been analyzed in patients with RRMS and secondary progressive MS (SPMS) by using a vision-based non-intrusive eye tracker [23]. In the study of De Santi et al. (2011), the POM frequency was significantly lower in pwMS compared with age- and gender-matched healthy controls. Interestingly, no relation between POM and the Expanded Disability Status Scale (EDSS) and no difference between RRMS and SPMS patients could be found [23].

Numerous studies have indicated that besides measuring oculomotor characteristics, eye-tracking tools reflect multifaceted cognitive information, contributing to the prediction of cognitive impairment and having the potential to assess disease progression even in the absence of aware clinical symptoms [28,31]. This opens the possibility to use these tracking tools to further develop diagnostic tools, and to use the results as digital biomarkers to evaluate disease progression and prognosis more precisely. By now, eye-tracking tools have been used to detect pathologic visuo-spatial viewing behavior in MS [32]. New approaches present short assessments to capture abnormalities of the oculomotor system, such as SONDA (Standardized Oculomotor and Neurological Disorder Assessment) which takes less than five minutes for the whole assessment and is also used in Parkinson's disease [33]. Quick and standardized assessments allow regular monitoring over time without overburdening patients, especially those suffering from fatigue.

Speech analysis: Speech and voice are frequently impaired in MS, with a prevalence of approximately 40–50% [34,35], within which dysarthria is the most frequent communication deficit [35]. Its presentation usually tends to be mild, so unintelligible speech is very rare [36,37]. The major dysarthric features are deficient loudness control, slowness, monopitch, increase in pauses, strained voice, imprecise consonants and decreased respirator capacity [13].

However, it is important to consider that impairment of speech may have negative effects on social participation and employment status, resulting in an overall reduced quality of life [13]. So far, the basic characteristics of pwMS with dysarthria related to prosody and articulation remain mostly unresearched [38]. Accordingly, regular screening for changes in speech may contribute to the gain of important new biomarkers of disease progression, wherefore further developments in technology make the quantitative acoustic assessment of speech possible [13,38]. Digital vocal biomarkers offer the possibility of a standardized measurement and monitoring of speech. As speech might also be influenced by fatigue, depression and impairment in verbal cognition [38–40], the evaluation of speech also enables us to screen for these aspects and expands the spectrum of measurable parameters.

Studies showed a statistically significant correlation between dysphonic symptoms and MS, and the odds for having MS were 2.2 times higher if dysphonic symptoms were present with high jitter and shimmer values as well as high soft phonation index (an indicator of vocal fold adduction; high values correlate with incomplete adduction of the vocal fold [41]) values [42,43]. The objective acoustic analysis of speech seems to be more sensitive for discrimination between affected patients and healthy controls (90% accuracy) than experienced raters (35% accuracy) are, and thus could be used as a biomarker for diagnosis and the monitoring of disease progression [13,35,44,45].

Speech analysis applications using artificial intelligence to evaluate acoustic speech and language measures via a tablet are thought to provide vocal biomarkers for diagnosis, risk prediction and regular monitoring not only in MS but also in Parkinson's or Alzheimer's disease, and are in general highly predictive for cerebellar dysfunctions [46,47]. The benefit of a standardized software-based evaluation of speech tasks is the avoidance of intra- and inter-individual deviations in perceptions [47], so that monitoring could also be possible outside of routine visits. Digital vocal biomarkers and their use in clinical practice are still facing challenges when it comes to different accents, ages, task complexities and individual cognitive abilities [47,48]. Signs of fatigue and depression are already detectable in healthy individuals or patients without neurological disease [39,49]. As fatigue, depression and cognitive impairment are common in MS, they could be detected by speech analyses [46]. Test batteries can be designed in such a way that they capture executive functions and processing speed (e.g., phonematic and semantic word fluency [50]), memory (e.g., the Wechsler Memory Scale and California Verbal Learning Test [51,52]), affect and fatigue (e.g., storytelling [53]), language (picture description [54]) and motoric function (Pa-ta-ka task [38,42]). To date, performing such speech and language tests might be limited to trials, but can be imagined to be used in the future during clinical visits of pwMS or even at home by the use of specific apps or recordings during telemedicine visits.

3.3. Upper Extremity Motor Function

At least 56% of pwMS have upper extremity impairment; 71% of those report limitations in hand and arm use that dramatically affect daily living activities [55–57]. Upper extremity impairment is mostly conditioned by weakness and/or impaired coordination/ataxia [58], and is likely to limit future ability to perform activities of daily living and further reduce quality of life.

Existing dysfunction increases with disease progression, especially in patients with progressive MS compared to patients with RRMS [56,59]. Due to their highly differentiated movement variability, a comprehensive assessment of the upper limb can be challenging, and thus assessments must address multiple subsystems, such as eye–hand coordination and intra-limb and inter-limb coordination, as increasing dysfunction is seen in patients after stroke or with other diseases affecting the coordination of the limbs [57,60–62].

One of the most popular functional outcome measures to examine upper extremity function is the Nine-Hole Peg Test (9HPT). The 9HPT has known deficiencies—it only assesses fine manual dexterity; other important upper extremity functions, such as proximal upper extremity movements, complex bimanual tasks or the manipulation of larger objects, are not captured [63]. Accordingly, there is an ongoing search for new, multidimensional, sensitive upper extremity performance tests that provide new biomarkers that may predict disease progression. Here, the widespread use and manual handling of smartphones make them a promising assessment device, especially with regard to their ever-increasing abilities. With smartphones containing sensors, such as a gyrometer, accelerometer, inclinometer, orientation and light sensors, the opportunities to develop new ways to measure neurological functions seem almost infinite [64].

Tanigawa et al. studied finger tapping via a smartphone-based app as an alternative outcome measure of upper extremity function in MS by an analogy to tapping as a useful outcome measure, e.g., in primary lateral sclerosis [65]. Finger taps correlated clearly with 9HPT results. Furthermore, a correlation between tap results and other raised measures of physical disability could be shown [64].

Several smartphone-based apps capturing different functional systems via digital tests and questionnaires have emerged, including the Floodlight app and Konectom (see Section 4.1). These apps contain tests for the upper extremities and use assessments to capture more than just fine motor skills. The pinching of balloons or tomatoes that emerge on different positions on the screen or the tracing of a figure with the index finger of both hands as quickly and accurately as possible measures, e.g., eye–hand coordination, fine motor function and the pressure of the fingers on the screen as well. Creagh et al. analyzed pwMS and healthy controls tracing a predefined shape on a smartphone, demonstrating an authentic prediction of 9HPT results [66].

The use of such apps on patients' smartphones enables a regular and continuous progression monitoring of upper limb function even outside of the clinic by patients' themselves, without supervision [64]. However, in order to fulfill the function of a monitoring tool and to influence therapy decisions, it must also be ensured that the test results are transmitted to the treating physician.

Additionally, depth camera systems together with machine learning algorithms were examined to objectively quantify changes in movement-related symptoms to discriminate between healthy, not healthy and disease progression, which still needs to be researched further [67].

Another possibility with which to measure impairments in upper limb function are questionnaires (patient-reported outcome measure, PROM) that address different aspects of daily usage of hands and arms in different situations, such as tying shoes, buttoning up shirts or opening bottles. A regular questioning of the patient regarding his or her impairments provides important indications of upper limb dysfunction and potential further examination. To date, no standardized upper limb PROM has been established.

3.4. Lower Extremity Motor Function/Gait

Lower extremity impairment and the resulting gait deficits are the most frequent and visible consequences of MS, caused by a variety of pathophysiologic conditions such as pyramidal, cerebellar or sensory dysfunction [68]. Approximately 85% of pwMS report impaired walking, with an often profound impact on daily life [69,70]. Compared to healthy controls, abnormal gait characteristics of pwMS are characterized by decreased walking speed, shorter step and stride length, prolonged double limb support time and increased step variability [70,71]—even without clinical evidence of gait disturbance early in the course of the disease [72]. Several factors are thought to contribute to gait impairment in pwMS, of which sensory changes and the resulting imbalance, weakness of the lower limbs or spasticity and cerebellar ataxia might have the biggest impact [73]. Depending on one's assessment goals, different tools can be used for the evaluation of gait impairment in pwMS, ranging from standardized clinical measures, timed measures, patient-reported outcomes, observational gait analysis, instrumented walkways or three-dimensional gait analysis, which all require different expertise of the examiner, time and equipment [73]. Each of them show advantages and disadvantages (Table 2).

Table 2. Advantages and disadvantages of various gait assessment methods (AmI = ambulation index; EDSS = Expanded Disability Status Scale; T25FW = Timed 25-Foot Walk test; 6MWT = 6-Minute Walk Test; MSWS-12 = 12-item Multiple Sclerosis Walking Scale; and EMIQ = Early Mobility Impairment Questionnaire) [73–75].

	Outcome Measures	Advantages	Disadvantages
Standardized clinical measures.	-Disability score (EDSS). -Time and degree of assistance required to walk 25 feet.	-Take into account the use of assistive devices. -EDSS: directly related to neurologic examination; used in clinical trials. -AmI: simple and quick.	-Require a skilled examiner. -Do not identify mechanisms underlying gait dysfunction. -EDSS and AmI have limited precision and responsiveness. -No normative data.
Timed measures (e.g., T25FW, 6MWT).	Quantified aspect of gait, such as speed and endurance.	-Simple. -Readily quantified. -Require limited training. -Published norms available.	Do not identify mechanisms underlying gait dysfunction.
Patient-based measures (e.g., MSWS-12; EMIQ).	Patient's perspective of their walking disability.	-Document the patient's perspective. -Require little time to complete.	Do not identify mechanisms underlying gait dysfunction.
Observational gait analysis (e.g., during T25FT or other walking conditions).	Gait pattern in terms of kinematic and spatiotemporal parameters.	-Identify mechanisms underlying gait dysfunction. -Requires limited time and equipment.	-Limited validity, reliability and precision. -Requires skilled examiner.
Sensor floor plates: (a) Instrumented walkways; (b) Force platform; (c) Balance boards.	(a) Spatial and temporal variables. (b) Ground reaction force pattern. -Kinematics. (c) Ground reaction force pattern.	(a) -Simple. -Clinical feasibility. -Objectivity. -Quantification. -Good sensitivity. (b) -Objectivity. -Quantification. -Good sensitivity. (c) -Objectivity. -Quantification. -Portability.	(a) Require equipment. -Do not identify mechanisms underlying gait dysfunction. -Restricted to clinic or laboratory environments. -Restricted to few steps at a time. (b) Restricted to laboratory environments. (c) Clinical, research and home.
Three-dimensional gait analysis (reflecting markers places on a person and recording movement with infrared cameras).	Detailed quantitative measures of kinematic, kinetic and spatiotemporal parameters.	-Identify mechanisms underlying gait dysfunction. -Provide precise kinematic, kinetic, and spatiotemporal data.	Require expensive equipment and skilled examiner.
Video-based: (a) Marker-based motion capture; (b) Marker-free motion capture.	(a) and (b): -Spatial and temporal variables. -Kinematics. -Joint range of motion.	(a) -Comprehensive analysis of the widest range of gait variables. -Power consumption is not an issue. -Little interference from external environmental factors. (b) -Objectivity. -Quantification. -High sensitivity. -Comprehensiveness. -Better suited to clinical environments than marker-based systems.	(a) -Expensive. -Must be used in a laboratory environment. -Markers and restricted space can hinder movement. (b) -Can be expensive. -Generally, cannot be used outside the clinic or laboratory environment. -Measures a restricted number of steps.
Wearable sensors: (a) Inertial sensors (research-oriented/consumer-driven); (b) Pressure sensors.	(a) -Spatiotemporal measures: -Joint range of motion. -Kinematics. -Balance. (b) Spatial and temporal variables.	(a) -Clinical feasibility. -Objectivity. -Quantification. -Good sensitivity. -Face validity. (b) -Clinical feasibility. -Objectivity. -Quantification. -Good sensitivity. -Can be used outside the clinic and laboratory.	(a) -Sensors can impede movement. -Battery power. -Susceptible to environmental interference. -May need technical operators. (b) -Sensors can impede movement. -Battery power.

In the following, these assessments are presented for the different settings of research, in-clinic monitoring assessment or functional tests to be performed at home, whereby the application of these tools is not always limited to one area. Wearables and smartphone apps, e.g., enable their use in several areas. As in 50% of pwMS with lower gait dysfunction also show upper limb impairment [76] this needs to be examined and addressed as well when therapy is considered.

3.4.1. Lower Extremity Function in MS Research

Research offers the possibility to use more advanced technologies for movement analysis than in common standardized clinical assessments providing a higher sensitivity for subtle impairments [75]. Therefore, not only a complex infrastructure is needed but also trained medical staff to accompany pwMS and to conduct the tests as well as to analyze the data. A selection of potential assessment technologies in MS and a selection of their associated outcomes is shown below (Table 3) [74].

Table 3. Potential gait assessment technologies in MS.

Assessment Technology	Method	Outcomes *	Device [+] (Manufacturer)
Video-based	(a) Marker-based (b) Marker-free	(a) Joint range of motion	(a) Vicon (Civon Motion Systems Ltd.); Miqus Hybrid (Qualisys AB) (b) Miqus Hybrid (Qaulisys AB)
Sensor floor plates	(a) Instrumented walkway (b) Force platform (c) Balance boards	(a) Spatiotemporal measures (b) Ground reaction force pattern (c) Ground reaction force pattern	(a) GAITRite (CIR Systems) (b) ProKin (Tecnobody); 3D Force Plate (Kistler Instruments AG (c) Wii Balance Board (Nintendo)
Wearable sensors	(a) Research-oriented ± (b) Consumer-driven ⁹	(a) Spatiotemporal measures, joint range of motion	(a) Mobility lab (APDM), XActiGraph GT9X Link (ActiGraph); GENEActiv Original (Activinsights) (b) Fitbit Charge 5 (fitbit), vívosport® (Garmin), Xiaomi Mi Band 6 (Xiaomi)

* Selection of key outcomes; [+] examples; ± devices developed primarily for research purposes: no direct patient feedback, no modifying of movement behavior through, e.g., motivation, raw data output; ⁹ devices developed primarily for consumer requirements: direct feedback of movement behavior on device display, no direct access to raw data (adapted from Trentzsch et al., 2020 [74]).

Video-based assessment technology captures so-called kinematics (motion sequences and range of motion) regarding time, place, speed and acceleration [77], either marker-based or marker-free. Marker-free systems show to be more user-friendly; however, marker-based systems are on the one hand more time consuming and involve extensive technological and human resources, but on the other hand offer higher accuracy and reproducibility [74,75].

Sensor floor plates allow for the measuring of spatiotemporal parameters (instrumented walkways such as GAITRite®), as well as information about ground reaction force (force platforms or balance boards). As such systems are mainly focused on muscle force, joint load and moment during initial contact and toe-off to evaluate gait impairment [78], other aspects of mobility are missed, such as swaying, rotation and balancing of the body, data which are needed to obtain a more precise movement pattern of pwMS. Therefore, all of these devices can be expanded by wearables.

Wearable sensors can also be used at home by patients themselves to measure their gait restrictions. One wearable for research use is the Mobility Lab system (APMD, Portland, OR, USA) which consists of Opal sensors that are fixed on specific body parts (e.g., wrist, sternum, lower lumbar spine and feet) [79]. Three-dimensional linear acceleration, angular velocity and magnetic field (for directional orientation) are captured by the use of onboard accelerometers, gyroscopes and magnetometers, and Mobility Lab software analyzes these data for gait parameters such as stride length, velocity, cadence, stand and swing time, etc. [79]. In addition, so-called consumer-driven wearables (e.g., GPS watches) are of interest as they can provide data collected in research, a clinical setting or at home.

Video-based and sensor floor plates assessments are only possible to perform in an in-clinic setting, whereas wearable sensors can also be used by pwMS themselves in their daily living over a longer period of time, thus providing an additional quantitative large dataset which better represents the mobility of pwMS. Spain et al. could also show that body-worn motion sensors could discriminate pwMS from healthy controls with a higher sensitivity than tests conducted using stopwatches, as wearables can also detect sway and axial rotation while the latter only captures speed, which might not show any impairment yet [80].

3.4.2. Lower Extremity Function in the Clinic

The most frequently used clinical assessment tool and outcome measure in MS, the Expanded Disability Status Scale (EDSS), considers general ambulation by rating gait impairment upon endpoints, e.g., requirements of rest, dependency on help or loss of walking ability/wheelchair [81]. Thereby, subtle functional impairment cannot be taken adequately into account, leading to an insensitive scoring concerning disease progression, especially in the early stages of the disease [68,82]. However, as subtle gait impairment and balance dysfunction are seen as precursors of mobility loss in MS [75], the need for suitable outcome measures, capable to detect even subtle gait impairments and to monitor disease progression during a clinical assessment and also out of the artificial clinical setting under real-life conditions of pwMS becomes clear [72]. Nevertheless, it is also necessary to monitor the worsening of gait and balance dysfunction throughout the whole disease course. Interventions (pharmacologic and/or non-pharmacologic) need to be started and/or optimized as soon as possible to prevent further or faster progression of disability. One test alone is not able to describe impairment in the many facets of walking of pwMS. A combination of standardized functional tests that capture walking speed, walking endurance and balance as well as the quality of walking, or standardized patient reported outcomes regarding mobility restrictions will lead to a broad and sensitive dataset to evaluate mobility, at best on a regular basis. Various digital tools can be used for this purpose. Many of the gait assessments available in the research are not possible, as not everyone can be transferred into a routine clinical setting due to a lack of infrastructure, time, space or well-trained staff [74]. For those who can afford to integrate a broad evaluation of mobility into their clinic, all of the above-mentioned assessments can be performed. It is recommended to implement a protocol to follow and, thus, enable a standardized measurement for pwMS. At the Multiple Sclerosis Center Dresden, we developed the Dresden Protocol for Multidimensional Walking Assessment (DMWA) [74] to capture mobility in all of our pwMS at least once a year. Thus, with this long-term monitoring, early walking impairments as well as development over time or even the response to certain gait-influencing drugs can also be recorded, and the current standard of clinical practice be improved [74]. Gait analysis can also be supplemented in the clinical setting with other (digital) functional tests that include, e.g., cognition, speech, vision, or PROMs. Therefore, we added the Multiple Sclerosis Performance Test (MSPT) to the clinical routine of pwMS.

The MSPT is a tablet-based (iPad Air® 2, Apple, Cupertino, CA, USA) digital assessment tool (app) designed to be used in a routine clinical setting without or with only minimal supervision [83]. Based on and extending the Multiple Sclerosis Functional Composite, the MSPT uses a digital adaption of the Symbol Digit Modalities Test (SDMT), the Sloan low-contrast visual acuity test, the 9HPT and the Timed-25 Foot Walk (T25FW) tests as well as a questionnaire regarding quality of life in neurologic diseases [58,84–87]. The MSPT includes all tasks to evaluate cognitive function (Processing Speed Test (PST), a digital adaption of the SDMT), contrast sensitivity, upper extremity function (9HPT) and walking speed/lower extremity function (T25FW) [83]. The aim is to assess the often-impacted neurologic functions of pwMS regularly and standardize them to create a longitudinal digital medical record, contributing to a better disease understanding and progression monitoring, which may contribute to more optimized patient care and management [83]. The MSPT is basically meant to be performed by pwMS without supervision, which allows data collection without consuming time and staff at the clinic. Data are available right after completion and can also be used for monitoring; therefore, a baseline MSPT should be performed at the time of diagnosis or treatment start/change to refer changes to. The benefit of using the MSPT is the availability of standardized functional testing and the possibility of having a great amount of pwMS performing the MSPT without the requirement of additional staff. Learning effects, such as for the paper-based SDMT [88], are excluded by randomly assigning numbers to symbols for every assessment [89]. Studies showed excellent test–retest reliability for the manual dexterity test (digital version of the 9HPT) and the walking speed test (T25FW), a significant (but only modest) correlation of the contrast seeing test with the standard Sloan low-contrast vision acuity [90] and an excellent test–retest reliability for the PST, with a high correlation with the SDMT and with cerebral T2 load (in contrast to the SDMT) [89].

The implementation of the tests in a digital format is user friendly as each test is explained by a video. The tablet is brought in an upright position. At first, information about current disease modifying therapy (DMT), relapses and Patient Determined Disease Steps is made before filling out the NeuroQoL [91–93]. The PST shows a random assignment of numbers to symbols and ten symbols at a time for which patients have to choose the correct number by tapping on one of the numbers shown at the bottom of the screen. For contrast vision, a certain distance and illumination are needed before the test can be started. At first, letters are shown at 100% and then at 2.5% contrast, whereas patients have to choose the letter they see out of a collection of letters at the bottom of the screen. In cases where a letter cannot be clearly identified patients can guess or tap "unclear". To perform the 9HPT, the MSPT needs to be lying flat on the table and the stand with the pegboard is folded down. Nine pegs are put in the row at the bottom and after activating the countdown patients are asked to take one peg at a time from the row and insert it into one of the holes of the pegboard. After all pegs have been inserted, they need to be removed, again, one at a time, and put back into the row. Time automatically stops when the last peg is put in the row at the bottom of the pegboard. Before performing the T25FW patients need to specify if they will use any gait support or if they wear any lower leg orthosis. If patients are rather unsteady on their feet, a nurse supports the patient to avoid any falls. At the end, an overview of the results can be seen on a dashboard, and the longitudinal course can be seen by tapping each test.

Despite the fact that the MSPT was designed for pwMS to be performed without support or supervision, we recommend pwMS to be supported if needed, and the provision of feedback to their results increases adherence to and understanding of monitoring.

3.4.3. Lower Extremity Function at Home

The collection of real-time data on a longitudinal basis becomes more and more important when monitoring chronic diseases in particular, such as MS, as they do not only state a condition at one point in time and thus allow for progress and follow-up control. In particular, accelerometers are used, and depending on their position on the body, allow for the partial documentation of the relevant mobility; however, not all physical activities are captured equally as well [94]. With the help of wearables, it is possible to focus on different aspects such as gait, upper or lower limb function, behavior or other body movement patterns; when used regularly, they provide information about mobility from outside a clinical setting and may correlate with disease-specific predictors, outcomes or interventions [95]. Various accelerometers can now be used, such as the already widely used fitness trackers (e.g., Fitbit, Garmin, Xiaomi, ActiGraph and others), which have been shown to be useful in an everyday setting and can even be used to collect data over several days [74,82,96]. By tracking the physical activity of pwMS continuously over one year, Block et al. (2019) could show an association between a reduction in average daily step count and the worsening of standard clinic-based and patient-reported metrics [97]. They also showed that patients with a lower baseline average daily step count were found to be at a higher risk of disability worsening one year later [97]. Other wearables, such as the skin-mounted inertial sensor BioStampRC (MC10, Inc., Cambridge, MA, USA), could support physicians in identifying gait pathology and in evaluating disability progression of gait in pwMS [98]. As wearables become more and more affordable and broadly accepted, they might work as an ambulatory, real-life and continuous gait monitoring system [98,99], allowing for increased sensitivity in regard to monitoring disease progression and the efficacy of immunomodulation [98].

Captured variables can include step count, active minutes, activity count, activity bouts and energy expenditure [97]. Compared to non-wearable laboratory/research systems, wearable sensors capture a smaller number of gait variables [75].

Smartphone-based apps that use functioning tests or record movement parameters are another way of tracking patients' mobility and activity. They will be discussed in Section 4.1.

3.5. Coordination/Balance

Deficits in balance are, even in early disease stages, common [72,100–102]. Overall, 50–80% of pwMS state balance problems over the course of the disease [103,104]. Balance can be defined as a skill of the nervous system, using several systems such as passive biomechanical elements, all available sensory systems and muscles as well as a multitude of different parts of the brain, instead of simply reacting reflex-like to perturbations [105]. As the heterogeneous demyelinating lesions in MS could also affect somatosensory or vestibular paths, visual input was shown to be necessary to maintain postural control in pwMS [106]. Postural control is defined as the act of maintaining, achieving or restoring a state of balance during any postures or activities [107], which a person tries to achieve by reactive, predictive or a combination of both behaviors [108]. Postural control is closely associated with falls in pwMS [106], which emphasizes the need for longitudinal evaluation during the course of the disease. As for today, postural perturbations are subjectively rated by neurologists as part of the cerebellar functional score of the EDSS [109]. To avoid subjective judgment of postural control in MS and to allow for follow-up evaluation of changes, objective, digital and quantifiable measurements are needed. In a clinical or research assessment, proprioceptive deficits can be evaluated, e.g., by using the Romberg test. To objectify its results, it may be connected with the use of body sensors (e.g., Mobility Lab system) that allow software-based calculation of deviations from the norm [110]. Static posturography is another method of assessing balance in which patients are asked to stand on a force platform with their feet closed and their eyes closed or open for 20 to 60 s to measure spontaneous body sway, which can be extended by more difficult stand trials (e.g., tandem stand or standing on one leg) [111]. Balance parameters that can be captured include average sway and speed as well as delineated area [106]. Inojosa et al. (2020) showed in their study that static posturography could detect balance impairment even if patients had no disability according to their neurological examination [106]. Special apps for smartphones also provide tests with which to perform the Romberg test for balance evaluation and other gait assessments to be performed at home by pwMS themselves (see Section 4.1). Additionally, the use of portable balance boards (e.g., Nintendo Wii) are under investigation to be used as an inexpensive alternative to force platforms for balance assessment in pwMS [112]. An interesting aspect here is whether balance training could have a positive impact on postural control in pwMS. In their review on balance improvement, Gunn et al. reported a positive influence of exercise interventions on balance in pwMS [113]. Other studies focusing on general motor rehabilitation in pwMS pointed at the issue that motor learning consists of three stages (cognitive, associative and autonomous phase), where the first stage depends on the person's cognitive abilities [114], and the fact that cognitive impairment is very common in pwMS thus connects cognitive and mobility dysfunction [115].

3.6. Cognition

Approximately 40–60% of pwMS report cognitive dysfunction, and it is not uncommon that the symptom onset is immediately after first disease manifestation or even before [116]. Impairment in cognition can occur at all stages of the disease and in all MS phenotypes [117]. Frequently impaired domains are working memory, verbal fluency, information processing speed, verbal and visual memory, executive functions [84,118] and, according to new findings, "the theory of mind domain" (the ability to conclude on the basis of nonverbal and verbal hints about other people's emotions) [119]. As cognitive impairment is a strong predictor of health-related quality of life (QoL) [120] and QoL in turn has a huge impact on adherence [121], together with the negative impact of cognitive dysfunction on employment [122] and many other aspects of life [123], a thorough and regular evaluation is necessary [118]. So far, cognitive monitoring is often a not-well-established part of standard care in MS. This is partly due to time and staff that are needed to allow for a routinely, longitudinal follow-up of pwMS. Therefore, digitalization of cognitive assessments where patients are able to perform these by themselves without supervision can enable long-term cognitive monitoring. Provided in a smartphone-based format, this monitoring could be done also at home, e.g., with the Floodlight app (Roche, Basel, Switzerland) to perform the SDMT or the MS Sherpa app (Orimaki personalized healthcare, Nijmegen, The Netherlands) to evaluate the cognitive signal processing speed (see also Section 4.1).

Implementing digital cognitive assessments in the monitoring of MS is challenging, given the fact that many pwMS show not only cognitive deficits but also physical impairments that are required for this kind of testing and need to be addressed when transforming paper-based tests into a digital form, as they can change what exactly is measured [124]. For clinical use, a number of simplified tests of cognition have been developed in MS, including test batteries such as the Brief Repeatable International Cognitive Assessment for MS [125], the Brief Repeatable Battery of Neuropsychological Tests [126] and the Minimal Assessment of Cognitive Function in MS [127,128]. The transformation of such tests into a digital form (computerized neuropsychological assessment device (CNAD)) is considered very controversial by some experts, stating that this transformation results in a new and different test: it has a different patient interface and is also available to examiners with no expertise in neuropsychological assessments or knowledge of psychometric principles, and thus no accurate interpretation of test results is achieved as other factors influencing performance are not considered, no observational interpretation of the examinee is possible, etc. [129]. Other review papers could show, e.g., for the PST, the Computerized Speed Cognitive Test and Computerized SDMT (C-SDMT), compared with the SDMT, a high test–retest reliability and validity, and for other tests acceptable psychometrics [130]. Before applying CNADs to clinical routine or trials, adequate test–retest reliability and sensitivity should be demonstrated [130].

Amato et al. (2001) already showed that if a follow-up was long enough, cognitive dysfunction was likely to emerge in a great proportion of pwMS, re-emphasizing the need for regular, standardized monitoring [123]. It has been shown that assessing cognitive function early in the course of the disease did not only identify cognitive impairment in individuals but could also predict future impairments, limitations and MS disease progression [131]. Thus, recommendations can be made to start cognitive assessments right from the start and re-assess cognitive functions in pwMS, thus enabling early treatment interventions.

As interactions between motor and cognitive functions are known in MS, linking them together (termed dual-tasking) can be used to evaluate the interference of performing a cognitive task during gait assessment [73,74,132–134].

Dual-Tasking

Coordinating two or more tasks simultaneously is an everyday requirement, and is increasingly recognized in the treatment and supervision of pwMS as having a major impact on employment status [135]. This makes it even more important to recognize early and subtle cognitive (executive) dysfunctions [136]. Up to now, dual-tasks are performed during walking or balancing and, e.g., showed a slowing of gait depending on MS disease severity [136–144]. Dual-task tests that are already able to detect subtle and early executive dysfunctions are still lacking in MS. A study investigated the use of a standard psychological refractory period (PRP) paradigm [145,146] in pwMS where two tasks (first stimulus—high or low tone; second stimulus—letter A or B) have to be performed which are presented in close succession and to which pwMS have to respond as quickly as possible (Figure 2) [136].

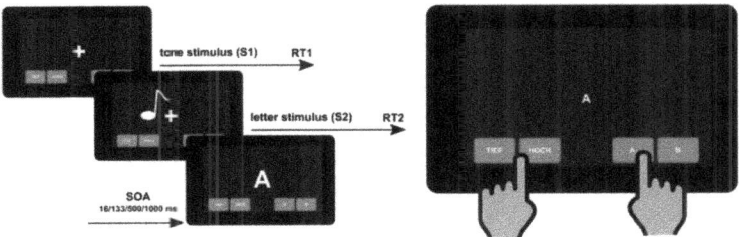

Figure 2. Illustration of the psychological refractory period paradigm as a dual-task assessment in MS. Stimulus 1 (tone) is always presented first, followed by stimulus 2 (letter) in a defined stimulus-onset asynchrony (SOA). PwMS are advised to respond first to stimulus 1 and as quickly as possible to stimulus 2 by pressing defined keys. RT: reaction time [147].

This dual-task test is still under further development, but the first results were promising. They showed that with this applied PRP paradigm, multitasking deficits, even in patients at an early stage of their MS disease course, could be detected [136]. Of course, such tests also face challenges, such as time required to perform the test, staff support and the test device. A follow-up study recently investigated the same dual-task test in an outpatient setting using a tablet [147]. Böttrich et al. could show that the accuracy parameter in tablet-based PRP implementations can be used in neuropsychological assessments to examine dual-tasking abilities in pwMS [147]. Such data are promising for the use of such devices for the diagnosis and monitoring of the MS disease course on a regular basis.

4. Collection of Digital Biomarkers

The longitudinal and multidimensional acquisition of digital biomarkers is already possible, and includes the use of smartphone-based apps as well as computer- or tablet-based functional tests and questionnaires.

4.1. Smartphones and Smartphone Applications

Smartphones are omnipresent everyday objects, and are usually provided with innovative high-quality nine-axis inertial motion sensors that are able to track motion and position in three-dimensional space [148]. These sensors enable basic measurements, such as acceleration or the calculation of data, to conclude how a person walks or to capture their daily step count; the sensing of geographic position, voice analyses and touchscreen pressure can often be measured, detecting falls, monitoring heart rate or daily activity parameters are further examples of what make smartphones today a more and more health-related product [148]. These features can be used when implementing digital assessment into MS patient care. Various applications (apps) use these sensors and extend them by different, other tests that evaluate the functional systems usually affected by MS (e.g., cognition, vision, mobility and fine motor function of the upper limbs). Part of this data collection is done actively, with pwMS performing specific assessments; passive data collection is also possible. Therefore, the pre-installed smartphone developer's own app (e.g., Health for iOS, Google Fit for Android, etc.) can be used in MS as well for monitoring, e.g., gait. When implementing such apps in research or clinical practice, the precision and accuracy of these sensors need to be considered [96]. To actively collect data from pwMS they need to be prompted either to perform a test or to fill out a questionnaire. Currently, several apps are available that offer a set of various functional tests. Apps such as Floodlight (Roche, Switzerland), Konectom$^{(TM)}$ (Biogen, Cambridge, MA, USA), MSCopilot® (Ad Scientiam, Paris, France) or MS Sherpa (Orikami, Nijmegen, The Netherlands), some of which are still in evaluation and only used in research, collect data regarding mobility (2- or 6-min-walk, U-turns, standing still: distance, speed, balance, etc.), cognition (matching symbols: cognitive processing speed), hand motor function (squeezing objects, drawing lines: coordination, pressure, speed and accuracy of hand and finger movement) and mood (questionnaires), or leaving options for patients to make notes [149–152]. The benefit of such apps lies in the collection of data from daily life, the possibility to perform functional tests independent of clinical visits, enabling patients to use them for self-evaluation or in cases where they feel as though they are experiencing a worsening of symptoms and, of course, for pwMS and treating neurologists in order to include these data in therapy decisions as well. A regular functional system that monitors and thus detects progression early can lead to early treatment decisions or treatment changes.

The implementation of such apps could overcome the challenge of often infrequent and rare clinic visits and capture all, sometimes daily, even subtle symptom changes. Thus, a more accurate monitoring of the individual disease course and associated optimized therapeutic decisions becomes achievable [66,148,150]. Furthermore, daily patient self-made tasks via a smartphone may contribute to more disease responsibility and informed discussions in clinical visits about subsequent therapeutic steps. PwMS acquire a more active, responsible part of progression monitoring, which might contribute to increased compliance. Adherence to the use of such apps is crucial to allow for longitudinal monitoring, especially in chronic diseases as MS, and will be a challenge.

Other smartphone apps that belong to the group of digital health applications (DIGAs) focus more on special symptoms and can already be prescribed in Germany. These apps aim, e.g., to help and support pwMS regarding fatigue (e.g., elevida by GAIA AG, Germany) and offer talks, exercises and informative material to enable help for self-help, independent of MS management. More DIGAs are already available for patients suffering from anxiety, depression, diabetes, stroke, etc. [153].

4.2. Digital Questionnaires in MS

Besides responsible MS management from the side of clinical staff, the patient's point of view, including quality of life together with subjective treatment and disease effects, is increasingly weighted and raised via PROMs. PROMs combine any information "of a patient's health condition that comes directly from the patient, without interpretation of the patient's response by a clinician or anyone else" [154], allowing the specification of whether patients' feelings/thoughts are congruent with those of clinicians [1,155,156]. With the aim of patient-centered therapeutic management, PROMs are collected directly from patients and contain items that subjectively rate functioning/activity limitations, symptoms, quality of life and health-related quality of life [157,158]. Existing PROMs focus on patients' subjective evaluation of dealing with fatigue (e.g., Fatigue Assessment Scale), depression (e.g., Hospital Anxiety and Depression Scale), quality of life (e.g., NeuroQoL), mobility (e.g., 12-Item Multiple Sclerosis Walking Scale) and many more. To date, few PROMs of sufficient psychometric quality are available, necessitating the development of standardized, high-quality MS-specific PROMs to collect robust, consistent and reliable real-world data [156,159]. Additionally, electronically answered questionnaires via app-based technologies such as tablets/smartphones, or via the Internet, enable more frequent PROM collection even in-between clinical visits, allowing a closer patient-centered view.

Combined with a transmission of patients' answers into an electronic health record system, it could function as an automated monitoring/notification system in the case of concerning symptoms [1,160]. To avoid long and burdensome questionnaires it would be desirable that PROMs become adaptive to each individual person with MS. The use of computerized adaptive testing is based on an item response theory to decrease administration time, still maintain accuracy, diminish the floor and ceiling effect and also improve the ability to detect the minimal clinically significant difference among patients [161–163]. This would lead to a higher patient adherence to perform PROMs on a regular basis, as well as more precise and individualized outcomes.

4.3. Digital Data Collection in MS

As there is already the possibility of data collection in many ways and areas, these data are of no use if they cannot be centrally stored, analyzed and made available to healthcare professionals and even patients. Especially when we think of the collection of big data to pave the way to a personalized treatment and consider MS as a lifelong disease that needs thorough and regular monitoring, quality care should enable a digitally supported quick response to any kind of disease worsening. Therefore, the Multiple Sclerosis Documentation System (MSDS) project group started to develop the MSDS software with the support of the Hertie Foundation in 1999, followed by the integrative patient management system MSDS3D, adapting to growing data collection and documentation needs [164]. The integration of a survey system for questionnaires, which not only can be made available on tablets while pwMS come to their visits but can also be sent by email with regular reminders, and thus immediately be documented in patients' medical records and visible for HCPs, became another feature of MSDS in recent years [165]. Documentation of medication plans, comedication and comorbidities, EDSS and relapses as well as pre-defined procedures for pwMS on a certain DMT, or even without any therapy, also support the monitoring and follow-up of meeting quality standards, and provide hints for improving medical care in the future. As pwMS are not only treated by neurologists alone, but by a variety of other HCPs, such as neuroradiologists, general practitioners, dermatologists, nursing services, psychiatrists, pain management therapists, etc., the integration of interfaces for using telemedicine services, digital communication and sharing medical data with patients, practitioners and caregivers play an increasingly crucial role in MS care [165]. These big data create a holistic picture of an individual patient and lead to specific therapy decisions. Additionally, from an economic point of view to avoid duplicate examinations and to enable high-quality treatment, all these data need to be exchanged between the parties involved. In the future, this need must be further met to provide holistic, high-quality and personalized care to pwMS.

4.4. Magnet Resonance Imaging

MRI scans are a standard investigation in MS and are essential both for diagnosis and as a monitoring tool, and are already documented digitally. MRI, in general, cannot only assist in the diagnostic process but is also crucial in regular monitoring to provide information about the treatment response as well as the efficacy and safety of DMTs [166]. Software systems that assist neuroradiologists in evaluating MRIs are already used in clinical trials and investigated regarding their ability to support neuroradiologists and enhance the evaluation of imaging. They can scan defined MRI sequences for the quantification of new or enlarging lesions, lesion volume and brain atrophy. Different companies are working on such software systems, which are partly already used in regular care [155]. Here, an inter-scanner reproducibility is of great importance [167]. Efforts have been made to provide consensus guidelines on the use of MRI in pwMS [168]. This is beyond this review on clinical, digital biomarkers in MS.

4.5. The Future of Digital Biomarkers

Much research is in progress regarding digital biomarkers in MS and other diseases, and studies are already evaluating the use of various devices for their collection (Konect-MS and Floodlight), those already available as DIGAs (elevida) or those about to be one (MS Sherpa, Emendia MS). Chronic diseases such as MS or Alzheimer's disease are complex and can show a diversity of symptoms. These symptoms can also emerge in other diseases, e.g., depression (speech and cognition). Therefore, there will not be "the ideal" digital biomarker with which a disease can be detected and monitored. Rather, it will be the case that different applications will be used, which can easily be installed on smartphones (MS Sherpa, Floodlight, Konectom, elevida, etc.) or integrated into telemedicine (e.g., speech analysis).

5. Data Analysis

The use of digital biomarkers creates different demands on data analysis than the traditional processing of data in everyday clinical practice and even than those on a more elaborate level in clinical trials. To fulfill the predictive purpose of a biomarker, real-time data transmission and analysis is the goal. This requires independence of location and data collection situation, i.e., data processing that can take place in clinical practice, but is not limited to the neurologist's premises, and the visits that take place at longer intervals. To accomplish this, data from a wide variety of sources must be digitally aggregated via standardized secure interfaces (see Section 4.3)—a task far beyond the capabilities of individual apps.

Isolated analyses can also be performed locally, offline, on individual end devices (e.g., the calculation of individual PROM scores) and, assuming timely transmission to the treating neurologist, fulfill targeted warning functions. Here, the general requirement for (automated) information processing systems is that they can reliably distinguish useful information (real medical needs) from noise, such as by applying established cut-off values. These are usually predefined values, which are usually applied population-wide, and the exceeding of which is associated with the presence of an indication. However, the full potential of digital biomarkers as part of a precision medicine approach can only be accessed by integrating a wide variety of data sources into an electronic repository. This is based on the insight that single biomarkers can hardly be used to control a disease as complex as MS, the disease activity of which is, to a large extent, pre-symptomatic, and that rigid, generalized thresholds often do not best reflect the individual situation.

The aim of an integrative evaluation of digital biomarkers in combination with other (clinical) data sources is the creation of a valid statistical model which evaluates prognostic tasks, such as selection and change recommendation regarding a DMT, as well as retrospective processing of information on progression assessment, therapy efficacy and safety aspects, and makes them applicable to individual cases. On the one hand, this results in the necessity of the highest possible data density with regard to the data diversity and the temporal distribution of the surveys. On the other hand, the requirements for the analysis also make it clear that this cannot be achieved with traditional statistical methods/models. The now-established solution for such concerns is found in the field of machine learning. Here, complex data structures are evaluated in a data-driven manner, and information of various types is processed jointly. The desired application situation in real-time and prognostic performance of the model can be extended by self-optimizing methods of deep learning. Schwab et al. chose an application situation for MS for this purpose, in which they aimed to achieve (retrospective) classification between pwMS and healthy controls by evaluating digital biomarkers from smartphone data using deep learning [169]. While this was not yet done as part of an established multiprofessional digital infrastructure for MS, they were able to successfully incorporate multi-layered data on mobility, upper limb functionality, cognition and affect.

However, the further the performance of such an analysis system goes, the more its ability to make recommendations and prognostic deductions comes into focus. This begins with immediate predictions of the general state of impairment from a current cross-sectional measurement of a patient [170], and increases through the consideration of individual longitudinal courses to the prediction of individual symptom areas and the competing effectiveness of therapies. At the same time, this increases the regulatory requirements for digital analysis systems for clinical practice, which in Germany, for example, are regulated by the Medical Devices Act. The end product of integrated digital data analysis is, in the best case, an approved product, which can be used by different HCPs as well as by the individual patient for recording as well as for evaluation, which remains self-updating on the best scientific level and derives understandable as well as useful parameters and overviews for all parties involved.

6. Digital Twins

Digital biomarkers are an important component of so-called digital twins. A digital twin in healthcare is a virtual copy of a patient that exactly matches that patient's characteristics and attributes, thus mirroring that patient. Using machine learning algorithms, the digital twin can be trained to predict disease progression and simulate treatments without risk to the patient. This involves using population data collected from previous patients and study cohorts to build and validate statistical and mechanistic models and to create a population-based digital twin, as well as analyzing data from the individual patient using the existing models and, in turn, integrating them into the patient's digital twin. The comparison and interaction between the digital twins provide valuable insights (e.g., phenotyping, risk assessment and the prediction of disease evolution) that are clinically interpreted and combined with traditional data to support clinical decision-making. In the process, the digital twin is constantly fed with new data so that it adapts and continuously improves [171]. To create the digital twin of a patient, a large and multidimensional amount of data is needed. A digital twin for MS (DTMS), due to the complexity and long-term nature of the disease, requires a particularly large and multidimensional amount of high-quality, high-frequency and structured data to propose a tailored therapy for the patient. These data are, in detail, physiological condition data of the patient (structured clinical data, paraclinical and multimicrobial data as well as patient-reported data) and procedures applied to the patient (diagnostic workup, treatment and monitoring, integrated in personalized clinical pathways). Many clinical and paraclinical data, including lab and imaging data, can be captured with digital biomarkers that can be transformed into interpretable outcome measures using algorithms. Digital twins also offer the possibility of visualizing a wide variety of parameters using a dashboard and mapping personalized clinical pathways. With the development of a DTMS, clinical treatment decisions, physician–patient communication and thus the quality of treatment can be improved. Even though there are still many challenges to be overcome on the way to the DTMS (effectiveness and safety, data protection, data security, data quality data management, creation of meaningful algorithms and ethical as well as individual concerns) and a DTMS need to be validated and tested before being used in practice, it is a valuable tool with which to make precision medicine and patient-centered care in MS part of everyday clinical practice [172].

7. Conclusions/Summary

The heterogeneous, multisymptomatic MS disease offers numerous possibilities for the acquisition of digital biomarkers. As the possibilities to collect digital data are continuously growing, such data can also be used for prognostic and diagnostic aspects as well as for the evaluation of disease activity and response to therapy. These digital biomarkers can be collected by devices available to everyone (e.g., wearables such as fitness trackers) or special devices created for specific examinations (e.g., vision, upper and lower limb function. MRI, cognition, PROMs, etc.). Therefore, they need to be validated, standardized, analyzed and made available to HCP to be used in pwMS care.

To our knowledge, older MS patients are becoming more and more familiar with using new technologies such as apps on smartphones or tablets [164]. Additionally, the in-clinic collection of digital biomarkers by a physician or escorting staff benefits all patients, regardless of their age.

As MS is a lifelong disease, pwMS should be integrated into their treatment. Here, smartphone applications can be used to document mood or specific problems (e.g., headache, fatigue, depression, etc.) or to check functional systems on a regular basis (such as vision, cognition, motor function of the extremities, etc.). The use of digital biomarkers may also be of interest to developing countries, where medical/neurological care is not widely available. For example, data could be collected from patients and transmitted to physicians as soon as Internet access is available, or a voice analysis could be performed via a telephone call. However, the establishment and validation procedures of digital biomarkers do not yet follow generally accepted standards. Developments according to the requirements of the Medical Devices Act are necessary, but are as complex as the development of classical biomarkers. Once the collection of standardized, validated digital biomarkers in all aspects of life (in-clinic and in daily life) is possible, the way is clear to develop digital twins and personalized treatment.

Author Contributions: Conceptualization, A.D. and M.L.W.; methodology, M.L.W. and A.D.; resources, M.L.W. and A.D.; writing—original draft preparation, A.D. and M.L.W.; writing—review and editing, M.L.W., A.D., T.Z., R.H., K.T., H.I., D.S., M.S. and I.V.; visualization, M.L.W. and A.D.; supervision, T.Z. and K.A. All authors have read and agreed to the published version of the manuscript.

Funding: This research received no external funding.

Conflicts of Interest: T.Z. received personal compensation from Biogen, Bayer, Celgene, Novartis, Roche, Sanofi and Teva for consulting services, and additional financial support for research activities from Bayer, BAT, Biogen, Novartis, Teva and Sanofi. K.A. received personal compensation from Novartis, Biogen Idec, Sanofi, Alexion, Celgene and Roche for consulting services and speaker honoraria. R.H. received travel grants by Celgene and Sanofi. A.D. received personal compensation and travel grants from Biogen, Celegene, Roche and Sanofi for speaker activity. M.L.W. received travel grants from Biogen. M.S. received travel grants from TEVA.

References

1. Ziemssen, T.; Kern, R.; Thomas, K. Multiple Sclerosis: Clinical Profiling and Data Collection as Prerequisite for Personal-ized Medicine Approach. *BMC Neurol.* **2016**, *16*, 124. [CrossRef] [PubMed]
2. Ziemssen, T. Multiple sclerosis beyond EDSS: Depression and fatigue. *J. Neurol. Sci.* **2009**, *277*, S37–S41. [CrossRef]
3. Kourtis, L.; Regele, O.B.; Wright, J.M.; Jones, G.B. Digital biomarkers for Alzheimer's disease: The mobile/wearable devices opportunity. *NPJ Digit. Med.* **2019**, *2*, 9. [CrossRef] [PubMed]
4. Gold, M.; Amatniek, J.; Carrillo, M.C.; Cedarbaum, J.M.; Hendrix, J.A.; Miller, B.B.; Robillard, J.; Rice, J.J.; Soares, H.; Tome, M.B.; et al. Digital technologies as biomarkers, clinical outcomes assessment, and recruitment tools in Alzheimer's disease clinical trials. *Alzheimer's Dement. Transl. Res. Clin. Interv.* **2018**, *4*, 234–242. [CrossRef]
5. Rykov, Y.; Thach, T.-Q.; Bojic, I.; Christopoulos, G.; Car, J. Digital Biomarkers for Depression Screening With Wearable Devices: Cross-sectional Study With Machine Learning Modeling. *JMIR mHealth uHealth* **2021**, *9*, e24872. [CrossRef] [PubMed]
6. Ziemssen, T.; Akgün, K.; Brück, W. Molecular biomarkers in multiple sclerosis. *J. Neuroinflamm.* **2019**, *16*, 272. [CrossRef]
7. Coravos, A.; Khozin, S.; Mandl, K.D. Erratum: Author Correction: Developing and Adopting Safe and Effective Digital Biomarkers to Improve Patient Outcomes. *NPJ Digit. Med.* **2019**, *2*, 40. [CrossRef]
8. Dorsey, E.R.; Papapetropoulos, S.; Xiong, M.; Kieburtz, K. The First Frontier: Digital Biomarkers for Neurodegenerative Disorders. *Digit. Biomark.* **2017**, *1*, 6–13. [CrossRef]
9. Wang, T.; Azad, T.; Rajan, R. The Emerging Influence of Digital Biomarkers on Healthcare. Available online: https://rockhealth.com/insights/the-emerging-influence-of-digital-biomarkers-on-healthcare/ (accessed on 18 October 2021).
10. Babrak, L.M.; Menetski, J.; Rebhan, M.; Nisato, G.; Zinggeler, M.; Brasier, N.; Baerenfaller, K.; Brenzikofer, T.; Baltzer, L.; Vogler, C.; et al. Traditional and Digital Biomarkers: Two Worlds Apart? *Digit. Biomark.* **2019**, *3*, 92–102. [CrossRef]
11. Bielekova, B.; Martin, R. Development of biomarkers in multiple sclerosis. *Brain* **2004**, *127*, 1463–1478. [CrossRef]
12. Ziemssen, T.; Medin, J.; Couto, C.A.; Mitchell, C.R. Multiple Sclerosis in the Real World: A Systematic Review of Fin-golimod as a Case Study. *Autoimmun. Rev.* **2017**, *16*, 355–376. [CrossRef] [PubMed]
13. Noffs, G.; Perera, T.; Kolbe, S.C.; Shanahan, C.J.; Boonstra, F.M.C.; Evans, A.; Butzkueven, H.; van der Walt, A.; Vogel, A.P. What speech can tell us: A systematic review of dysarthria characteristics in Multiple Sclerosis. *Autoimmun. Rev.* **2018**, *17*, 1202–1209. [CrossRef]
14. Hoff, J.M.; Dhayalan, M.; Midelfart, A.; Tharaldsen, A.R.; Bo, L. Visual Dysfunction in Multiple Sclerosis. *Tidsskr. Nor. Legeforening* **2019**, *139*. [CrossRef]

15. Green, A.J.; McQuaid, S.; Hauser, S.L.; Allen, I.V.; Lyness, R. Ocular pathology in multiple sclerosis: Retinal atrophy and inflammation irrespective of disease duration. *Brain* **2010**, *133*, 1591–1601. [CrossRef] [PubMed]
16. Martínez-Lapiscina, E.H.; Arnow, S.; Wilson, J.A.; Saidha, S.; Preiningerova, J.L.; Oberwahrenbrock, T.; Brandt, A.U.; Pablo, L.E.; Guerrieri, S.; González-Suárez, I.; et al. Retinal thickness measured with optical coherence tomography and risk of disability worsening in multiple sclerosis: A cohort study. *Lancet Neurol.* **2016**, *15*, 574–584. [CrossRef]
17. Britze, J.; Frederiksen, J.L. Optical coherence tomography in multiple sclerosis. *Eye* **2018**, *32*, 884–888. [CrossRef]
18. Balcer, L.J.; Raynowska, J.; Nolan, R.; Galetta, S.L.; Kapoor, R.; Benedict, R.; Phillips, G.; LaRocca, N.; Hudson, L.; Rudick, R.; et al. Validity of low-contrast letter acuity as a visual performance outcome measure for multiple sclerosis. *Mult. Scler. J.* **2017**, *23*, 734–747. [CrossRef]
19. Fisher, J.B.; Jacobs, D.A.; Markowitz, C.E.; Galetta, S.L.; Volpe, N.J.; Nano-Schiavi, M.L.; Baier, M.L.; Frohman, E.M.; Winslow, H.; Frohman, T.C. Relation of Visual Function to Retinal Nerve Fiber Layer Thickness in Multiple Sclerosis. *Ophthalmology* **2006**, *113*, 324–332. [CrossRef]
20. Maggio, M.G.; Russo, M.; Cuzzola, M.F.; Destro, M.; La Rosa, G.; Molonia, F.; Bramanti, P.; Lombardo, G.; De Luca, R.; Calabrò, R.S. Virtual reality in multiple sclerosis rehabilitation: A review on cognitive and motor outcomes. *J. Clin. Neurosci.* **2019**, *65*, 106–111. [CrossRef]
21. Frohman, E.M.; Frohman, T.C.; Zee, D.S.; McColl, R.; Galetta, S. The neuro-ophthalmology of multiple sclerosis. *Lancet Neurol.* **2005**, *4*, 111–121. [CrossRef]
22. Niestroy, A.; Rucker, J.; Leigh, R.J. Neuro-ophthalmologic aspects of multiple sclerosis: Using eye movements as a clinical and experimental tool. *Clin. Ophthalmol.* **2007**, *1*, 267–272. [PubMed]
23. De Santi, L.; Lanzafame, P.; Spano', B.; D'Aleo, G.; Bramanti, A.; Bramanti, P.; Marino, S. Pursuit ocular movements in multiple sclerosis: A video-based eye-tracking study. *Neurol. Sci.* **2010**, *32*, 67–71. [CrossRef] [PubMed]
24. Gibaldi, A.; Vanegas, M.; Bex, P.J.; Maiello, G. Evaluation of the Tobii EyeX Eye tracking controller and Matlab toolkit for research. *Behav. Res. Methods* **2017**, *49*, 923–946. [CrossRef] [PubMed]
25. Sheehy, C.K.; Beaudry-Richard, A.; Bensinger, E.; Theis, J.; Green, A.J. Methods to Assess Ocular Motor Dysfunction in Multiple Sclerosis. *J. Neuro-Ophthalmol.* **2018**, *38*, 488–493. [CrossRef]
26. Reulen, J.P.; Sanders, E.A.; Hogenhuis, L.A. Eye Movement Disorders in Multiple Sclerosis and Optic Neuritis. *Brain* **1983**, *106*, 121–140. [CrossRef]
27. Nygaard, G.O.; Benavent, S.A.D.R.; Harbo, H.F.; Laeng, B.; Sowa, P.; Damangir, S.; Nilsen, K.B.; Etholm, L.; Tønnesen, S.; Kerty, E.; et al. Eye and hand motor interactions with the Symbol Digit Modalities Test in early multiple sclerosis. *Mult. Scler. Relat. Disord.* **2015**, *4*, 585–589. [CrossRef] [PubMed]
28. Fielding, J.; Kilpatrick, T.; Millist, L.; White, O. Antisaccade performance in patients with multiple sclerosis. *Cortex* **2009**, *45*, 900–903. [CrossRef]
29. Fielding, J.; Kilpatrick, T.; Millist, L.; White, O. Control of visually guided saccades in multiple sclerosis: Disruption to higher-order processes. *Neuropsychology* **2009**, *47*, 1647–1653. [CrossRef]
30. Finke, C.; Pech, L.M.; Sömmer, C.; Schlichting, J.; Stricker, S.; Endres, M.; Ostendorf, F.; Ploner, C.J.; Brandt, A.U.; Paul, F. Dynamics of Saccade Parameters in Multiple Sclerosis Patients with Fatigue. *J. Neurol.* **2012**, *259*, 2656–2663. [CrossRef]
31. Tao, L.; Wang, Q.; Liu, D.; Wang, J.; Zhu, Z.; Feng, L. Eye tracking metrics to screen and assess cognitive impairment in patients with neurological disorders. *Neurol. Sci.* **2020**, *41*, 1697–1704. [CrossRef]
32. Fielding, J.; Kilpatrick, T.; Millist, L.; White, O. Multiple sclerosis: Cognition and saccadic eye movements. *J. Neurol. Sci.* **2009**, *277*, 32–36. [CrossRef]
33. Grillini, A.; Renken, R.J.; Vrijling, A.C.; Heutink, J.; Cornelissen, F.W. Eye Movement Evaluation in Multiple Sclerosis and Parkinson's Disease Using a Standardized Oculomotor and Neuro-Ophthalmic Disorder Assessment (Sonda). *Front. Neurol.* **2020**, *11*, 971. [CrossRef]
34. Merson, R.M.; Rolnick, M.I. Speech-language Pathology and Dysphagia in Multiple Sclerosis. *Phys. Med. Rehabil. Clin. N. Am.* **1998**, *9*, 631–641. [CrossRef]
35. Hartelius, L.; Runmarker, B.; Anderser, O. Prevalence and Characteristics of Dysarthria in a Multiple-Sclerosis Incidence Cohort: Relation to Neurological Data. *Folia Phoniatr. Logop.* **2000**, *52*, 160–177. [CrossRef] [PubMed]
36. Beukelman, D.R.; Kraft, G.H.; Freal, J. Expressive Communication Disorders in Persons with Multiple Sclerosis: A Survey. *Arch. Phys. Med. Rehabil.* **1985**, *66*, 675–677.
37. Stipancic, K.L.; Tjaden, K.; Wilding, G. Comparison of Intelligibility Measures for Adults with Parkinson's Disease, Adults with Multiple Sclerosis, and Healthy Controls. *J. Speech Lang. Hear. Res.* **2016**, *59*, 230–238. [CrossRef] [PubMed]
38. Rusz, J.; Benova, B.; Ruzickova, H.; Novotny, M.; Tykalova, T.; Hlavnicka, J.; Uher, T.; Vaneckova, M.; Andelova, M.; Novotna, K.; et al. Characteristics of motor speech phenotypes in multiple sclerosis. *Mult. Scler. Relat. Disord.* **2018**, *19*, 62–69. [CrossRef]
39. Greeley, H.P.; Friets, E.; Wilson, J.P.; Raghavan, S.; Picone, J.; Berg, J. Detecting Fatigue from Voice Using Speech Recognition. Proceedings 2006 IEEE International Symposium on Signal Processing and Information Technology, Vancouver, BC, Canada, 27–30 August 2006; pp. 567–571. [CrossRef]
40. Amunts, J.; Camilleri, J.A.; Eickhoff, S.B.; Heim, S.; Weis, S. Executive functions predict verbal fluency scores in healthy participants. *Sci. Rep.* **2020**, *10*, 11141. [CrossRef] [PubMed]

41. Mathew, M.M.; Bhat, J.S. Soft Phonation Index—A Sensitive Parameter? *Indian J. Otolaryngol. Head Neck Surg.* **2009**, *61*, 127–130. [CrossRef]
42. Feijó, A.V.; Parente, M.A.; Behlau, M.; Haussen, S.; De Veccino, M.C.; Martignago, B.C.D.F. Acoustic analysis of voice in multiple sclerosis patients. *J. Voice* **2004**, *18*, 341–347. [CrossRef] [PubMed]
43. Dogan, M.; Midi, I.; Yazıcı, M.A.; Kocak, I.; Günal, D.; Sehitoglu, M.A. Objective and Subjective Evaluation of Voice Quality in Multiple Sclerosis. *J. Voice* **2007**, *21*, 735–740. [CrossRef]
44. Hartelius, L.; Buder, E.H.; Strand, E.A. Long-Term Phonatory Instability in Individuals with Multiple Sclerosis. *J. Speech Lang. Hear. Res.* **1997**, *40*, 1056–1072. [CrossRef] [PubMed]
45. Vizza, P.; Mirarchi, D.; Tradigo, G.; Redavide, M.; Bossio, R.B.; Veltri, P. Vocal signal analysis in patients affected by Multiple Sclerosis. *Procedia Comput. Sci.* **2017**, *108*, 1205–1214. [CrossRef]
46. Noffs, G.; Boonstra, F.M.C.; Perera, T.; Kolbe, S.C.; Stankovich, J.; Butzkueven, H.; Evans, A.; Vogel, A.; Van Der Walt, A. Acoustic Speech Analytics Are Predictive of Cerebellar Dysfunction in Multiple Sclerosis. *Cerebellum* **2020**, *19*, 691–700. [CrossRef]
47. Fagherazzi, G.; Fischer, A.; Ismael, M.; Despotovic, V. Voice for Health: The Use of Vocal Biomarkers from Research to Clinical Practice. *Digit. Biomark.* **2021**, *5*, 78–88. [CrossRef]
48. Zhang, L.; Duvvuri, R.; Chandra, K.K.L.; Nguyen, T.; Ghomi, R.H. Automated Voice Biomarkers for Depression Symp-toms Using an Online Cross-Sectional Data Collection Initiative. *Depress Anxiety* **2020**, *37*, 657–669. [CrossRef]
49. Cummins, N.; Scherer, S.; Krajewski, J.; Schnieder, S.; Epps, J.; Quatieri, T.F. A review of depression and suicide risk assessment using speech analysis. *Speech Commun.* **2015**, *71*, 10–49. [CrossRef]
50. Henry, J.D.; Beatty, W.W. Verbal fluency deficits in multiple sclerosis. *Neuropsychology* **2006**, *44*, 1166–1174. [CrossRef] [PubMed]
51. Barcellos, L.F.; Bellesis, K.H.; Shen, L.; Shao, X.; Chinn, T.; Frndak, P.; Drake, A.; Bakshi, N.; Marcus, J.; Schaefer, C.; et al. Remote assessment of verbal memory in MS patients using the California Verbal Learning Test. *Mult. Scler. J.* **2017**, *24*, 354–357. [CrossRef] [PubMed]
52. Fischer, J.S. Using the wechsler memory scale-revised to detect and characterize memory deficits in multiple sclerosis. *Clin. Neuropsychol.* **1988**, *2*, 149–172. [CrossRef]
53. Krajewski, J.; Wieland, R.; Batliner, A. *An Acoustic Framework for Detecting Fatigue in Speech Based Hu-man-Computer-Interaction*; Springer: Berlin/Heidelberg, Germany, 2008; pp. 54–61.
54. Wallace, G.L.; Holmes, S. Cognitive-linguistic assessment of individuals with multiple sclerosis. *Arch. Phys. Med. Rehabil.* **1993**, *74*, 637–643. [CrossRef]
55. Yozbatıran, N.; Baskurt, F.; Baskurt, Z.; Ozakbas, S.; Idiman, E. Motor assessment of upper extremity function and its relation with fatigue, cognitive function and quality of life in multiple sclerosis patients. *J. Neurol. Sci.* **2006**, *246*, 117–122. [CrossRef] [PubMed]
56. Holper, L.; Coenen, M.; Weise, A.; Stucki, G.; Cieza, A.; Kesselring, J. Characterization of functioning in multiple sclerosis using the ICF. *J. Neurol.* **2009**, *257*, 103–113. [CrossRef]
57. Pellegrino, L.; Coscia, M.; Muller, M.; Solaro, C.; Casadio, M. Evaluating upper limb impairments in multiple sclerosis by exposure to different mechanical environments. *Sci. Rep.* **2018**, *8*, 2110. [CrossRef]
58. Kraft, G.H.; Amtmann, D.; Bennett, S.E.; Finlayson, M.; Sutliff, M.H.; Tullman, M.; Sidovar, M.; Rabinowicz, A.L. As-sessment of Upper Extremity Function in Multiple Sclerosis: Review and Opinion. *Postgrad. Med.* **2014**, *126*, 102–108. [CrossRef] [PubMed]
59. Kahraman, T. Performance Measures for Upper Extremity Functions in Persons with Multiple Sclerosis. *Arch. Neuropsychiatry* **2018**, *55*, S41–S45. [CrossRef]
60. Mollà-Casanova, S.; Llorens, R.; Borrego, A.; Salinas-Martínez, B.; Serra-Añó, P. Validity, reliability, and sensitivity to motor impairment severity of a multi-touch app designed to assess hand mobility, coordination, and function after stroke. *J. Neuroeng. Rehabil.* **2021**, *18*, 70. [CrossRef]
61. Cirstea, M.C.; Mitnitski, A.B.; Feldman, A.G.; Levin, M.F. Interjoint coordination dynamics during reaching in stroke. *Exp. Brain Res.* **2003**, *151*, 289–300. [CrossRef]
62. Ivry, R.; Diedrichsen, J.; Spencer, R.; Hazeltine, E.; Semjen, A. A Cognitive Neuroscience Per-spective on Bimanual Coordination and Interference. In *Neuro-Behavioral Determinants of Interlimb Coordination*; Springer: Boston, MA, USA, 2004; pp. 259–295.
63. Lamers, I.; Feys, P. Assessing upper limb function in multiple sclerosis. *Mult. Scler. J.* **2014**, *20*, 775–784. [CrossRef]
64. Tanigawa, M.; Stein, J.; Park, J.; Kosa, P.; Cortese, I.; Bielekova, B. Finger and foot tapping as alternative outcomes of upper and lower extremity function in multiple sclerosis. *Mult. Scler. J. Exp. Transl. Clin.* **2017**, *3*, 2055217316688930. [CrossRef]
65. Floeter, M.K.; Mills, R. Progression in Primary Lateral Sclerosis: A Prospective Analysis. *Amyotroph. Lateral Scler.* **2009**, *10*, 339–346. [CrossRef]
66. Creagh, A.; Simillion, C.; Scotland, A.; Lipsmeier, F.; Bernasconi, C.; Belachew, S.; Van Beek, J.; Baker, M.; Gossens, C.; Lindemann, M.; et al. Smartphone-based remote assessment of upper extremity function for multiple sclerosis using the Draw a Shape Test. *Physiol. Meas.* **2020**, *41*, 054002. [CrossRef] [PubMed]
67. Kontschieder, P.; Dorn, J.F.; Morrison, C.; Corish, R.; Zikic, D.; Sellen, A.; D'Souza, M.; Kamm, C.P.; Burggraaff, J.; Tewarie, P.; et al. Quantifying Pro-gression of Multiple Sclerosis Via Classification of Depth Videos. In *International Conference on Medical Image Computing and Computer-Assisted Intervention*; Springer: Cham, Switzerland, 2014; pp. 429–437.
68. Flachenecker, F.; Gassner, H.; Hannik, J.; Lee, D.H.; Flachenecker, P.; Winkler, J.; Eskofier, B.; Linker, R.A.; Klucken, J. Ob-jective Sensor-Based Gait Measures Reflect Motor Impairment in Multiple Sclerosis Patients: Reliability and Clinical Valida-tion of a Wearable Sensor Device. *Mult. Scler. Relat. Disord.* **2019**, *39*, 101903. [CrossRef]

69. Larocca, N.G. Impact of Walking Impairment in Multiple Sclerosis: Perspectives of Patients and Care Partners. *Patient* **2011**, *4*, 189–201. [CrossRef] [PubMed]
70. Bethoux, F. Gait Disorders in Multiple Sclerosis. *Contin. Lifelong Learn. Neurol.* **2013**, *19*, 1007–1022. [CrossRef]
71. Sosnoff, J.J.; Sandroff, B.M.; Motl, R.W. Quantifying Gait Abnormalities in Persons with Multiple Sclerosis with Minimal Disability. *Gait Posture* **2012**, *36*, 154–156. [CrossRef]
72. Martin, C.L.; Phillips, B.A.; Kilpatrick, T.; Butzkueven, H.; Tubridy, N.; McDonald, E.; Galea, M. Gait and balance impairment in early multiple sclerosis in the absence of clinical disability. *Mult. Scler. J.* **2006**, *12*, 620–628. [CrossRef] [PubMed]
73. Cameron, M.H.; Wagner, J.M. Gait Abnormalities in Multiple Sclerosis: Pathogenesis, Evaluation, and Advances in Treatment. *Curr. Neurol. Neurosci. Rep.* **2011**, *11*, 507–515. [CrossRef]
74. Trentzsch, K.; Weidemann, M.L.; Torp, C.; Inojosa, H.; Scholz, M.; Haase, R.; Schriefer, D.; Akgün, K.; Ziemssen, T. The Dresden Protocol for Multidimensional Walking Assessment (DMWA) in Clinical Practice. *Front. Neurosci.* **2020**, *14*, 582046. [CrossRef]
75. Shanahan, C.J.; Boonstra, F.M.C.; Lizama, L.E.C.; Strik, M.; Moffat, B.A.; Khan, F.; Kilpatrick, T.J.; Van Der Walt, A.; Galea, M.P.; Kolbe, S.C. Technologies for Advanced Gait and Balance Assessments in People with Multiple Sclerosis. *Front. Neurol.* **2018**, *8*, 708. [CrossRef]
76. Coghe, G.; Corona, F.; Pilloni, G.; Porta, M.; Frau, J.; Lorefice, L.; Fenu, G.; Cocco, E.; Pau, M. Is There Any Relationship between Upper and Lower Limb Impairments in People with Multiple Sclerosis? A Kinematic Quantitative Analysis. *Mult. Scler. Int.* **2019**, *2019*, 9149201. [CrossRef] [PubMed]
77. Willimczik, K.; Roth, K. *Bewegungslehre*; Rowohlt-Taschenbuch-Verlag: Reinbek, Germany, 1988.
78. Fang, X.; Liu, C.; Jiang, Z. Reference values of gait using APDM movement monitoring inertial sensor system. *R. Soc. Open Sci.* **2018**, *5*, 170818. [CrossRef] [PubMed]
79. Washabaugh, E.P.; Kalyanaraman, T.; Adamczyk, P.; Claflin, E.S.; Krishnan, C. Validity and repeatability of inertial measurement units for measuring gait parameters. *Gait Posture* **2017**, *55*, 87–93. [CrossRef] [PubMed]
80. Spain, R.I.; George, R.J.S.; Salarian, A.; Mancini, M.; Wagner, J.M.; Horak, F.B.; Bourdette, D. Body-Worn Motion Sensors Detect Balance and Gait Deficits in People with Multiple Sclerosis Who Have Normal Walking Speed. *Gait Posture* **2012**, *35*, 573–578. [CrossRef]
81. Kurtzke, J.F. Rating neurologic impairment in multiple sclerosis: An expanded disability status scale (EDSS). *Neurology* **1983**, *33*, 1444–1452. [CrossRef]
82. Block, V.J.; Lizée, A.; Crabtree-Hartman, E.; Bevan, C.J.; Graves, J.S.; Bove, R.; Green, A.J.; Nourbakhsh, B.; Tremblay, M.; Gourraud, P.-A.; et al. Continuous daily assessment of multiple sclerosis disability using remote step count monitoring. *J. Neurol.* **2017**, *264*, 316–326. [CrossRef] [PubMed]
83. Rhodes, J.K.; Schindler, D.; Rao, S.M.; Venegas, F.; Bruzik, E.T.; Gabel, W.; Williams, J.; Phillips, G.A.; Mullen, C.C.; Freiburger, J.L.; et al. Multiple Sclerosis Performance Test: Technical Development and Usability. *Adv. Ther.* **2019**, *36*, 1741–1755. [CrossRef]
84. Rao, S.M.; Leo, G.J.; Bernardin, L.; Unverzagt, F. Cognitive dysfunction in multiple sclerosis: I. Frequency, patterns, and prediction. *Neurology* **1991**, *41*, 685–691. [CrossRef]
85. Kaufman, M.; Moyer, D.; Norton, J. The Significant Change for the Timed 25-Foot Walk in the Multiple Sclerosis Functional Composite. *Mult. Scler.* **2000**, *6*, 286–290. [CrossRef]
86. Baier, M.L.; Cutter, G.R.; Rudick, R.A.; Miller, D.; Cohen, J.A.; Weinstock-Guttman, B.; Mass, M.; Balcer, L.J. Low-contrast letter acuity testing captures visual dysfunction in patients with multiple sclerosis. *Neurology* **2005**, *64*, 992–995. [CrossRef] [PubMed]
87. Rudick, R.A.; Miller, D.; Bethoux, F.; Rao, S.M.; Lee, J.C.; Stough, D.; Reece, C.; Schindler, D.; Mamone, B.; Alberts, J. The Multiple Sclerosis Performance Test (Mspt): An Ipad-Based Disability Assessment Tool. *J. Vis. Exp.* **2014**, *88*, e51318. [CrossRef]
88. Sumowski, J.F.; Benedict, R.; Enzinger, C.; Filippi, M.; Geurts, J.J.; Hamalainen, P.; Hulst, H.; Inglese, M.; Leavitt, V.M.; Rocca, M.A.; et al. Cognition in Multiple Sclerosis: State of the Field and Priorities for the Future. *Neurology* **2018**, *90*, 278–288. [CrossRef] [PubMed]
89. Rao, S.M.; Losinski, G.; Mourany, L.; Schindler, D.; Mamone, B.; Reece, C.; Kemeny, D.; Narayanan, S.; Miller, D.M.; Bethoux, F.; et al. Processing Speed Test: Validation of a Self-Administered, Ipad((R))-Based Tool for Screening Cognitive Dysfunction in a Clinic Setting. *Mult. Scler.* **2017**, *23*, 1929–1937. [CrossRef] [PubMed]
90. Rao, S.M.; Galioto, R.; Sokolowski, M.; McGinley, M.; Freiburger, J.; Weber, M.; Dey, T.; Mourany, L.; Schindler, D.; Reece, C.; et al. Multiple Sclerosis Performance Test: Validation of Self-Administered Neuroperformance Modules. *Eur. J. Neurol.* **2020**, *27*, 878–886. [CrossRef] [PubMed]
91. Learmonth, Y.C.; Motl, R.W.; Sandroff, B.M.; Pula, J.H.; Cadavid, D. Validation of patient determined disease steps (PDDS) scale scores in persons with multiple sclerosis. *BMC Neurol.* **2013**, *13*, 37. [CrossRef]
92. Medina, L.D.; Torres, S.; Alvarez, E.; Valdez, B.; Nair, K.V. Patient-Reported Outcomes in Multiple Sclerosis: Validation of the Quality of Life in Neurological Disorders (Neuro-Qol) Short Forms. *Mult. Scler. J. Exp. Transl. Clin.* **2019**, *5*, 2055217319885985. [CrossRef]
93. Cella, D.; Lai, J.S.; Nowinski, C.J.; Victorson, D.; Peterman, A.; Miller, D.; Bethoux, F.; Heinemann, A.; Rubin, S.; Cavazos, J.E.; et al. Neuro-Qol: Brief Measures of Health-Related Quality of Life for Clinical Research in Neurology. *Neurology* **2012**, *78*, 1860–1867. [CrossRef]
94. Weidemann, M.L.; Trentzsch, K.; Torp, C.; Ziemssen, T. Enhancing Monitoring of Disease Progression-Remote Sensoring in Multiple Sclerosis. *Nervenarzt* **2019**, *90*, 1239–1244. [CrossRef]

95. Block, V.A.; Pitsch, E.; Tahir, P.; Cree, B.A.; Allen, D.D.; Gelfand, J.M. Remote Physical Activity Monitoring in Neuro-logical Disease: A Systematic Review. *PLoS ONE* **2016**, *11*, e0154335. [CrossRef]
96. Balto, J.M.; Kinnett-Hopkins, D.; Motl, R.W. Accuracy and precision of smartphone applications and commercially available motion sensors in multiple sclerosis. *Mult. Scler. J. Exp. Transl. Clin.* **2**, 2055217316634754. [CrossRef] [PubMed]
97. Block, V.J.; Bove, R.; Zhao, C.; Garcha, P.; Graves, J.; Romeo, A.R.; Green, A.J.; Allen, D.D.; Hollenbach, J.A.; Olgin, J.E.; et al. Association of Continuous Assessment of Step Count by Remote Monitoring With Disability Progression Among Adults With Multiple Sclerosis. *JAMA Netw. Open* **2019**, *2*, e190570. [CrossRef]
98. Moon, Y.; McGinnis, R.S.; Seagers, K.; Motl, R.W.; Sheth, N.; Wright, J.A., Jr.; Ghaffari, R.; Sosnoff, J.J. Monitoring gait in multiple sclerosis with novel wearable motion sensors. *PLoS ONE* **2017**, *12*, e0171346. [CrossRef] [PubMed]
99. Chitnis, T.; Glanz, B.I.; Gonzalez, C.; Healy, B.C.; Saraceno, T.J.; Sattarnezhad, N.; Diaz-Cruz, C.; Polgar-Turcsanyi, M.; Tummala, S.; Bakshi, R.; et al. Quantifying Neurologic Disease Using Bi-osensor Measurements in-Clinic and in Free-Living Settings in Multiple Sclerosis. *NPJ Digit. Med.* **2019**, *2*, 123. [CrossRef]
100. Daley, M.L.; Swank, R.L. Changes in postural control and vision induced by multiple sclerosis. *Agressologie* **1983**, *24*, 327–329.
101. Cameron, M.H.; Lord, S. Postural Control in Multiple Sclerosis: Implications for Fall Prevention. *Curr. Neurol. Neurosci. Rep.* **2010**, *10*, 407–412. [CrossRef]
102. Matsuda, P.N.; Shumway-Cook, A.; Ciol, M.A.; Bombardier, C.H.; Kartin, D.A. Understanding Falls in Multiple Scle-rosis: Association of Mobility Status, Concerns About Falling, and Accumulated Impairments. *Phys. Ther.* **2012**, *92*, 407–415. [CrossRef] [PubMed]
103. Gunn, H.; Newell, P.; Haas, B.; Marsden, J.F.; Freeman, J.A. Identification of Risk Factors for Falls in Multiple Sclerosis: A Systematic Review and Meta-Analysis. *Phys. Ther.* **2013**, *93*, 504–513. [CrossRef]
104. Mazumder, R.; Murchison, C.; Bourdette, D.; Cameron, M. Falls in People with Multiple Sclerosis Compared with Falls in Healthy Controls. *PLoS ONE* **2014**, *9*, e107620. [CrossRef]
105. Horak, F.B.; Henry, S.M.; Shumway-Cook, A. Postural Perturbations: New Insights for Treatment of Balance Disor-ders. *Phys. Ther.* **1997**, *77*, 517–533. [CrossRef]
106. Inojosa, H.; Schriefer, D.; Trentzsch, K.; Kloditz, A.; Ziemssen, T. Visual Feedback and Postural Control in Multiple Scle-rosis. *J. Clin. Med.* **2020**, *9*, 1291. [CrossRef] [PubMed]
107. Pollock, A.S.; Durward, B.R.; Rowe, P.J.; Paul, J.P. What Is Balance? *Clin. Rehabil.* **2000**, *14*, 402–406. [CrossRef]
108. Maki, B.E.; McIlroy, W.E. The Role of Limb Movements in Maintaining Upright Stance: The "Change-in-Support" Strategy. *Phys. Ther.* **1997**, *77*, 488–507. [CrossRef] [PubMed]
109. Inojosa, H.; Schriefer, D.; Kloditz, A.; Trentzsch, K.; Ziemssen, T. Balance Testing in Multiple Sclerosis-Improving Neuro-logical Assessment with Static Posturography? *Front. Neurol.* **2020**, *11*, 135. [CrossRef] [PubMed]
110. APDM Wearable Technologies Inc. Comprehensive Gait and Balance Analysis. Available online: https://apdm.com/mobility/ (accessed on 18 October 2021).
111. Heilmann, F. *Dynamische Posturographie—Entwicklung Und Validierung Einer Testbatterie Zur Gleichgewichtsdiagnostik Unter Verwendung Des Posturomeds*; Monograph; Martin–Luther–Universität Halle–Wittenberg: Halle, Germany, 2019.
112. Clark, R.A.; Mentiplay, B.; Pua, Y.-H.; Bower, K.J. Reliability and validity of the Wii Balance Board for assessment of standing balance: A systematic review. *Gait Posture* **2018**, *61*, 40–54. [CrossRef]
113. Gunn, H.; Markevics, S.; Haas, B.; Marsden, J.; Freeman, J. Systematic Review: The Effectiveness of Interventions to Reduce Falls and Improve Balance in Adults With Multiple Sclerosis. *Arch. Phys. Med. Rehabil.* **2015**, *96*, 1898–1912. [CrossRef]
114. Al-Sharman, A.; Khalil, H.; El-Salem, K.; Alghwiri, A.A.; Khazaaleh, S.; Khraim, M. Motor performance improvement through virtual reality task is related to fatigue and cognition in people with multiple sclerosis. *Physiother. Res. Int.* **2019**, *24*, e1782. [CrossRef]
115. Schreck, L.M.; Ryan, S.P.P.; Monaghan, P.G. Cerebellum and cognition in multiple sclerosis. *J. Neurophysiol.* **2018**, *120*, 2707–2709. [CrossRef]
116. Lovera, J.; Kovner, B. Cognitive Impairment in Multiple Sclerosis. *Curr. Neurol. Neurosci. Rep.* **2012**, *12*, 618–627. [CrossRef]
117. Langdon, D.W. Cognition in Multiple Sclerosis. *Curr. Opin. Neurol.* **2011**, *24*, 244–249. [CrossRef]
118. Rao, S.M.; Leo, G.J.; Ellington, L.; Nauertz, T.; Bernardin, L.; Unverzagt, F. Cognitive Dysfunction in Multiple Sclerosis. Ii. Impact on Employment and Social Functioning. *Neurology* **1991**, *41*, 692–696. [CrossRef]
119. Banati, M.; Sandor, J.; Mike, A.; Illes, E.; Bors, L.; Feldmann, A.; Herold, R.; Illes, Z. Social cognition and Theory of Mind in patients with relapsing-remitting multiple sclerosis. *Eur. J. Neurol.* **2010**, *17*, 426–433. [CrossRef]
120. Mitchell, A.J.; Benito-León, J.; González, J.M.; Rivera-Navarro, J. Quality of Life and Its Assessment in Multiple Sclero-sis: Integrating Physical and Psychological Components of Wellbeing. *Lancet Neurol.* **2005**, *4*, 556–566. [CrossRef]
121. Bruce, J.M.; Hancock, L.M.; Arnett, P.; Lynch, S. Treatment Adherence in Multiple Sclerosis: Association with Emotion-al Status, Personality, and Cognition. *J. Behav. Med.* **2010**, *33*, 219–227. [CrossRef] [PubMed]
122. Honarmand, K.; Akbar, N.; Kou, N.; Feinstein, A. Predicting Employment Status in Multiple Sclerosis Patients: The Util-ity of the Ms Functional Composite. *J. Neurol.* **2011**, *258*, 244–249. [CrossRef]
123. Amato, M.P.; Ponziani, G.; Siracusa, G.; Sorbi, S. Cognitive Dysfunction in Early-Onset Multiple Sclerosis: A Reappraisal after 10 Years. *Arch. Neurol.* **2001**, *58*, 1602–1606. [CrossRef]

124. Middleton, R.M.; Pearson, O.R.; Ingram, G.; Craig, E.M.; Rodgers, W.J.; Downing-Wood, H.; Hill, J.; Tuite-Dalton, K.; Roberts, C.; Watson, L.; et al. A Rapid Electronic Cognitive Assessment Measure for Multiple Sclerosis: Validation of Core (Cognitive Reaction), an Electronic Version of the Symbol Digit Modalities Test. *J. Med Internet. Res.* **2020**, *22*, e18234. [CrossRef]
125. Langdon, D.W.; Amato, M.P.; Boringa, J.; Brochet, B.; Foley, F.; Fredrikson, S.; Hämäläinen, P.; Hartung, H.P.; Krupp, L.; Penner, I.K.; et al. Recommendations for a Brief International Cognitive Assessment for Multiple Scle-rosis (Bicams). *Mult. Scler.* **2012**, *18*, 891–898. [CrossRef]
126. Bever, C.T.; Grattan, L.; Panitch, H.S.; Johnson, K.P. The Brief Repeatable Battery of Neuropsychological Tests for Mul-tiple Sclerosis: A Preliminary Serial Study. *Mult. Scler. J.* **1995**, *1*, 165–169. [CrossRef] [PubMed]
127. Benedict, R.H.; Fischer, J.S.; Archibald, C.J.; Arnett, P.A.; Beatty, W.W.; Bobholz, J.; Chelune, G.J.; Fisk, J.D.; Langdon, D.; Caruso, L.; et al. Minimal Neuropsychological Assessment of MS Patients: A Consensus Approach. *Clin. Neuropsychol.* **2002**, *16*, 381–397. [CrossRef] [PubMed]
128. Benedict, R.H.; Cookfair, D.; Gavett, R.; Gunther, M.; Munschauer, F.; Garg, N.; Weinstock-Guttman, B. Validity of the minimal assessment of cognitive function in multiple sclerosis (MACFIMS). *J. Int. Neuropsychol. Soc.* **2006**, *12*, 549–558. [CrossRef]
129. Bauer, R.M.; Iverson, G.; Cernich, A.N.; Binder, L.M.; Ruff, R.M.; Naugle, R.I. Computerized Neuropsychological Assess-ment Devices: Joint Position Paper of the American Academy of Clinical Neuropsychology and the National Academy of Neuropsychology. *Arch. Clin. Neuropsychol.* **2012**, *27*, 362–373. [CrossRef] [PubMed]
130. Wojcik, C.M.; Beier, M.; Costello, K.; DeLuca, J.; Feinstein, A.; Goverover, Y.; Gudesblatt, M.; Jaworski, M.; Kalb, E.; Kostich, L.; et al. Computerized Neuropsychological Assessment Devices in Multiple Sclerosis: A Systematic Review. *Mult. Scler.* **2019**, *25*, 1848–1869. [CrossRef] [PubMed]
131. Kalb, R.; Beier, M.; Benedict, R.H.; Charvet, L.; Costello, K.; Feinstein, A.; Gingold J.; Goverover, Y.; Halper, J.; Harris, C.; et al. Recommendations for Cognitive Screening and Man-agement in Multiple Sclerosis Care. *Mult. Scler.* **2018**, *24*, 1665–1680. [CrossRef]
132. Etemadi, Y. Dual task cost of cognition is related to fall risk in patients with multiple sclerosis: A prospective study. *Clin. Rehabil.* **2016**, *31*, 278–284. [CrossRef]
133. Woollacott, M.; Shumway-Cook, A. Attention and the control of posture and gait: A review of an emerging area of research. *Gait Posture* **2002**, *16*, 1–14. [CrossRef]
134. Fritz, N.E.; Kloos, A.D.; Kegelmeyer, D.A.; Kaur, P.; Nichols-Larsen, D.S. Supplementary motor area connectivity and dual-task walking variability in multiple sclerosis. *J. Neurol. Sci.* **2019**, *396*, 159–164. [CrossRef]
135. Krause, I.; Kern, S.; Horntrich, A.; Ziemssen, T. Employment status in multiple sclerosis: Impact of disease-specific and non-disease-specific factors. *Mult. Scler. J.* **2013**, *19*, 1792–1799. [CrossRef]
136. Beste, C.; Mückschel, M.; Paucke, M.; Ziemssen, T. Dual-Tasking in Multiple Sclerosis—Implications for a Cognitive Screening Instrument. *Front. Hum. Neurosci.* **2018**, *12*, 24. [CrossRef]
137. Hamilton, F.; Rochester, L.; Paul, L.; Rafferty, D.; O'Leary, C.P.; Evans, J.J. Walking and talking: An investigation of cognitive—motor dual tasking in multiple sclerosis. *Mult. Scler. J.* **2009**, *15*, 1215–1227. [CrossRef]
138. Butchard-MacDonald, E.; Paul, L.; Evans, J.J. Balancing the Demands of Two Tasks: An Investigation of Cognitive–Motor Dual-Tasking in Relapsing Remitting Multiple Sclerosis. *J. Int. Neuropsychol. Soc.* **2018**, *24*, 247–258. [CrossRef]
139. Monticone, M.; Ambrosini, E.; Fiorentini, R.; Rocca, B.; Liquori, V.; Pedrocchi, A.; Ferrante, S. Reliability of spatial–temporal gait parameters during dual-task interference in people with multiple sclerosis. A cross-sectional study. *Gait Posture* **2014**, *40*, 715–719. [CrossRef]
140. Holtzer, R.; Wang, C.; Verghese, J. Performance Variance on Walking While Talking Tasks: Theory, Findings, and Clini-cal Implications. *Age* **2014**, *36*, 373–381. [CrossRef]
141. Learmonth, Y.C.; Ensari, I.; Motl, R.W. Cognitive Motor Interference in Multiple Sclerosis: Insights from a Systematic Quantitative Review. *Arch. Phys. Med. Rehabil.* **2017**, *98*, 1229–1240. [CrossRef]
142. Downer, M.B.; Kirkland, M.C.; Wallack, E.M.; Ploughman, M. Walking impairs cognitive performance among people with multiple sclerosis but not controls. *Hum. Mov. Sci.* **2016**, *49*, 124–131. [CrossRef] [PubMed]
143. Wajda, D.A.; Sosnoff, J.J. Cognitive-Motor Interference in Multiple Sclerosis: A Systematic Review of Evi-dence, Correlates, and Consequences. *BioMed Res. Int.* **2015**, *2015*, 720856. [CrossRef] [PubMed]
144. Holtzer, R.; Mahoney, J.; Verghese, J. Intraindividual Variability in Executive Functions but Not Speed of Processing or Conflict Resolution Predicts Performance Differences in Gait Speed in Older Adults. *J. Gerontol. Ser. A Biol. Sci. Med. Sci.* **2014**, *69*, 980–986. [CrossRef]
145. Welford, A. The "Psychological Refractory Period" and the Timing of High Speed Performance: A Review and a Theory. *Br. J. Psychol. Gen. Sect.* **2011**, *43*, 2–19. [CrossRef]
146. Pashler, H. Dual-task interference in simple tasks: Data and theory. *Psychol. Bull.* **1994**, *116*, 220–244. [CrossRef]
147. Böttrich, N.; Mückschel, M.; Dillenseger, A.; Lange, C.; Kern, R.; Ziemssen, T.; Beste, C. On the Reliability of Examining Dual-Tasking Abilities Using a Novel E-Health Device—A Proof of Concept Study in Multiple Sclerosis. *J. Clin. Med.* **2020**, *9*, 3425. [CrossRef] [PubMed]
148. Sim, I. Mobile Devices and Health. *N. Engl. J. Med* **2019**, *381*, 956–968. [CrossRef] [PubMed]

149. Maillart, E.; Labauge, P.; Cohen, M.; Maarouf, A.; Vukusic, S.; Donzé, C.; Gallien, P.; De Sèze, J.; Bourre, B.; Moreau, T.; et al. MSCopilot, a new multiple sclerosis self-assessment digital solution: Results of a comparative study versus standard tests. *Eur. J. Neurol.* **2020**, *27*, 429–436. [CrossRef]
150. Montalban, X.; Graves, J.; Midaglia, L.; Mulero, P.; Julian, L.; Baker, M.; Schadrack, J.; Gossens, C.; Ganzetti, M.; Scotland, A.; et al. A Smartphone Sensor-Based Digital Outcome Assessment of Multiple Sclero-sis. *Mult. Scler. J.* **2021**, 13524585211028561. [CrossRef]
151. Healthcare, Orikami Personalized. Ms Sherpa. Available online: https://www.mssherpa.nl/en/ (accessed on 18 October 2021).
152. Biogen. Validation of Digicog and Konectom Tools to Support Digitalized Clinical Assessment in Multiple Sclerosis (Digi-toms). Available online: https://www.clinicaltrials.gov/ct2/show/NCT04756700?term=biogen&recrs=a&cond=Multiple+Sclerosis&draw=2 (accessed on 18 October 2021).
153. Medizinprodukte, Bundesinstitut für Arzneimittel und. Diga-Verzeichnis. Available online: https://diga.bfarm.de/de/verzeichnis (accessed on 20 October 2021).
154. Klose, K.; Kreimeier, S.; Tangermann, U.; Aumann, I.; Damm, K. RHO Group Patient- and person-reports on healthcare: Preferences, outcomes, experiences, and satisfaction—An essay. *Health Econ. Rev.* **2016**, *6*, 18. [CrossRef] [PubMed]
155. Heesen, C.; Bohm, J.; Reich, C.; Kasper, J.; Goebel, M.; Gold, S.M. Patient Perception of Bodily Functions in Multiple Scle-rosis: Gait and Visual Function Are the Most Valuable. *Mult. Scler.* **2008**, *14*, 988–991. [CrossRef] [PubMed]
156. D'Amico, E.; Haase, R.; Ziemssen, T. Review: Patient-reported outcomes in multiple sclerosis care. *Mult. Scler. Relat. Disord.* **2019**, *33*, 61–66. [CrossRef]
157. Wiklund, I. Assessment of patient-reported outcomes in clinical trials: The example of health-related quality of life. *Fundam. Clin. Pharmacol.* **2004**, *18*, 351–363. [CrossRef] [PubMed]
158. Van Munster, C.E.; Uitdehaag, B.M. Outcome Measures in Clinical Trials for Multiple Sclerosis. *CNS Drugs* **2017**, *31*, 217–236. [CrossRef]
159. Ziemssen, T.; Hillert, J.; Butzkueven, H. The Importance of Collecting Structured Clinical Information on Multiple Scle-rosis. *BMC Med.* **2016**, *14*, 81. [CrossRef]
160. Kern, R.; Haase, R.; Eisele, J.C.; Thomas, K.; Ziemssen, T. Designing an Electronic Patient Management System for Multi-ple Sclerosis: Building a Next Generation Multiple Sclerosis Documentation System. *Interact. J. Med. Res.* **2016**, *5*, e4549. [CrossRef]
161. Ho, B.; Houck, J.R.; Flemister, A.S.; Ketz, J.; Oh, I.; DiGiovanni, B.F.; Baumhauer, J.F. Preoperative PROMIS Scores Predict Postoperative Success in Foot and Ankle Patients. *Foot Ankle Int.* **2016**, *37*, 911–918. [CrossRef] [PubMed]
162. Gausden, E.B.; Levack, A.; Nwachukwu, B.U.; Sin, D.; Wellman, D.S.; Lorich, D.G. Computerized Adaptive Testing for Patient Reported Outcomes in Ankle Fracture Surgery. *Foot Ankle Int.* **2018**, *39*, 1192–1198. [CrossRef] [PubMed]
163. Hung, M.; Hon, S.D.; Cheng, C.; Franklin, J.D.; Aoki, S.K.; Anderson, M.B.; Kapron, A.L.; Peters, C.L.; Pelt, C.E. Psychometric Evaluation of the Lower Extremity Computerized Adaptive Test, the Modified Harris Hip Score, and the Hip Outcome Score. *Orthop. J. Sports Med.* **2014**, *2*, 2325967114562191. [CrossRef]
164. Haase, R.; Scholz, M.; Dillenseger, A.; Kern, R.; Akgün, K.; Ziemssen, T. Improving multiple sclerosis management and collecting safety information in the real world: The MSDS3D software approach. *Expert Opin. Drug Saf.* **2018**, *17*, 369–378. [CrossRef]
165. Ziemssen, T.; Kern, R.; Voigt, I.; Haase, R. Data Collection in Multiple Sclerosis: The MSDS Approach. *Front. Neurol.* **2020**, *11*, 445. [CrossRef]
166. Wattjes, M.P.; Rovira, À.; Miller, D.; Yousry, T.A.; Sormani, M.P.; de Stefano, M.P.; Tintoré, M.; Auger, C.; Tur, C.; Filippi, M.; et al. Evidence-Based Guidelines: Magnims Consensus Guidelines on the Use of Mri in Multiple Sclerosis–Establishing Disease Prognosis and Monitoring Patients. *Nat. Rev. Neurol.* **2015**, *11*, 597–606.
167. Manjón, J.V.; Coupé, P. volBrain: An Online MRI Brain Volumetry System. *Front. Aging Neurosci.* **2016**, *10*, 30. [CrossRef]
168. Rovira, À.; on behalf of the MAGNIMS study group; Wattjes, M.P.; Tintoré, M.; Tur, C.; Yousry, T.A.; Sormani, M.P.; De Stefano, N.; Filippi, M.; Auger, C.; et al. MAGNIMS consensus guidelines on the use of MRI in multiple sclerosis—clinical implementation in the diagnostic process. *Nat. Rev. Neurol.* **2015**, *11*, 471–482. [CrossRef]
169. Schwab, P.; Karlen, W. A Deep Learning Approach to Diagnosing Multiple Sclerosis from Smartphone Data. *IEEE J. Biomed. Health Inform.* **2021**, *25*, 1284–1291. [CrossRef]
170. Zhao, Y.; Wang, T.; Bove, R.; Cree, B.; Henry, R.; Lokhande, H.; Polgar-Turcsanyi, M.; Anderson, M.; Bakshi, R.; Weiner, H.L.; et al. Ensemble learning predicts multiple sclerosis disease course in the SUMMIT study. *NPJ Digit. Med.* **2020**, *3*, 135. [CrossRef] [PubMed]
171. Corral-Acero, J.; Margara, F.; Marciniak, M.; Rodero, C.; Loncaric, F.; Feng, Y.; Gilbert, A.; Fernandes, J.F.; Bukhari, H.A.; Wajdan, A.; et al. The 'Digital Twin' to Enable the Vision of Precision Cardiology. *Eur. Heart J.* **2020**, *41*, 4556–4564. [CrossRef] [PubMed]
172. Voigt, I.; Inojosa, H.; Dillenseger, A.; Haase, R.; Akgün, K.; Ziemssen, T. Digital Twins for Multiple Sclerosis. *Front. Immunol.* **2021**, *12*, 669811. [CrossRef] [PubMed]

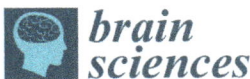

Article

The Potential Impact of Digital Biomarkers in Multiple Sclerosis in the Netherlands: An Early Health Technology Assessment of MS Sherpa

Sonja Cloosterman [1,*], Inez Wijnands [1], Simone Huygens [2], Valérie Wester [2,3], Ka-Hoo Lam [4], Eva Strijbis [4], Bram den Teuling [1] and Matthijs Versteegh [2]

1. Orikami Digital Health Products, Ridderstraat 29, 6511 TM Nijmegen, The Netherlands; inez@orikami.nl (I.W.); bram@orikami.nl (B.d.T.)
2. Institute for Medical Technology Assessment (iMTA), Erasmus University of Rotterdam, Burgemeester Oudlaan 50, 3062 PA Rotterdam, The Netherlands; huygens@imta.eur.nl (S.H.); wester@eshpm.eur.nl (V.W); versteegh@imta.eur.nl (M.V.)
3. Erasmus School for Health Policy & Management, Erasmus University of Rotterdam, Burgemeester Oudlaan 50, 3062 PA Rotterdam, The Netherlands
4. Department of Neurology, MS Center Amsterdam, Amsterdam University Medical Centers, Location VUmc, De Boelelaan, 1117 HV Amsterdam, The Netherlands; k.lam1@amsterdamumc.nl (K.-H.L.); e.strijbis@amsterdamumc.nl (E.S.)
* Correspondence: sonja@orikami.nl; Tel.: +31-24-3010100

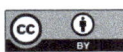

Citation: Cloosterman, S.; Wijnands, I.; Huygens, S.; Wester, V.; Lam, K.-H.; Strijbis, E.; den Teuling, B.; Versteegh, M. The Potential Impact of Digital Biomarkers in Multiple Sclerosis in the Netherlands: An Early Health Technology Assessment of MS Sherpa. *Brain Sci.* **2021**, *11*, 1305. https://doi.org/10.3390/brainsci11101305

Academic Editors: Tjalf Ziemssen, Rocco Haase and Moussa Antoine Chalah

Received: 30 July 2021
Accepted: 26 September 2021
Published: 30 September 2021

Publisher's Note: MDPI stays neutral with regard to jurisdictional claims in published maps and institutional affiliations.

Copyright: © 2021 by the authors. Licensee MDPI, Basel, Switzerland. This article is an open access article distributed under the terms and conditions of the Creative Commons Attribution (CC BY) license (https://creativecommons.org/licenses/by/4.0/).

Abstract: (1) *Background*: Monitoring of Multiple Sclerosis (MS) with eHealth interventions or digital biomarkers provides added value to the current care path. Evidence in the literature is currently scarce. MS sherpa is an eHealth intervention with digital biomarkers, aimed at monitoring symptom progression and disease activity. To show the added value of digital biomarker-based eHealth interventions to the MS care path, an early Health Technology Assessment (eHTA) was performed, with MS sherpa as an example, to assess the potential impact on treatment switches. (2) *Methods*: The eHTA was performed according to the Dutch guidelines for health economic evaluations. A decision analytic MS model was used to estimate the costs and benefits of MS standard care with and without use of MS sherpa, expressed in incremental cost-effectiveness ratios (ICERs) from both societal and health care perspectives. The efficacy of MS sherpa on early detection of active disease and the initiation of a treatment switch were modeled for a range of assumed efficacy (5%, 10%, 15%, 20%). (3) *Results*: From a societal perspective, for the efficacy of 15% or 20%, MS sherpa became dominant, which means cost-saving compared to the standard of care. MS sherpa is cost-effective in the 5% and 10% scenarios (ICERs EUR 14,535 and EUR 4069, respectively). From the health care perspective all scenarios were cost-effective. Sensitivity analysis showed that increasing the efficacy of MS sherpa in detecting active disease early leading to treatment switches be the most impactful factor in the MS model. (4) *Conclusions*: The results indicate the potential of eHealth interventions to be cost-effective or even cost-saving in the MS care path. As such, digital biomarker-based eHealth interventions, like MS sherpa, are promising cost-effective solutions in optimizing MS disease management for people with MS, by detecting active disease early and helping neurologists in decisions on treatment switch.

Keywords: digital biomarkers; eHealth; digital health; AI; (early) Health Technology Assessment; multiple sclerosis; home monitoring; MS disease activity; MS disease progression; early detection; disease modelling; digital therapeutics

1. Introduction

eHealth interventions play a growing role in shaping the future healthcare system. The integration of eHealth interventions can enhance the efficiency and quality of patient management and optimize the course of treatment for chronically ill patients [1] by alleviating pressure on health care systems when productivity of labor is restricted [2]. In this paper, we investigate the benefits of adding a digital biomarker–based eHealth intervention to the standard of care of multiple sclerosis (MS).

MS is the most prevalent chronic neurological disorder among young adults [3]. The severity and nature of symptoms and disability in MS depend on the location and extent of inflammatory demyelination and axonal loss in the central nervous system due to inflammation. Therefore, MS shows a highly individualized trajectory and large day-to-day variation [4]. Fatigue, decline in cognitive functions, impaired vision, motor and sensory deficits are the most common symptoms in persons with MS (pwMS) [4,5]. There is no cure for MS, but treatment is aimed at reducing neuroinflammation (and indirectly neurodegeneration) to prevent relapses and slow down disability progression. These disease modifying therapies (DMTs) are costly and the choice is plentiful. Current consensus recommends no evidence of disease activity (NEDA) as the treatment goal [6,7].

In the Netherlands, pwMS are under treatment by a neurologist, preferably complemented by a specialized MS nurse [8,9]. They usually have around one or two visits a year. Using MRI of the brain (and if necessary, the spinal cord), the presence of inflammatory disease activity is assessed, generally presenting as new or enlarged T2 lesions. The functioning of pwMS may be monitored by a variety of patient-reported (PRO) or performance-based outcome measures, such as test batteries to assess cognitive function and walking tests for ambulatory function for instance. The Expanded Disability Status Scale (EDSS) is the standard measure for how a person is affected by their MS. This combination of assessments of functioning, degree of disability and treatment effects, enable the determination of whether a pwMS is experiencing disease progression, a relapse or whether NEDA is maintained [6,7].

Typically, pwMS only remember certain days or periods that stand out, and the time in between is not recalled and the physician will not hear all information [10]. eHealth interventions and specifically those with objective measures, like digital biomarkers, in addition to PROs, can help monitor disease and symptom progression, and potentially disease activity [1,10].

Especially for persons with relapse-remitting MS, there are several treatment options and pwMS react differently to the different available drugs [6]. It is often a trade-off between the effectiveness of the drug and occurrence and severity of side effects, i.e., possibly overtreating or undertreating the patient. It is currently not possible to determine which treatment is the most appropriate for an individual pwMS. The disease course is highly heterogeneous and although we are able to assess the effectivity of a treatment according to NEDA [6], it is not yet possible to predict if and when pwMS will reach severe disability or secondary-progressive MS right at the moment after diagnosis. Additionally, subtle changes in functioning or symptoms and day-to-day variation are difficult to capture with the low frequent hospital visits that are currently the standard of care [6,7].

Because eHealth interventions can be applied in the home situation and this enables monitoring on a more frequent basis, the monitoring extends to the period between consultations and shows the individual course of symptoms. Therefore, the results can be used to detect disease activity early and find the optimal disease management for the individual patient.

1.1. eHealth Interventions in MS

Several eHealth interventions are currently developed and under investigation in MS [1]. These interventions support different aspects of the MS care path, like social, single use case, integrated and complex support, but with the common intention to improve the care path of pwMS leading to better outcomes. Social eHealth interventions (e.g., My Support Plus [11–13]) are usually meant for pwMS to get connected to other pwMS, to obtain information or to get in contact with their neurologist. Single use case solutions focus more on the disease and usually contain one or more measurement methods, which may be digital biomarkers or biomarker components. Scholz et al. [1] distinguish these interventions from the more integrated eHealth interventions, such as Floodlight (Genentech,

Inc., Basel, Switzerland), MSCopilot (Ad Scientiam, Paris, France), MSPT (Cleveland Clinic Foundation & Biogen, Cleveland, OH, USA), etc. These digital biomarker–based eHealth interventions aim at enhancing MS monitoring and to better detect disease activity and progression so that better therapy can be applied.

Another example of an integrated eHealth intervention containing digital biomarkers for MS, is MS sherpa (Orikami Digital Health Products, Nijmegen, The Netherlands). MS sherpa is a CE-certified eHealth intervention (medical device) intended to support the monitoring of persons with MS with the help of digital biomarkers, in order to give pwMS and their health care professionals personalized insight into the presence and progress of MS-related symptoms. The digital biomarkers are embedded in a smartphone application for pwMS and consist of tests that pwMS can perform regularly. The results are directly available for their neurologist via a web-based portal for caregivers, integrating MS sherpa into the MS care path. The Orikami Digital Biomarker platform on which the app and portal are built consists of several components to combine the sensors of the smartphone and user input with proprietary algorithms into digital biomarkers and of supporting modules such as a customer support, subscription and consent management and modules for regulatory compliance and authentication. A graphical presentation of MS sherpa concept is given in Figure 1.

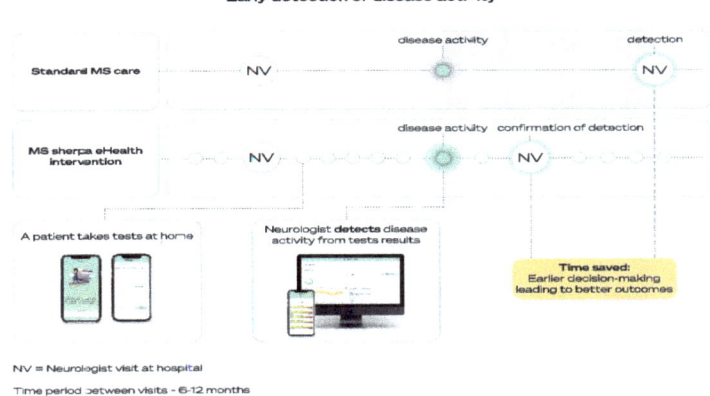

Figure 1. Graphical representation of the MS sherpa concept.

The current MS sherpa digital biomarkers are validated to reliably measure cognitive processing speed and walking function [14–16]. These digital biomarkers represent relevant MS symptoms that are selected based on their relevance in MS and relation with disease activity and relapses. eHealth interventions require the willingness of the users to adhere to the intervention and to include the insights in disease management, therefore it is important to tailor the designs of eHealth interventions to the needs of the different users and to involve them in the development [17–19]. During the development of MS sherpa, input of different users, both pwMS and neurologists, were included via co-creation. Additionally, the designs have been tested via usability testing methods [18]. Adherence to eHealth interventions with digital biomarkers show promising results. MS Sherpa has shown in a one-month study that there was >90% adherence to the scheduled tasks [20]. This is in line with high adherence figures of other digital biomarker–based e-health interventions like Floodlight, which shows 70% adherence in a 24-week study [21], and an acceptability study with MSCopilot that shows that 85% of questioned pwMS are willing to use the intervention more than once a month and that 68% prefer the digital biomarkers over the MSFC [22], supporting the believe that adoption of and adherence to such interventions can be reasonably expected.

As eHealth interventions, and digital biomarkers more specifically, are a very nascent field, there are currently no RCTs that show their impact to personalized treatment. However, the potential impact of digital biomarker–based integrated eHealth interventions like MS sherpa in the MS care path is more and more being investigated in clinical trials. MS sherpa has multiple clinical trials in preparation or under investigation.

The Dutch Ministry of Health, Welfare and Sport and the iMTA institute aimed to show the potential impact of AI in healthcare, and MS sherpa was selected as a suitable eHealth intervention for Health Technology Assessment by both organizations, because of its already accumulated evidence and the availability of a model for MS to map the impact of an intervention on the care path.

1.2. (Early) Health Technology Assessment ((e)HTA)

To estimate the impact of health technologies, in terms of costs and benefits that fall upon the health care system and wider society, Health Technology Assessments (HTA) are conducted [23]. Cost-effectiveness analysis (CEA) is a central component of HTA. When a CEA is conducted before all effectiveness estimates have been collected in studies, the analysis is referred to as 'early HTA'.

The result of an early HTA (eHTA) is an estimate of incremental costs and benefits with and without a new technology. The ratio between these increments gives the incremental cost-effectiveness ratio (ICER), which is compared with some reference value reflecting if the technology should be adopted in the basic benefit package [23]. Benefits are expressed in quality adjusted life years (QALYs). In the Netherlands, the National Health Care Institute determines the reference value for cost-effectiveness, based on the disease burden of the health care problem under study [24]. For MS, this value is set at EUR 50,000 per QALY [25].

In this article, we describe an eHTA analysis for the potential impact of MS sherpa, both from the societal and health care perspective using a recently published decision analytic model for MS treatments [25]. The analysis focused on the impact of MS sherpa on treatment decisions, and more specifically on switches of MS medication based on disease insights achieved with MS sherpa. The impact of digital biomarkers on treatment decisions is one of the important concepts to be tested for the MS field.

2. Materials and Methods

2.1. Early Health Technology Assesment (HTA), Concept and Analyses

This eHTA was performed according to the Dutch guidelines for economic evaluations [26]. The MS model was used to estimate the costs and benefits of MS standard care with and without the use of MS sherpa and expressed in an ICER.

$$\text{ICER} = (\text{costs new intervention} - \text{costs standard care})/(\text{health gains new intervention} - \text{health gains standard care}) = \text{€ per QALY}$$

This ICER is compared to the reference value for the maximum costs that the society is willing to pay for 1 additional QALY within MS in the Netherlands [25].

These calculations were performed from both a societal and a health care perspective. In a societal perspective, all relevant costs and benefits related to MS are included in the cost-effectiveness analysis (CEA), regardless of who bears the costs or enjoys the benefits. The costs of an intervention are therefore not limited to costs within health care, but costs outside health care are also included in the CEA. Costs outside of health care include the costs of informal caregivers and reduced productivity in paid and unpaid work due to health problems. This is the standard perspective as prescribed by the National Health Care Institute [26]. In a health care perspective, costs outside healthcare (i.e., costs of informal care and productivity losses) are not included.

2.2. MS Model and Clinical, Costs and Quality of Life Input

The CEA was performed using the MS model developed by Huygens and Versteegh [25]. This model describes the lifetime of a pwMS based on MS relapses (Annual Relapse Rate (ARR)) and MS disease progression (EDSS). The rate of progression and relapses are influenced by the efficacy of the MS medication. Treatment switching was allowed for up to five lines of treatment. Besides disease progression and relapse, adverse events of MS medication, the option of discontinuing MS medication, health-related quality of life (HRQoL) and mortality rate were included in the model. All costs related to the treatment of MS (MS medication, other health care costs, informal care, productivity loss) were included in the model. During the development of this model, neurologists were involved to confirm clinical assumptions and decisions in this model. A graphical representation of the model is given in Figure 2.

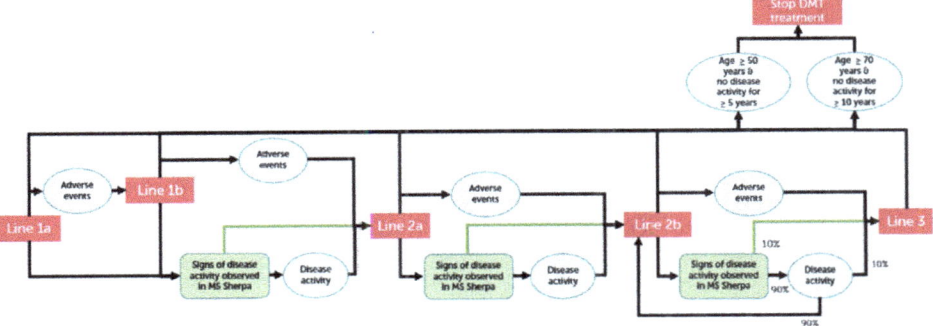

Figure 2. Schematic representation of the MS model.

The output of the MS model are the lifetime costs and subsequent the lifetime clinical MS outcomes ('benefits') represented as EDSS and ARR for pwMS, both for MS care with and without MS sherpa. These modeled costs and benefits are used for the CEA and ICER calculations.

To assess uncertainty of the model and tested intervention, univariate sensitivity analyses were performed, in which the value of one key parameter at a time is changed into a higher and lower value than assumed in the base-case analysis. The results of this analysis, which will be presented in a tornado diagram, give insight in which parameters have the most impact on the cost-effectiveness of MS sherpa. This might serve as input for future improvements of MS sherpa or for other eHealth interventions that share the same or equivalent components or digital biomarkers. The cost-effectiveness in this analysis is presented as the net health benefit, calculated with the following formula:

Net Health Benefit = Total QALYs − (total costs/Cost-effectiveness threshold (€50,000/QALY))

2.3. MS Sherpa and Potential Effects

MS sherpa is a CE Class I Medical Device under MDD consisting of a smartphone application for pwMS and a web-based portal for caregivers. For this eHTA, MS sherpa version 1.12 was used. The MS sherpa 1.12 app for pwMS contains two digital biomarkers: one as an indicator for cognitive processing speed, an adaptation of the Symbol Digit Modalities Test (SDMT); and one for walking speed, an adaptation of the two-minute walking test (2MWT). Both are smartphone adaptations of standardized tests that assess important symptoms of MS and are suitable for frequent self-administration. The SDMT was chosen because of its sensitivity to changes in mental status during clinical relapses, and during isolated cognitive relapses without changes on EDSS [27–29]. The 2MWT was chosen because of its strong correlation with EDSS [30]. Both digital biomarkers showed robust concurrent validity and test–retest reliability [14–16], and for the SDMT also the construct validity was shown by distinguishing pwMS from healthy controls [15]. As such, these digital biomarkers are reliable tools for monitoring relevant MS symptoms, enabling pwMS to monitor their symptoms objectively and more frequently in their home situation.

In addition to the objective measurements, pwMS can answer a daily questionnaire in MS sherpa, containing several Likert-scale questions on fatigue, pain, stress, memory, concentration and the impact of MS on the day. PwMS can also leave notes in the app on events and symptoms as deemed relevant by the patients. The clinician portal contains a dashboard for caregivers that shows their pwMS' results from the MS sherpa app. They can see the SDMT and 2MWT scores as individual data points, but also informative curves over time using multiple measurements to model individualized performance trajectories. This is giving more detailed insights in MS symptom changes over time than during clinical visits. Recent results [31] showed that more frequent monitoring in combination with smart algorithms significantly reduces signal-to-noise ratio of the measurements and the ability to follow individualized trajectories (patent pending: N2028255). For the MS field these innovations make it possible to detect more subtle changes with the potential to detect disease progression and relapses earlier. Moreover, the answers to the questionnaire and the notes that pwMS write can also be viewed, giving context to the measurements. This can improve the shared decision-making process between the neurologist and pwMS. The information from MS sherpa can help tailor the care path to the individual pwMS, resulting in earlier treatment switches to other, more effective treatment.

The MS sherpa solution and its effect on treatment decisions was operationalized in the MS model as shown in Figure 2: with the use and insights of MS sherpa, pwMS and neurologists will have insight into active disease sooner and, as a consequence, will switch to the next treatment line earlier than without MS sherpa. Second line treatments are generally considered to be more effective, but also more expensive treatments. Timely switches to these treatments could prevent disease progression and relapses, which will subsequently lead to health and quality of life benefits and potential cost savings. It is assumed that all pwMS with an EDSS below 7 will use the MS sherpa app, as pwMS with an EDSS of 7 and higher are wheelchair-dependent and not able to use the app in the intended way [32]. As the effect of MS sherpa on treatment switches is not yet known and is dependent of the efficacy in the detection of disease activity, different assumptions of the efficacy of MS sherpa were tested in the eHTA. MS sherpa's efficacy is defined as the proportion of pwMS who are detected early by MS sherpa to have disease progression or relapse that will switch to a next line treatment prior to that disease progression or relapse occurring. Four scenarios for MS sherpa's efficacy in detecting disease activity earlier than standard care were chosen: 5, 10, 15 and 20 percent. As the effect size of MS sherpa is not yet known, and effects of comparable eHealth interventions are also not available, the effect sizes were discussed with neurologists who are involved in the ongoing clinical studies with MS sherpa. They are familiar with the insights provided by MS sherpa and the role of the digital biomarkers in MS sherpa, which are smartphone adaptations of commonly used clinical outcome measures (i.e., SDMT and 2MWT). They indicated that it is currently difficult to estimate the efficacy of MS sherpa for early detection of disease activity, but they confirmed that the chosen range seems plausible given the current development stage of MS sherpa.

The cost of MS sherpa is currently estimated to be EUR 480 per patient per year.

3. Results

3.1. Clinical Effects (Benefits) of MS Sherpa (Modeled)

Based on the MS model, the clinical outcomes for MS care both with and without MS sherpa were modeled. Figures 3 and 4 demonstrate the reduction in disease progression and relapse rates of MS sherpa use, under the assumption of 5% efficacy. Figure 3 shows that, under this assumption, the use of MS sherpa slows down disease progression: a larger proportion of pwMS have mild disability due to MS (EDSS 0–3) for a longer period of time, a smaller proportion of pwMS develop severe disability (EDSS 7–9), and severe disability develops later than without the use of MS sherpa. For example, 10 years after the diagnosis of MS, the proportion of pwMS who still have mild disability due to MS is higher with use of MS sherpa (63.5%) compared to without (51.7%). The number of pwMS who had progressed to moderate disability 10 years after MS diagnosis is lower with the use of MS sherpa (22.8%) than without the use of MS sherpa (23.4%). The same is true for the percentage of pwMS with severe disability: 13.0% with MS sherpa compared to 14.2%, without MS sherpa.

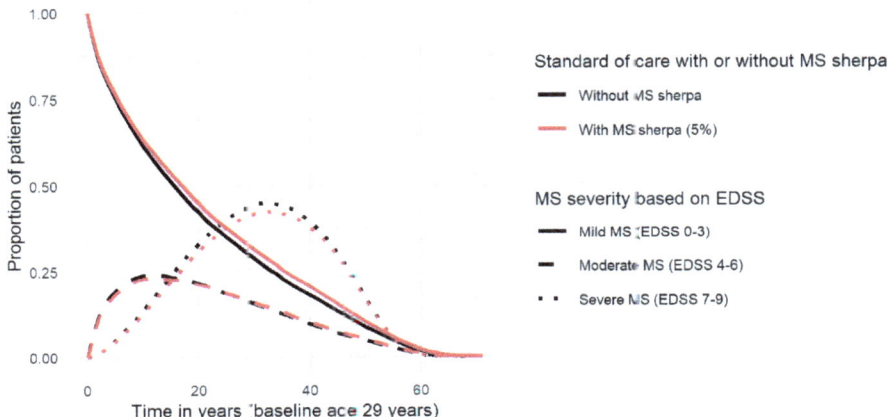

Figure 3. Progression in MS severity over time measured with EDSS over time, with and without use of MS Sherpa.

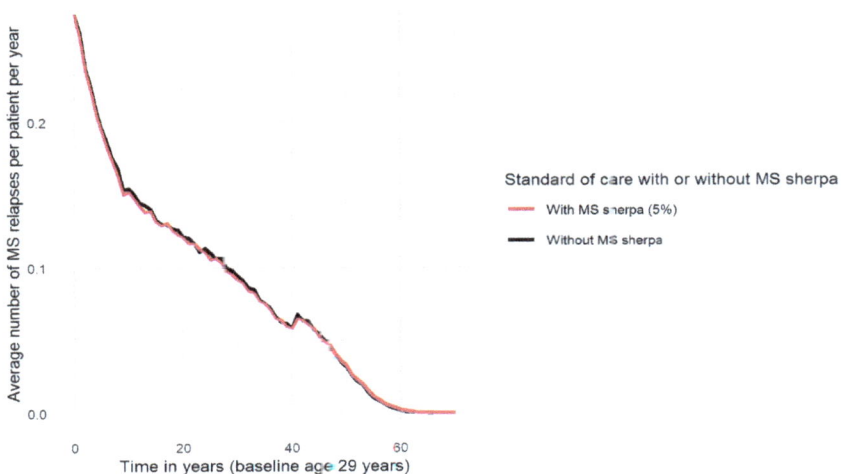

Figure 4. Average number of MS relapses per patient per year over time, with and without use of MS sherpa. The hiccup at t = 41 can be explained by the rule in the MS model (see Figure 2) that pwMS will discontinue DMTs at age 70 in the absence of disease activity ≥10 years and the risk of relapses is not reduced by the DMT anymore.

In addition, Figure 4 shows that the ARR is slightly lower among users of MS sherpa. Ten years after the diagnosis of MS, the probability of an MS relapse without the use of MS sherpa is 15.7% compared to 15.3% with the use of MS sherpa.

3.2. Cost-Effectiveness of MS Sherpa, Societal Perspective

The cost-effectiveness results for MS sherpa compared to standard of care without MS sherpa for each of the MS sherpa efficacy scenarios from a societal perspective are shown in Table 1. When assuming 5% and 10% efficacy of MS sherpa, QALYS were gained (0.43 and 0.87, respectively), but this was associated with higher costs. Compared to the reference value of EUR 50,000 per QALY, MS sherpa is cost-effective in these scenarios. In the scenarios where the assumed effect of MS sherpa was 15% or 20%, MS sherpa became dominant, which means costs are saved while pwMS yielded 1.33 or 1.78 additional QALYs.

Table 1. Cost-effectiveness results of MS sherpa versus standard care from a societal perspective.

Scenario	Total		Difference between Standard Care and MS Sherpa		
	Costs	QALYs	Costs	QALYs	ICER
MS standard Care	€614,732	20.51			
MS sherpa 5%	€620,990	20.94	€6258	0.43	€14,535
MS sherpa 10%	€618,288	21.38	€3556	0.87	€4069
MS sherpa 15%	€614,538	21.84	€−194	1.33	D
MS sherpa 20%	€611,073	22.29	€−3659	1.78	D

QALY = Quality Adjusted Life Year. D = Dominant (lower costs and more benefits).

3.3. Cost-Effectiveness of MS Sherpa, Health Care Perspective

Table 2 presents the cost-effectiveness results from a health care perspective (i.e., without costs of informal care and productivity loss). The results show that total costs are lower, but that the difference in costs between standard of care with and without MS sherpa is larger because some of the benefits of using MS sherpa, such as reducing informal care and productivity loss due to less disease progression and relapses, are no longer included in the cost calculations. Nevertheless, the ICER is still below the reference value of EUR 50,000.

Table 2. Cost-effectiveness results of MS sherpa versus standard care from a health care perspective.

Scenario	Total		Difference between Standard Care and MS Sherpa		
	Costs	QALYs	Costs	QALYs	ICER
MS Standard Care	€540,345	20.51			
MS sherpa 5%	€539,528	20.94	€9183	0.43	€21,328
MS sherpa 10%	€539,803	21.38	€9458	0.87	€10,822
MS sherpa 15%	€539,101	21.84	€8756	1.33	€6574
MS sherpa 20%	€538,703	22.29	€8358	1.78	€4696

3.4. Sensitivity Analysis, Tornado Diagram

The results of the univariate sensitivity analyses are shown in Figure 5. The vertical line represents the net health benefit (this is the number of QALYs reduced with the total costs, in which the QALY has a value of EUR 50,000) in the base-case analysis (i.e., 5% efficacy of MS sherpa). The bars represent the impact of the different parameters on the cost-effectiveness results.

These results show that the assumed effect of MS sherpa has substantial impact on the net health benefit. The higher the efficacy of MS sherpa in detecting disease activity, the higher the effect on treatment switches and the higher the net health benefit. This means that it would be worthwhile to focus on further improving the efficacy of MS sherpa. In addition, the diagram shows that quality of life and health care costs of pwMS with mild MS (EDSS 0–3) have substantial impact on the net health benefit. This is not surprising as pwMS spend a large part of their life with mild MS, and this period is prolonged when using MS sherpa.

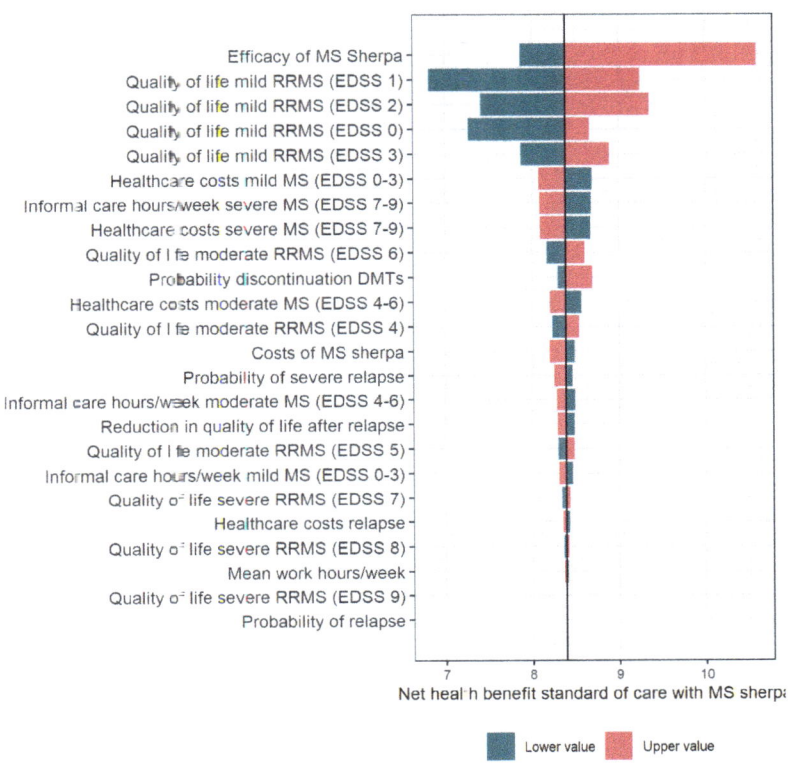

Figure 5. Tornado diagram with results of the univariate sensitivity analysis.

All other key parameters showed to have less influence on the outcomes of the model when assuming a 5% efficacy of MS sherpa. For instance, when the annual costs of MS sherpa per patient were increased to EUR 1000, even with 5% efficacy, it is still cost-effective.

4. Discussion

4.1. Principal Results and Implications for Clinical Practice and MS Society

MS sherpa is an eHealth intervention aimed at enabling (home) monitoring of pwMS with the help of digital biomarkers, in order to give pwMS and their caregivers individual insights into the presence and progress of MS-related symptoms and disease activity. In this research, we modeled how with the insights from digital biomarker interventions like MS sherpa (efficacy), neurologists together with pwMS have the potential to decide earlier to switch to more effective MS medication, with the intention to prevent or slow down disability worsening and disease progression. The recent Huygens and Versteegh MS model [25] that simulates the disease progress over the lifetime of a patient was used to show whether using MS sherpa to support treatment decisions would be cost-effective. The eHTA showed that under all efficacy assumptions MS sherpa is cost-effective from both a societal and health care perspective in the MS care path. Moreover, in the societal perspective MS sherpa can become dominant and cost saving when the efficacy of detecting disease activity early is 15% or higher and higher proportions of pwMS switch medication.

The eHTA as performed in this research gives valuable insight into the potential cost and benefits of digital biomarkers in MS and supports the use of new solutions like MS sherpa by neurologists to detect early symptom progression and disease activity of pwMS. While the effect of a digital biomarker-based eHealth intervention on clinical outcome can seem moderate from this analysis, it should be placed in the right context. First of all, the effect on clinical outcomes can be strong for an individual pwMS where preventing one relapse with the associated brain damage can mean the difference between years with or without work or physical dysfunction on the long term. Second, cost-effectiveness of current DMTs has long been debated and health gains come at a high costs. For example, it was shown that cost-effectiveness of MS DMTs in the US far exceeded USD 800,000/QALY [33]. The results of the current analysis on an ICER of EUR 14,535/QALY gives another dimension to more appropriate investment and reimbursement decisions. At this moment, the literature is lacking a strong benchmark of cost-effectiveness of monitoring solutions in MS. It would be relevant for future research to show how self-monitoring with digital biomarker–based eHealth interventions benchmarks with other monitoring solutions like MRI, test batteries administered by a clinician and recent blood-based biomarkers.

The presented eHTA was performed both from a societal and health care perspective. As MS usually onsets in early adult life, when persons are still active and taking part in the working life, developing MS will affect not only health care costs but especially also the non-health care costs like employability. Therefore, we feel that the presented eHTA with a societal perspective is the most comprehensive. The health care perspective is of importance for hospitals or health insurance companies in adopting digital biomarker–based eHealth interventions and gives them more insights where costs and benefits are falling within the health care setting. Reimbursement decisions based on health care perspective alone might not be appropriate for eHealth interventions; therefore, this confirms that it is advisable to include the societal perspective in reimbursement models for such interventions.

4.2. Relation to Previous Work

The efficacy of MS sherpa in detecting disease activity and enable optimal disease management earlier compared to standard care, is now varied between 5% and 20%. Digital biomarker–based eHealth interventions for monitoring MS, like MS sherpa, are relatively new in the MS field. The current literature gives us no guidance in the potential clinical impact of these solutions. A benchmark for integrated eHealth interventions and digital biomarkers on MS outcomes is not (yet) available. As explained, the impact of MS sherpa insights on treatment decisions are thought to achieve at least the assumed efficacy of 5%, based on the described evidence and setting. Additionally, a minimum efficacy of 5% as a starting point seems plausible according to interviewed neurologists involved in testing the MS Sherpa solution.

The MS model was used to calculate the costs and clinical benefits, and was used in the eHTA. While all models require assumptions, this model is shown to be a good predictor for short-term switch behavior when validated against external data [25]. Moreover, this is the first model that takes into account subsequent medication steps, as a complete treatment sequence cost-utility model for MS. As the presented concept of MS sherpa is mainly focused on treatment decisions, this MS model seems currently the best basis to test the potential effects of an eHealth intervention like MS sherpa. As such, we believe that the chosen model is both fit for purpose and state-of-the-art in showing impact by treatment decisions on switching medication.

4.3. Considerations and Limitations

Next to the abovementioned assumptions in the model, some aspects can still be considered. Firstly, in the effectiveness of MS sherpa on treatment switches, the entire MS population with an EDSS below 7 is included. The adoption rate of an eHealth intervention might be a smaller proportion of this population. Moreover, subgroups may be identified in which a higher or lower effect is to be expected; for instance, neurologists may be able to identify pwMS for whom a higher gain from using MS sherpa is expected.

Secondly, the MS model is based on the MS care path in the Netherlands and the CEA is based on guidelines from the National Health Care Institute [26], which may not be applicable in other countries. Naturally, changes in the MS field in the future (e.g., new treatment options become available) can also influence the underlying assumptions in the MS model.

Besides the efficacy of MS sherpa in the MS care path, adherence to and acceptance of these kind of interventions is also important. Using eHealth interventions during a lifetime (or until EDSS is 7 or higher as modeled) might be challenging, which might reduce its impact. Usually, pwMS show their first symptoms at the age of 20 to 40 years; consequently, they live with this chronic disease for several decades, which is why these patients may be important early adopters of emerging eHealth trends [1,34]. A part of the pwMS indicated that using eHealth tools confront them with their disease. On the other hand, pwMS that start using MS sherpa showed high adherence to scheduled tests and valued the insights [20].

Next to the adherence of pwMS to the eHealth intervention, the adoption of MS sherpa by neurologists and its use in treatment decisions is an important factor [20]. The current model assumes that the efficacy of MS sherpa is directly related to treatment switch. It is expected that neurologists perform additional clinical assessments before switching treatment. Growing evidence, improved user experience, training of clinicians and algorithm improvements will help tackle this challenge.

4.4. Further Research

The key assumption that should be further investigated is the efficacy of the MS sherpa intervention in detecting disease activity early. Especially a clinical study that determines the sensitivity and specificity of the intervention in early detection of disease activity compared to standard care would be valuable. A multi-center RCT with MS sherpa as integrated eHealth intervention is scheduled presently.

In the meantime, the eHTA results show that by increasing the effect of MS sherpa on treatment switches, more benefits could be gained and as such the ICER becomes more favorable for MS sherpa. Increasing the MS sherpa efficacy is shown to be the most sensitive parameter of the model and therefore confirms that this should be the main focus in further development. As there are no univocal criteria for reimbursement of eHealth interventions in current reimbursement models, the sensitivity analyses provide us with helpful insights into which aspects of the eHealth intervention to focus on. Improving the efficacy can be achieved by improving the algorithms in the MS sherpa tool or adding measurements, so that disease progression, subclinical disease activity and relapses can be detected or predicted earlier.

Besides earlier detection of disease activity and subsequent treatment switches, MS sherpa potentially has other benefits within the MS care path, like supporting stopping of MS treatment in stable pwMS, earlier diagnosis of SPMS, improved self-efficacy and patient empowerment, monitoring effects of therapies other than DMTs, etc. The use of eHealth interventions might substitute clinical procedures with home/remote testing, leading to cost and efficiency gains. Especially for pwMS, not only disease outcomes are important, but self-efficacy and patient empowerment might be more relevant drivers for them to adopt eHealth interventions like MS sherpa [20]. Future research will also focus on a broader spectrum of benefits than the impact on earlier treatment switch alone.

5. Conclusions

eHealth interventions hold the promise of alleviating pressure on the health care labor force and improve the lives of patients. Several eHealth initiatives are underway in the MS field, but the evidence on their impact on pwMS, MS care path and wider society is still lacking. Digital biomarker interventions for home-monitoring of pwMS like MS sherpa are promising. This research showed positive impact from using a digital biomarker–based eHealth intervention for early detection of active disease and switching treatment accordingly. This eHTA for MS sherpa is the first to combine a complex decision analytical model which captures lifetime treatment sequences with an MS-specific eHealth intervention. The results indicate the potential of MS sherpa to be cost-effective or even cost-saving. It is shown that its use may increase costs within the health care setting, but that these costs are offset by savings outside the health care setting. Dependent on the efficacy of the solution in early detection of active disease, MS sherpa has the potential to become dominant. The results of future and ongoing research should validate the assumptions on efficacy of MS sherpa incorporated in the model. Moreover, improving MS sherpa may further increase benefits.

Author Contributions: Conceptualization, S.C., I.W., B.d.T., M.V., V.W., S.H., E.S. and K.-H.L.; methodology, S.C., I.W., B.d.T., M.V., V.W. and S.H.; software, S.C., I.W. and B.d.T.; validation, M.V., V.W. and S.H.; formal analysis, M.V., V.W. and S.H.; investigation, M.V., V.W. and S.H.; resources, M.V., V.W. and S.H.; data curation, M.V., V.W. and S.H.; writing—original draft preparation, S.C. and I.W.; writing—review and editing, M.V., V.W., S.H., E.S., K.-H.L. and B.d.T.; visualization, M.V., V.W. and S.H.; supervision, M.V. and B.d.T.; project administration, M.V., V.W. and S.H.; funding acquisition, M.V. All authors have read and agreed to the published version of the manuscript.

Funding: iMTA received project funding from the Ministry of Health, Welfare and Sport for performing this eHTA for an eHealth/AI application. MS sherpa was chosen as example by the Ministry. The MS health economic model was developed with an unrestricted research grant from the Erasmus Medical Center.

Institutional Review Board Statement: Not applicable.

Informed Consent Statement: Not applicable.

Data Availability Statement: The data presented in this study are available in Huygens & Versteegh. Modelling the cost-utility of treatment sequences for multiple sclerosis. Value in Health. Accepted for publication May 2021.

Conflicts of Interest: Orikami is the provider of MS sherpa; the eHTA analyses were performed independently by iMTA. iMTA has received payments outside the scope of this manuscript for activities related to patient preferences in multiple sclerosis from EMD-Serono and Merck KgGA in the past 36 months, with the last payments in 2018 and 2019, respectively. The MS centre Amsterdam authors are involved in MS sherpa studies. The presented eHTA analysis was performed by iMTA; during the preparations the MS centre Amsterdam authors were interviewed by iMTA. The involved affiliations have no financial relationship with each other for the presented analysis.

References

1. Scholz, M.; Haase, R.; Schriefer, D.; Voigt, I.; Ziemssen, T. Electronic Health Interventions in the Case of Multiple Sclerosis: From Theory to Practice. *Brain Sci.* **2021**, *11*, 180. [CrossRef]
2. Baumol, W.J. Health care, education and the cost disease. A looming crisis for public choice. *Public Choice* **1993**, *77*, 17–28. Available online: https://www.jstor.org/stable/30027203 (accessed on 15 June 2021). [CrossRef]
3. Embrey, N. Multiple sclerosis: Managing a complex neurological disease. *Nurs. Stand.* **2014**, *29*, 49–58. [CrossRef] [PubMed]
4. Compston, A.; Coles, A. Multiple sclerosis. *Lancet* **2002**, *359*, 1221–1231. [CrossRef]
5. Tillery, E.; Clements, J.; Howard, Z. What's new in multiple sclerosis? *Ment. Health Clin.* **2017**, *7*, 213–220. [CrossRef]
6. Gasperini, C.; Prosperini, L.; Tintofe, M.; Sormani Filippi, M.; Rio, J.; Palace, J.; Rocca, M.A.; Ciccarelli, O.; Barkhof, F.; Sastre-Garriga, J.; et al. MAGNIMS Study Group. Unraveling treatment response in multiple sclerosis: A clinical and MRI challenge. *Neurology* **2019**, *92*, 180–192. [CrossRef] [PubMed]
7. Giovannoni, G.; Butzkueven, H.; Dhib-Jalbut, S.; Hobart, J.; Kobelt, G.; Pepper, G.; Sormani, M.P.; Thalheim, C.; Traboulsee, A.; Vollmer, T. *Brain Health, Time Matters in Multiple Sclerosis*; Oxford Pharma Genesis Ltd.: Oxford, UK, 2015; Reprinted 2017; pp. 46–47. Available online: https://www.msbrainhealth.org/wp-content/uploads/2021/05/brain-health-time-matters-in-multiple-sclerosis-policy-report-1-1.png (accessed on 29 July 2021).
8. The Dutch Society for Neurology. 2012. Available online: https://richtlijnendatabase.nl/richtlijn/multipele_sclerose_2012/multipele_sclerose_-_startpagina_2012.html (accessed on 29 July 2021).
9. The Dutch Society for Neurology. 2020. Available online: https://richtlijnendatabase.nl/richtlijn/ziektemodulerende_behandeling_van_multiple_sclerose_bij_volwassenen/radiologically_isolated_syndrome.html (accessed on 29 July 2021).
10. Marziniak, M.; Brichetto, G.; Feys, P.; Meyding-Lamadé, U.; Vernon, K.; Meuth, S.G. The Use of Digital and Remote Communication Technologies as a Tool for Multiple Sclerosis Management: Narrative Review. *JMIR Rehabil. Assist. Technol.* **2018**, *5*, e5. [CrossRef] [PubMed]
11. Landtblom, A.M.; Guala, D.; Martin, C.; Olsson-Hau, S.; Haghighi, S.; Jansson, L.; Fredrikson, S. RebiQoL: A randomized trial of telemedicine patient support program for health-related quality of life and adherence in people with MS treated with Rebif. *PLoS ONE* **2019**, *14*, e0218453. [CrossRef] [PubMed]

12. Mercier, H.W.; Ni, P.; Houlihan, B.V.; Jette, A.M. Differential impact and use of a telehealth intervention by persons with MS or SCI. *Am. J. Phys. Med. Rehabil.* **2015**, *94*, 987–999. [CrossRef] [PubMed]
13. Kahraman, T.; Savci, S.; Ozdogar, A.T.; Gedik, Z.; Idiman, E. Physical, cognitive and psychosocial effects of telerehabilitation-based motor imagery training in people with multiple sclerosis: A randomized controlled pilot trial. *J. Telemed. Telecare* **2020**, *26*, 251–260. [CrossRef]
14. Van Oirschot, P.; Heerings, M.; Wendrich, K.; Den Teuling, B.; Martens, M.; Jongen, P.J. Symbol Digit Modalities Test Variant in a Smartphone App for Persons With Multiple Sclerosis: Validation Study. *JMIR Mhealth Uhealth* **2020**, *8*, e18160. [CrossRef]
15. Lam, K.H.; Van Oirschot, P.; Den Teuling, B.; Hulst, H.; De Jong, B.; Uitdehaag, B.; De Groot, V.; Killestein, J. Reliability, construct and concurrent validity of a smartphone-based cognition test in multiple sclerosis. *Mult. Scler. J.* **2021**. [CrossRef] [PubMed]
16. Van Oirschot, P.; Heerings, M.; Wendrich, K.; Den Teuling, B.; Dorssers, F.; Van Ee, R.; Martens, M.; Jongen, P.J. Two Minute Walking Test with a Smartphone App for Persons with Multiple Sclerosis: Validation Study. *JMIR Mhealth Uhealth* **2021**. submitted.
17. International Electrotechnical Commission, IEC 62366-1: 2015 Medical Devices—Part 1: Application of Usability Engineering to Medical Devices. Available online: https://webstore.iec.ch/publication/67220 (accessed on 30 July 2021).
18. International Electrotechnical Commission, IEC TR 62366-2: 2016 Medical Devices—Part 2: Guidance on the Application of Usability Engineering to Medical Devices. Available online: https://webstore.iec.ch/publication/24664 (accessed on 30 July 2021).
19. Conway, N.; Webster, C.; Smith, B.; Wake, D. eHealth and the use of individually tailored information: A systematic review. *Health Inform. J.* **2017**, *23*, 218–233. [CrossRef]
20. Wendrich, K.; Van Oirschot, P.; Martens, M.; Heerings, M.; Jongen, P.; Krabbenborg, L. Toward Digital Self-monitoring of Multiple Sclerosis: Investigating First Experiences, Needs, and Wishes of People with MS. *Int. J. MS Care* **2019**, *21*, 282–291. [CrossRef]
21. Midalgia, L.; Mulero, P.; Montalban, X.; Graves, J.; Hauser, S.L.; Julian, L.; Baker, M.; Schadrack, J.; Gossens, C.; Scotland, A.; et al. Adherence and satisfaction of smartphone- and smartwatch-based remote active testing and passive monitoring in people with multiple sclerosis: Nonrandomized interventional feasibility study. *J. Med. Int. Res.* **2019**, *21*, e14863.
22. Maillart, E.; Labauge, P.; Cohen, M.; Maarouf, A.; Vukusic, S.; Donze, C.; De Seze, J.; Bourre, B.; Moreau, T.; Bieuvelet, S.; et al. Acceptability in clinical practice of MSCopilot®, a smartphone application for the digital self-assessment of patients living with MS. *ECTRIMS Online Libr.* **2018**, E228545, P702.
23. Brouwer, W.; Van Baal, P.; Van Exel, J.; Versteegh, M. When is it too expensive? Cost-effectiveness thresholds and health care decision-making. *Eur. J. Health Econ.* **2019**, *20*, 175–180. [CrossRef] [PubMed]
24. National Health Care Institute. Ziektelast in de Praktijk De theorie en Praktijk Van Het Berekenen Van Ziektelast Bij Pakketbeoordelingen. 2018. Available online: https://www.zorginstituutnederland.nl/binaries/zinl/documenten/rapport/2018/05/07/ziektelast-in-de-praktijk/Ziektelast+in+de+praktijk_definitief.pdf (accessed on 29 July 2021).
25. Huygens, S.; Versteegh, M. Modeling the cost-utility of treatment sequences for multiple sclerosis. *Value Health* **2021**. [CrossRef]
26. National Health Care Institute. Richtlijn Voor Het Uitvoeren Van Economische Evaluaties in De Gezondheidszorg. 2016. Available online: https://www.zorginstituutnederland.nl/binaries/zinl/documenten/publicatie/2016/02/29/richtlijn-voor-het-uitvoeren-van-economische-evaluaties-in-de-gezondheidszorg/richtlijn-voor-het-uitvoeren-van-economische-evaluaties-in-de-gezondheidszorg.pdf (accessed on 15 May 2021).
27. Benedict, R.H.; De Luca, J.; Phillips, G.; LaRocca, N.; Hudson, L.; Rudick, R. Multiple Sclerosis Outcome Assessments Consortium. Validity of the Symbol Digit Modalities Test as a cognition performance outcome measure for multiple sclerosis. *Mult. Scler. J.* **2017**, *23*, 721–733. [CrossRef]
28. Pardini, M.; Uccelli, A.; Grafman, J.; Yaldizli, O.; Mancardi, G.; Roccatagliata, L. Isolated cognitive relapses in multiple sclerosis. *J. Neurol. Neurosurg. Psychiatry* **2014**, *85*, 1035–1037. [CrossRef] [PubMed]
29. Morrow, S.; Jurgensen, S.; Forrestal, F.; Munchauer, F.; Benedict, R. Effects of acute relapses on neuropsychological status in multiple sclerosis patients. *J. Neurol.* **2011**, *258*, 1603–1608. [CrossRef] [PubMed]
30. Bethoux, F.; Bennett, S. Evaluating walking in patients with multiple sclerosis: Which assessment tools are useful in clinical practice? *Int. J. MS Care* **2011**, *13*, 4–14. [CrossRef] [PubMed]
31. Lam, K.H.; Bucur, I.G.; Oirschot, P.; de Graaf, F.; Weda, H.; Uitdehaag, B.; Heskes, T.; Killestein, J.; de Groot, V. Smartphone-based monitoring of cognition in multiple sclerosis. 2021; in preparation.
32. Kurtzke, J.F. Rating neurologic impairment in multiple sclerosis: An expanded disability status scale (EDSS). *Neurology* **1983**, *33*, 1444–1452. [CrossRef]
33. Noyes, K.; Bajorska, A.; Chappel, A.; Schwid, S.R.; Mehta, L.R.; Weinstock-Guttman, B.; Holloway, R.G.; Dick, A.W. Cost-effectiveness of disease-modifying therapy for multiple sclerosis, A population-based study. *Neurology* **2011**, *77*, 355–363. [CrossRef]
34. Nielsen, A.S.; Halamka, J.D.; Kinkel, R.P. Internet portal use in an academic multiple sclerosis center. *J. Am. Med. Inform. Assoc. JAMIA* **2012**, *19*, 128–133. [CrossRef] [PubMed]

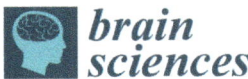

Article

Health Economic Impact of Software-Assisted Brain MRI on Therapeutic Decision-Making and Outcomes of Relapsing-Remitting Multiple Sclerosis Patients—A Microsimulation Study

Diana M. Sima [1,2,*], Giovanni Esposito [1], Wim Van Hecke [1,2], Annemie Ribbens [1], Guy Nagels [1,2,3] and Dirk Smeets [1,2]

1 icometrix, 3012 Leuven, Belgium; giovanni.esposito@icometrix.com (G.E.); wim.vanhecke@icometrix.com (W.V.H.); annemie.ribbens@icometrix.com (A.R.); guy.nagels@vub.be (G.N.); dirk.smeets@icometrix.com (D.S.)
2 AI Supported Modelling in Clinical Sciences (AIMS), Vrije Universiteit Brussel, 1050 Brussels, Belgium
3 Department of Engineering, University of Oxford, Oxford OX1 3PJ, UK
* Correspondence: diana.sima@icometrix.com

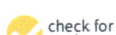

Citation: Sima, D.M.; Esposito, G.; Van Hecke, W.; Ribbens, A.; Nagels, G.; Smeets, D. Health Economic Impact of Software-Assisted Brain MRI on Therapeutic Decision-Making and Outcomes of Relapsing-Remitting Multiple Sclerosis Patients—A Microsimulation Study. *Brain Sci.* 2021, 11, 1570. https://doi.org/10.3390/brainsci11121570

Academic Editors: Tjalf Ziemssen and Rocco Haase

Received: 20 October 2021
Accepted: 25 November 2021
Published: 27 November 2021

Publisher's Note: MDPI stays neutral with regard to jurisdictional claims in published maps and institutional affiliations.

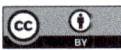

Copyright: © 2021 by the authors. Licensee MDPI, Basel, Switzerland. This article is an open access article distributed under the terms and conditions of the Creative Commons Attribution (CC BY) license (https://creativecommons.org/licenses/by/4.0/).

Abstract: Aim: To develop a microsimulation model to assess the potential health economic impact of software-assisted MRI in detecting disease activity or progression in relapsing-remitting multiple sclerosis (RRMS) patients. Methods: We develop a simulated decision analytical model based on a hypothetical cohort of RRMS patients to compare a baseline decision-making strategy in which only clinical evolution (relapses and disability progression) factors are used for therapy decisions in MS follow-up, with decision-making strategies involving MRI. In this context, we include comparisons with a visual radiologic assessment of lesion evolution, software-assisted lesion detection, and software-assisted brain volume loss estimation. The model simulates clinical (EDSS transitions, number of relapses) and subclinical (new lesions and brain volume loss) disease progression and activity, modulated by the efficacy profiles of different disease-modifying therapies (DMTs). The simulated decision-making process includes the possibility to escalate from a low efficacy DMT to a high efficacy DMT or to switch between high efficacy DMTs when disease activity is detected. We also consider potential error factors that may occur during decision making, such as incomplete detection of new lesions, or inexact computation of brain volume loss. Finally, differences between strategies in terms of the time spent on treatment while having undetected disease progression/activity, the impact on the patient's quality of life, and costs associated with health status from a US perspective, are reported. Results: The average time with undetected disease progression while on low efficacy treatment is shortened significantly when using MRI, from around 3 years based on clinical criteria alone, to 2 when adding visual examination of MRI, and down to only 1 year with assistive software. Hence, faster escalation to a high efficacy DMT can be performed when MRI software is added to the radiological reading, which has positive effects in terms of health outcomes. The incremental utility shows average gains of 0.23 to 0.37 QALYs over 10 and 15 years, respectively, when using software-assisted MRI compared to clinical parameters only. Due to long-term health benefits, the average annual costs associated with health status are lower by $1500–$2200 per patient when employing MRI and assistive software. Conclusions: The health economic burden of MS is high. Using assistive MRI software to detect and quantify lesions and/or brain atrophy has a significant impact on the detection of disease activity, treatment decisions, health outcomes, utilities, and costs in patients with MS.

Keywords: relapsing-remitting multiple sclerosis (RRMS); magnetic resonance imaging (MRI); brain MRI analysis software; non-evidence of disease activity (NEDA); Markov model

1. Introduction

There are almost 25,000 newly diagnosed Multiple Sclerosis (MS) cases in the US each year, and nearly 1 million people are living with MS in the US (Atlas of MS, 2020, www.atlasofms.org, accessed on 15 October 2021). Relapsing-remitting multiple sclerosis (RRMS) is the most prevalent type of MS at diagnosis, with about 85% of people with MS being initially diagnosed with relapsing MS and approximately three times more females than males (Atlas of MS, 2020, www.atlasofms.org, accessed on 15 October 2021).

When a person is diagnosed with MS, the therapy goal is to stop or slow down the natural course of disease evolution, while balancing at the same time an acceptable level of burden, risks of side effects, and costs. Currently, there are more than twenty FDA-approved disease-modifying therapies (DMTs) available for RRMS patients (nationalmssociety.org/Treating-MS/Medications, accessed on 15 October 2021). These are intended to reduce the disease burden, disease activity, and progression, but they do not cure the underlying disease. The current treatment guidelines state that any evidence of disease activity while on consistent treatment should prompt the consideration of an alternative regimen to optimize therapeutic benefit [1]. Therapy selection, either immediately after diagnosis or in further follow-up, is made on a case-by-case basis and depends on the perceived level of clinical and subclinical disease activity and progression.

Evidence of clinical disease activity and progression are new relapses and disability worsening, as often measured by the Kurtzke Expanded Disability Status Scale (EDSS). Subclinical disease activity and progression are evaluated on brain (and spinal cord) magnetic resonance imaging (MRI) scans, by measuring the number of new and enlarging lesions as well as brain atrophy [2]. Though relapses and EDSS are considered primary endpoints in pivotal clinical trials and are an important therapeutic target in MS, yearly MRI scans have become part of standard MS monitoring and are crucial for clinical decision-making. In addition, "silent" progression due to brain atrophy has been found to be associated with long term disability accumulation in patients without relapses, suggesting that the process that underlies secondary progressive MS likely begins far earlier than is generally recognized [3].

Though MRI measures of new and enlarging lesions and brain atrophy are essential for therapeutic decision-making in MS, the typical radiological report is qualitative and based on a visual assessment. Detecting and quantifying disease activity based on brain MRI scans visually is a difficult and tedious task, and it is known that around 24% of radiological reports of brain MRI scans contain discrepancies [4]. Fortunately, thanks to recent imaging artificial intelligence (AI) innovations, reliable regulatory cleared software solutions for MRI volumetry are being increasingly used in clinical practice to enhance radiological reporting [5]. This technology brings potential advantages in terms of enhanced sensitivity for detecting subclinical pathologic aspects, as well as increased reproducibility compared to visual radiological evaluation [4,6,7].

In this paper, we focus on the potential health economic impact of using brain MRI reading and analysis software during decision-making in MS. To this end, a novel approach is proposed, where a cohort of RRMS patients is simulated based on a hidden state of disease activity, which is assessed with different decision-making strategies. The impact of these decisions over time is evaluated in terms of health outcomes and costs.

Evaluating the health economic impact of treatment decisions in MS is very relevant, as, in the US, MS is the second most costly chronic condition (after congestive heart failure), with more than $4 million in total lifetime costs per patient [8–10]. With several MS therapies available, it has been shown that adopting a more personalized medicine in MS, including data-driven clinical decision-making, has the potential to increase the health impact of existing treatments by over 50%, and therefore significantly reduce the costs [11].

The present simulated decision analytical model compares a baseline decision-making strategy for RRMS follow-up, in which only clinical evolution (relapses and EDSS progression) factors are used, with decision-making strategies involving MRI actively. In addition, the health economic analysis is simulated in the case of visual inspection of

MRIs vs. using assistive software that detects new lesions and estimates the rate of brain atrophy. We run the model on a simulated cohort of RRMS patients from the moment they are prescribed a low efficacy DMT and evaluate the impact of the therapeutic decision-making path on outcomes, health utilities, and related costs, thereby adopting the US healthcare perspective.

2. Materials and Methods

2.1. Model Structure

We construct a decision-analytic model as a Markov model in which the states and state transitions are based on disability progression as measured with the EDSS, similar to previous widely used model structures of disability progression in RRMS [12–14]. In addition to these classical EDSS-based Markov models, the simulated patients can experience both clinical and subclinical disease activity, in the form of EDSS progression, relapses, new lesions, and/or brain atrophy; see Figure 1. The cycle duration is one year, which is the maximally recommended duration between neurological (including MRI) examinations for RRMS patients [15].

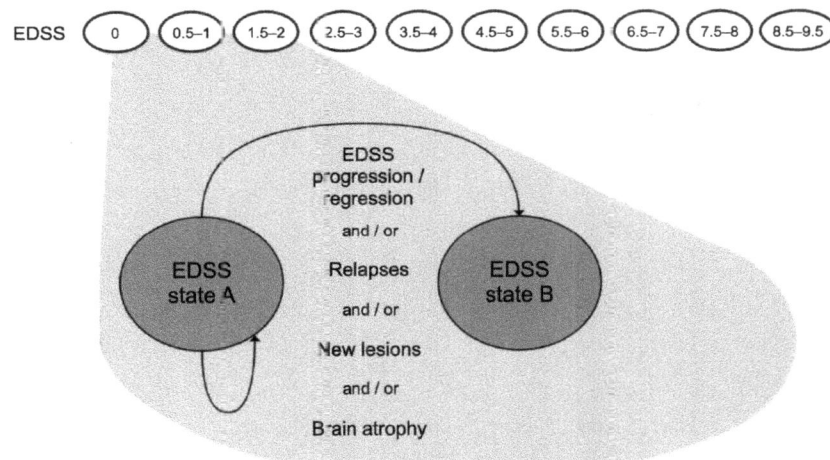

Figure 1. Schematic representation of the Markov model for disease progression. EDSS = Kurtzke Expanded Disability Status Scale; state A = EDSS state at the start of a model cycle; state B = EDSS state at the end of a model cycle. EDSS progression (B > A), regression (B < A) or stability (B = A) are possible. Clinical and subclinical disease activity may occur during each cycle.

A hypothetical cohort of 1000 RRMS patients (female to male ratio 3:1) is simulated from the moment they start therapy on a low efficacy DMT. During each model cycle over a certain horizon (here, 10- or 15-years horizons are considered), patients can experience disease progression in terms of EDSS, relapses, lesion evolution, and/or brain volume loss. EDSS transition probabilities are defined based on historical data of natural disease progression in RRMS under the "best supportive care" [16], modulated by the efficacy of various DMTs in slowing down disease progression. The number of annual relapses (aR) and the annual number of new lesions (aNL) are randomly drawn from discrete probability distributions, constructed based on the same two factors: (1) natural history data of annualized relapse rates and new lesions in untreated "best supportive care" RRMS, and (2) the efficacy of various DMTs in suppressing relapses or new lesion formation, respectively. Brain volume loss is modeled as an annualized percentage of brain volume change (aPBVC), which is simulated from a Gaussian distribution with mean and standard deviation parameters that depend on DMT efficacy in slowing down brain atrophy. Details regarding all simulation parameters are presented in Section 2.3.

These 4 parameters characterize each patient during each cycle, and, by applying appropriate thresholds (defined in Table 1 in Section 2.2), these parameters define the hidden state of disease activity for each patient at the end of each model cycle. If any one of the 4 parameters exceeds its respective threshold, then we refer to the patient's hidden state as "true disease activity", which might signify a suboptimal response to therapy if the patient is on a DMT. Else, we label the patient as stable since there is no evidence of disease activity.

Table 1. Observation strategies and choice of decision parameters.

Strategy	Criteria for Detecting Disease Activity	Parameter Choices *
without MRI	at least $n^{relapse}$ clinical relapses or EDSS disability progression **	$n^{relapse}$: {1, 2, 3}
NEDA-3 (visual)	same as "without MRI" or at least n^{lesion} new lesions, but only a proportion p^{lesion} of true lesions are caught	n^{lesion}: {1, 2, **3**, 4} p^{lesion}: **33%**, 66%
NEDA-3 (software)	same as "NEDA-3 (visual)"	n^{lesion}: {1, 2, **3**, 4} p^{lesion}: 90%, **100%**
NEDA-4 (software)	same as "NEDA-3 (software)" or annualized whole brain volume loss > α% measurement error between two consecutive scans: $\pm\varepsilon$%	α: {0.4, **0.52**, 0.72} ε: {0.1, **0.2**, 0.3}

* Default values used in the Section 3 are in bold; alternative parameter choices are discussed in Appendix C. ** EDSS disability progression is defined here as one of the following: if baseline EDSS 0, EDSS increase $\geq$ 1.5 points; if baseline EDSS $\geq$ 1, EDSS increase $\geq$ 1 point; if baseline EDSS > 5, EDSS increase $\geq$ 0.5 points. Abbreviations: EDSS, Expanded Disability Status Scale; NEDA, No Evidence of Disease Activity.

Additionally, we consider a clinical observation model that simulates how a clinician reads and interprets the (partially) available disease activity/progression information, and how this translates into therapy decisions (see Figure 2). In this context, four different clinical decision strategies are compared:

1. clinical examination without MRI: disease activity or progression is established solely on clinical relapses and/or EDSS progression;
2. NEDA-3 (visual): clinical criteria (as above) are complemented by visually inspected MRI to detect lesion evolution;
3. NEDA-3 (software): NEDA-3 (visual) criteria as above are complemented by software-assisted lesion detection;
4. NEDA-4 (software): NEDA-3 (software) criteria as above are complemented by software-assisted brain volume loss computation.

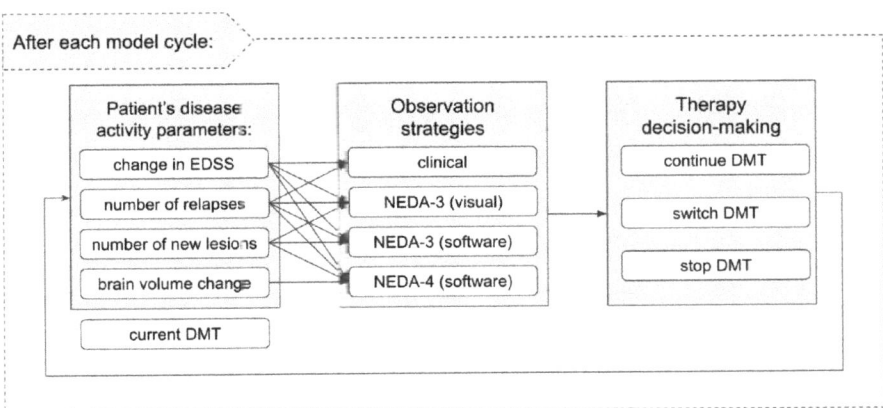

Figure 2. Schematic representation of the interaction between the hidden patient state, defined by the disease activity parameters, the considered observation strategies, and the therapy decision-making options after each model cycle.

Under the considered observation strategies, not all parameters are available or are used. Thus, different observation strategies might lead to different therapeutic decisions. The options are to either continue the current DMT or to stop/switch it (see Figures 2 and 3). For simplicity, we group DMTs in two families of "low efficacy DMTs" and "high efficacy DMTs", where the grouping reflects differences in the efficacy profile [17]. All patients start on a low efficacy DMT, with the possibility to escalate to a high efficacy DMT.

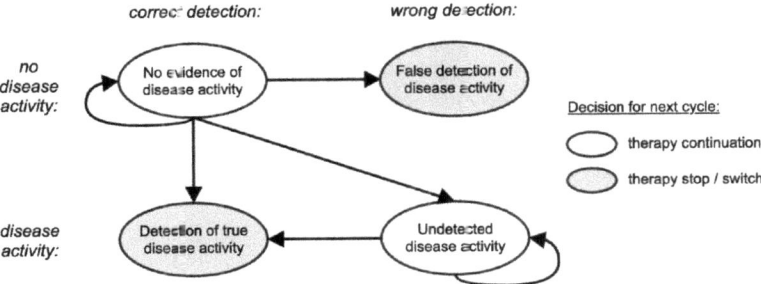

Figure 3. Schematic representation of the clinical decision-making process for a particular decision-making strategy. The disease activity status is either correctly or wrongly detected depending on the available information. At the next cycle, a patient stays on the same therapy if no disease activity is detected or can stop/switch therapy if disease activity is detected.

2.2. Simulation of Observation and Therapy Decision Strategies

At the end of a model cycle, each therapy decision-making strategy is applied to each simulated patient. Table 1 presents the specific criteria defining detection of disease activity/progression for each strategy. The same thresholds are also applied for deciding the "ground truth" status based on the simulated hidden disease activity parameters. An increase in EDSS, the occurrence of relapses, the occurrence of new lesions, or abnormal brain volume loss, with the thresholds described in Table 1, thus indicate disease activity/progression.

For the EDSS and aR values, which are used identically in all strategies, it is assumed that the true values are available, without measurement error. Inter-rater variability and other uncertainties are not modeled for these clinical parameters. For aNL, it is known that visual detection of lesion activity on MRI follow-up scans can be imperfect, and is also highly dependent on radiologists' experience and specialization [7,18]. Detection is significantly enhanced by assistive software, e.g., by tools that align MRI scans from different time points, or highlight new lesion candidates using a color code, with the rate of new lesion detection shown to be around 3–4 times higher when using assistive software compared to visual inspection of MRI scans [7,18–21].

In addition, visual MRI assessment is non-quantitative and precludes the use of a numerical threshold on the annualized brain volume loss, as this is impossible to assess with the naked eye. Specialized MRI volumetric software becomes a necessity to quantify subtle changes, which are typical of the order of -0.5%/year in MS patients [22]. However, aPBVC estimation with state-of-the-art software may suffer from measurement error of 0.1% (median absolute error) or higher, depending on the MRI machines, imaging sequences, use of different scanners for follow-up, etc [23]. In our model, we simulate measurement error on the aPBVC between two consecutive MRIs in the "NEDA-4 (software)" strategy by adding a zero-mean random error term on the ground truth aPBVC (see parameter choices in Table 1). However, when MRI scans are available for multiple years in a row, the brain volume loss computation would become more precise, because random measurement errors can be averaged out. To model this aspect, the standard deviation of the error term decreases in time with a factor equalling the square root of the number of available consecutive pairs of follow-up scans.

Based on these assumptions, true disease progression can be correctly or wrongly detected at the end of each cycle with any strategy, leading to a transition towards the "true detection of disease activity" or "undetected disease activity" states (i.e., the 2 bottom nodes in Figure 3), respectively. However, due to the nature of the simulation, only the "NEDA-4 (software)" strategy can lead to a wrong detection of disease activity (top-right node in Figure 3), which happens when there is no disease activity (i.e., all ground truth clinical and subclinical parameters correspond to a NEDA-4 status), but aPBVC gets slightly beyond the considered pathological threshold due to measurement error. In Section 3, we evaluate how often this happens, and what health economic consequences can be attributed to that. We also show the frequency of all other decision-making reasons per strategy and cycle.

Finally, if disease activity is detected based on the available parameters and the considered strategy, a patient on low efficacy DMT can switch to a high efficacy DMT. Whether the new DMT is successful or not is then evaluated at the end of the next model cycle under the same decision-making strategy.

If a patient with detected disease activity was already on high efficacy DMT, then a random switch within the high efficacy DMT family is allowed once, after which the patient is kept on the latest DMT until the end of the simulation or until it reaches EDSS greater than or equal to 7. In the latter case, it is assumed that the patient is taken off DMTs; the patient remains in the Markov model and follows a natural course of the disease but is ignored in the therapy decision-making model, meaning that no therapy decision state changes occur in the next model cycles.

2.3. Model Inputs—Simulation Details

2.3.1. MS Disease Progression Parameters

As mentioned above, the hidden state parameters (EDSS, aR, aNL, and aPBVC) are simulated for each patient at each cycle. They are randomly sampled from appropriate probabilistic distributions, learned from untreated "best supportive care" RRMS natural history data, but modulated by relative efficacy gains characterizing each DMT family. Efficacy gains for EDSS progression and aR are taken from a network meta-analysis of 33 unique randomized trials with 21,768 patients presented in [17] evaluating more than 10 FDA-approved DMTs, which we recombine into 2 wide intervals corresponding to low and high efficacy DMT families (Table 2). To simulate how well a particular DMT suppresses disease activity in a particular simulated patient, a percentile score is randomly chosen for each patient on DMT and defines the efficacy gain factors for each hidden parameter. This percentile score stays in principle constant for each patient during model cycles until a change in DMT occurs for that patient. However, the model assumes that undetected patients with MRI activity experience a faster EDSS progression than stable patients. This is penalized by including an acceleration parameter (AP = 1.484) in the model to increase the probability of future progression prior to adjustment for the effect of DMT, as described in [24].

2.3.2. EDSS

The disability states in the model are defined using steps 0 (normal) through 9.5 (help-less patient confined to bed and unable to communicate effectively or eat/swallow) of the EDSS. Each patient in the simulated cohort is initially assigned a random starting value for EDSS, uniformly sampled from 0 to 3 (Appendix A Table A1). In each model cycle, patients may stay in the same disability state, progress to a higher (worse) disability state, or regress to a lower (better) disability state. The unmodulated EDSS transition probability matrix is based on the British Columbia Multiple Sclerosis longitudinal observational cohort [16,25] and is presented in Appendix A Table A2. This "natural course" EDSS transition probability matrix is based on a mixed-sex cohort, therefore it is first modified for each patient by a sex-specific risk factor (1.05 for males and 0.97 for females, corresponding to an increased chance of EDSS progression in males, as observed in an analysis of the MSBase Registry data [26]). Then it is further modified for each patient by a relative risk factor based on the efficacy gain percentile score assigned to that particular patient and the assigned DMT:

- first, the relative risk factor is obtained from the interval corresponding to the patient's DMT family (see Table 2, second column) assuming a uniform distribution and using the patient's fixed percentile score;
- secondly, a new EDSS transition matrix is constructed by multiplying all transitions going from the patient's current EDSS state towards states higher than the current EDSS state by f. For f < 1, this leads to less chance of EDSS progression. The remaining transition probabilities corresponding to EDSS states lower than or equal to the current state are scaled proportionally in order to ensure that all probabilities sum to 1 in each row.

At the end of a cycle, a new EDSS state is randomly generated based on the current EDSS state and the adapted transition probability matrix.

2.3.3. Relapses and New Lesions

Both lesion activity and relapses are simulated as discrete random counts from zero-inflated distributions. The most widely accepted statistical model for annual counts of relapses or new lesions in MS is the negative binomial distribution, which is defined based on an average value μ and an over-dispersion parameter θ [27]. For aR, the mean μ is around 0.6–0.8 and varies with EDSS. We use estimates from [17], see Appendix A Table A3. The dispersion parameter is fixed at $\theta = 0.5$. For aNL, we use experimental lesion count fitting results in untreated MS MRI datasets [28], to get approximate estimates for μ and θ as 10 and 0.5, respectively.

In order to simulate treatment effects on aR and aNL, the mean value is modulated by the efficacy improvement expected for low or high efficacy DMTs, respectively. Aban et al. [29], among others, argued that the dispersion parameter θ can be kept constant, regardless of the treatment, and only the mean μ should be modulated by the treatment effect as $f * \mu$ with f < 1. It remains to define the specific efficacy factors f for aR and aNL, respectively. For aR, there are various sources (including the meta-analysis in [17]) that provide these factors for a range of currently available DMTs for RRMS. Moreover, the patient's sex is an additional modifier for the mean relapse rate, with the relapse frequency 17.7% higher in females compared with males [30]. We group the low and the high efficacy DMTs and express the efficacy gain in terms of a rate ratio (see Table 2, middle column). For the effect of DMTs on new lesions, we did not find efficacy gain estimates expressed similarly in the literature. However, we rely on the relationship between treatment effects on lesions and relapses uncovered in a comprehensive meta-analysis of MRI outcomes from 54 comparative randomized trials in more than 25,000 patients with RRMS [31]. The mean cumulative number of new or active T2 lesions, or gadolinium-enhancing lesions on monthly scans, counted over the follow-up period was extracted from each trial as the MRI endpoint for the analysis. The ratio between the average number of MRI lesions per patient in the experimental and the control groups was used to summarise the treatment effect on MRI lesions (lesions_effect) in each trial, and the effect on relapses (relapse_effect) was similarly computed. The treatment effect on lesions was found to be well correlated to the treatment effect on annual relapse rates, with log (relapse_effect) = 0.53 log (lesions_effect), $R^2 = 0.76$. We apply this relationship to the rate ratios available from [17] for aR in order to obtain rate ratios for new lesions; see Table 2 (4th column).

Table 2. Effectiveness of disease-modifying therapies on EDSS disability progression, relapses, new lesions, and brain volume loss.

Therapy Family	Relative Risk of Disability Progression [c]	Rate Ratio for Relapse Rate [c]	Rate Ratio for New Lesions [d]	aPBVC [e]
low efficacy [a]	0.52–1.23	0.55–0.94	0.32–0.89	−0.51% ± 0.27%
high efficacy [b]	0.25–0.90	0.22–0.63	0.06–0.42	−0.27% ± 0.15%

[a] Beta interferon, glatiramer acetate, teriflunomide are included. [b] Alemtuzumab, natalizumab, ocrelizumab are included. [c] Values are pooled from [17], taking the minimum and maximum bounds from the intervals given for different DMTs in the 2 considered DMT families. See also Appendix A Table A4. [d] Values are estimated based on the relationship between the relative treatment effect on MRI lesions and the relative treatment effect on relapses, log (relapse_effect) = 0.53 log (lesions_effect) [31]; in other words, the values in columns 3 and 4 are linked through this equation. [e] Mean ± standard deviation of Gaussian distributions are taken from [22].

2.3.4. Brain Atrophy

Annual brain volume loss is simulated based on 2 Gaussian distributions that can be attributed to low efficacy and high efficacy DMT profiles. It is known that the distribution of aPBVC is highly overlapping between healthy subjects and untreated MS groups [22] and that brain volume loss is age-dependent [32]. High efficacy DMTs are able to bring the average annual volume loss down to values seen in healthy controls, while the distribution of brain atrophy rates in patients treated with low efficacy DMTs is significantly more pronounced and often at the same rates as in untreated MS [22,33,34]. Mean aPBVC values observed in the placebo arms and treatment arms across about a dozen MS clinical trials range from −0.43% to −0.78% for placebo, −0.44% to −0.60% for low efficacy DMT and −0.22% to −0.36% for high efficacy DMT (see [34] (Table 4)). Since we consider only two DMT families (low and high efficacy), the Gaussian model parameters used for aPBVC simulation in our model are taken from [22] and shown in Table 2 (right-most column).

The probabilistic distributions used to simulate aR, aNL, and aPBVC, as well as to perform EDSS state transitions, are illustrated in Appendix C Figure A1.

2.4. Outcome Measures, Utilities, and Costs

For each strategy, the total number of years (cycles) spent by each patient in the "undetected disease progression" state while on low efficacy DMT is computed. This number gives an indication about the potential time lost before escalating to a high efficacy DMT.

The simulation also keeps track of utilities and costs for each patient by assuming them to be conditional on the EDSS state and the number of relapses occurring in each model cycle. Mean utility (in QALYs) by EDSS state is sourced from [25] (see Appendix B Table A5) and ranges from 0.9248 at EDSS 0, which is close to the value 1 corresponding to perfect health, to a negative value of −0.2304 at EDSS 9 (a state that is subjectively deemed as being worse than dead). For each cycle spent in a certain EDSS state, the utility value corresponding to that EDSS state is added to the total utility of the simulation. Disutility values per relapse vary widely in the literature and are usually dependent on relapse severity. For simplicity, we consider only an average relapse disutility of −0.0437 per relapse as in [12,35]. No disutility is considered for the occurrence of new lesions or brain atrophy during a cycle. Based on these (dis)utility values, the annual QALYs averaged over the considered 10-years horizon can be computed for each strategy. As a 14.67-years horizon was used in [13] to evaluate the effect of DMTs, the QALY and cost analysis was also performed for 15 years.

The costs of conventional care due to disease progression, i.e., annual health state costs conditional on EDSS state, are taken from ([17] Table 20), see Appendix B Table A6. Also, an average cost per relapse of US$3069 is applied, cfr. [17,36]. All costs are inflated to 2021 US dollars and are allowed to vary by ±20% for each occurrence. In order to focus purely on costs driven by the patients' health state, no DMT costs are explicitly included in the simulation, neither are costs for acquiring and reading MRI scans, or other factors such as adverse effects.

3. Results

3.1. Effect of Decision-Making Strategy on Detecting Disease Progression

Depending on the decision-making strategy, different proportions of patients having or not having disease activity at the end of each one-year cycle are observed. These proportions are illustrated per cycle in Figure 4 and reported as averages over the first 1, 5, and 10 cycles in Table 3. As expected, the proportion of patients with undetected disease activity decreases when increasing the complexity of the decision-making strategy, because there are more criteria that can lead to a detection of disease activity or progression. After the first model cycle, the simulation revealed 22% truly stable patients and 78% patients with disease activity. The 22% stable patients were correctly identified by all strategies, except for 4% wrongly perceived as having brain atrophy. However, among the 78% active/progressive patients, large proportions were missed by the clinical strategy without MRI (50%) and the NEDA-3 (visual) (36%). Averaged over more cycles, the two software-assisted strategies continue to take the lead in detecting more disease activity/progression compared to the clinical strategy without MRI and the NEDA-3 (visual) strategy. With the cumulation of more MRI follow-up data, the atrophy computation becomes less prone to measurement error, leading to a relatively low number (2%) of simulated decisions over the whole horizon that falsely indicates disease progression in the "NEDA-4 (software)" strategy. Since in our model all patients start on low efficacy DMT, there is more disease activity at the beginning of the simulation, and thus more chance to detect it, especially with the more sensitive strategies. Once patients switch to high efficacy DMT, the proportion of truly active patients, as well as those detected as such by the different strategies, decreases with time, until a stabilization takes place because only two switches are allowed in the high efficacy DMT family.

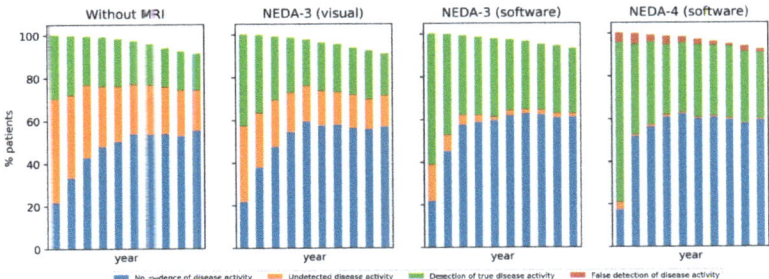

Figure 4. Comparison of decision-making strategies in terms of the proportion of patients in each model state according to the decision-making state transition model in Figure 2. Patients who reached EDSS 7 and are no longer on DMT are excluded.

Table 3. The proportion of patients detected as stable or active in the four decision-making strategies. Results are reported for several model horizons, namely after the first cycle, and averaged over the first 5, and 10 cycles/years. No decisions are reported for patients who reached EDSS 7, but their respective proportions are listed for each strategy.

Year	Decision	Clinical without MRI	NEDA-3 (Visual)	NEDA-3 (Software)	NEDA-4 (Software)
1	stable	72%	58%	40%	22%
	- truly stable	22%	22%	22%	18%
	- undetected disease activity	50%	36%	18%	4%
	active	28%	42%	60%	78%
	- true disease activity	28%	42%	60%	74%
	- false detection of disease activity	-	-	-	4%
	reached EDSS 7	0%	0%	0%	0%
5	stable	74%	71%	60%	59%
	- truly stable	38%	50%	55%	58%
	- undetected disease activity	36%	21%	5%	1%
	active	24%	28%	39%	41%
	- true disease activity	24%	28%	39%	37%
	- false detection of disease activity	-	-	-	4%
	reached EDSS 7	2%	1%	1%	0%
10	stable	75%	72%	62%	60%
	- truly stable	46%	54%	59%	59%
	- undetected disease activity	29%	18%	3%	1%
	active	20%	25%	35%	38%
	- true disease activity	20%	25%	35%	35%
	- false detection of disease activity	-	-	-	3%
	reached EDSS 7	5%	3%	3%	2%

As a consequence of detecting more patients with active disease in the first cycles of the simulation, a faster escalation to high efficacy DMT occurs in the decision-making strategies assisted by MRI. This is illustrated in the DMT distribution per strategy in Figure 5. Note the difference in escalation speed between the strategies.

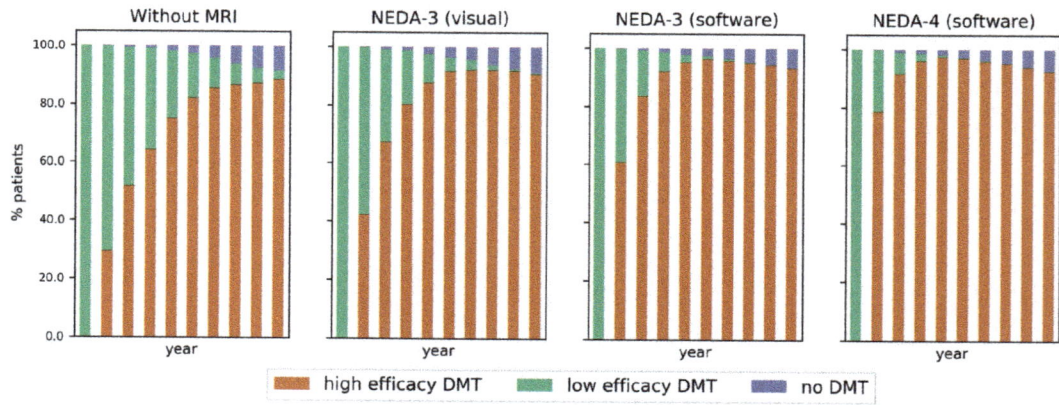

Figure 5. The proportion of patients for each strategy and cycle according to the family of DMT used. Patients who reached EDSS 7 are no longer on DMT.

3.2. Health Outcomes

On average, the simulation indicates that the considered cohort of RRMS patients stays on low efficacy DMT for:
- 3.2 ± 2.4 years for the clinical strategy without MRI,
- 2.3 ± 1.6 years for the NEDA-3 (visual) strategy,
- 1.7 ± 1.1 years for the NEDA-3 (software) strategy,
- 1.3 ± 0.7 years for the NEDA-4 (software) strategy.

While on this first-line therapy, the average time per patient in "undetected disease activity" state, which includes the year prior to the first decision moment, is:
- 2.8 ± 2.3 years for the clinical strategy without MRI,
- 1.9 ± 1.4 years for the NEDA-3 (visual) strategy,
- 1.3 ± 0.8 years for the NEDA-3 (software) strategy,
- 1.0 ± 0.2 years for the NEDA-4 (software) strategy.

There were no differences in these numbers when comparing the male and female subgroups, except for a mean difference of 0.1 years in detecting disease activity in males faster than in females with the clinical strategy; this can be attributed to the fact that there were proportionally more simulated male patients with EDSS progression than females. On the other hand, the slightly higher relapse rate in females did not influence these findings.

3.3. Utilities and Costs

Utilities per patient for each strategy are on average 6.48 to 6.71 QALYs over a 10-years horizon and 9.45 to 9.83 over a 15-years horizon for the different strategies (Table 4). The incremental comparisons between strategies in terms of the computed utilities presented in Table 4 indicate gains of up to 0.37 QALYs over the considered 15-years horizon compared to the clinical strategy without MRI.

Table 4. Utilities (in QALYs) and incremental utilities per patient compared between strategies.

Strategy	Utility	Incremental Utility Compared to		
		Clinical without MRI	NEDA-3 (Visual)	NEDA-3 (Software)
		over a 10-year horizon		
Clinical without MRI	6.48 ± 4.49	-	-	-
NEDA-3 (visual)	6.50 ± 4.63	0.03 ± 2.81	-	-
NEDA-3 (software)	6.67 ± 4.53	0.19 ± 2.80	0.16 ± 2.83	-
NEDA-4 (software)	6.71 ± 4.42	0.23 ± 2.79	0.20 ± 2.80	0.04 ± 2.81
		over a 15-year horizon		
Clinical without MRI	9.45 ± 4.83	-	-	-
NEDA-3 (visual)	9.48 ± 4.97	0.03 ± 4.71	-	-
NEDA-3 (software)	9.78 ± 4.85	0.32 ± 4.68	0.29 ± 4.75	-
NEDA-4 (software)	9.83 ± 4.78	0.37 ± 4.63	0.34 ± 4.69	0.05 ± 4.67

The annualized costs per patient for each strategy over the considered 10-years and 15-years horizons, as well as incremental comparisons between the strategies, are presented in Table 5. These costs are driven by each patient's health status (EDSS value per cycle) and disease activity (relapses per cycle). The maximal annual savings average is $2155 after 10 years and $2267 after 15 years when increasing the complexity of the decision-making strategy by adding both the MRI lesions and brain atrophy criteria to the clinical criteria.

Table 5. Annual costs related to health status (in US$ 2021) and incremental costs per patient compared between strategies.

Strategy	Cost	Incremental Cost Compared to		
		Clinical without MRI	NEDA-3 (Visual)	NEDA-3 (Software)
		in a 10-years horizon		
Clinical without MRI	$33,809 ± $15,918	-	-	-
NEDA-3 (visual)	$33,176 ± $16,056	−$633 ± $18,606	-	-
NEDA-3 (software)	$32,272 ± $15,470	−$1538 ± $18,759	−$905 ± $18,686	-
NEDA-4 (software)	$31,655 ± $15,104	−$2155 ± $18,764	−$1521 ± $18,661	−$617 ± $18,384
		in a 15-years horizon		
Clinical without MRI	$35,142 ± $17,304	-	-	-
NEDA-3 (visual)	$34,567 ± $17,437	−$576 ± $21,718	-	-
NEDA-3 (software)	$33,341 ± $16,565	−$1800 ± $21,366	−$1225 ± $21,348	-
NEDA-4 (software)	$32,875 ± $16,567	−$2267 ± $21,380	−$1691 ± $21,467	−$466 ± $20,831

4. Discussion and Conclusions

As many disease modifying treatments are available for MS patients, it is crucial to optimize therapeutic decision-making, especially as it has been shown that a more personalized medicine in MS has the potential to increase the health impact of existing treatments by over 50% [11]. In this context, a common paradigm is to aim for 'no evidence of disease activity' in each patient at each time point of evaluation. Depending on the definition, and the preference of the treating physician, disease activity is defined as a combination of relapses, disability (EDSS), new/enlarging lesions, and brain atrophy. However, it is known that, in a daily clinical routine setting, each of these has a measurement error as well as different sensitivities and specificities, resulting in a significant variation in decision-making.

The introduction of DMTs in the early nineties improved the lives of people with MS with about 0.5 QALYs accumulated in 15 years [13]. Our simulations (see Table 4) demonstrate that the introduction of a software-supported treatment paradigm (NEDA-4 with software) has the potential to add 0.34 QALYs compared to a visual analysis of brain MRI scans in 15 years, representing a relative improvement of 68% compared to the introduction of disease-modifying therapies.

To the best of our knowledge, this paper evaluates for the first time the effect of different treatment strategies in MS, as well as the availability of clinical and subclinical information in a microsimulation-based health economic setting. To this end, we modeled 1000 early MS patients, thereby simulating clinical and subclinical progression based on natural history data, modulated by treatment effect. These processes are assumed to be weakly correlated (e.g., the number of relapses per year differs across the EDSS spectrum; see Appendix A Table A3 for the employed mean rates), but the correlations are weak, because of high individual variability. We used a natural history EDSS transition matrix and applied a relative risk for each DMT family, in order to derive adapted transition probabilities between EDSS states. Furthermore, we included treatment effects in the simulation of relapse rates, new lesion rates, and brain atrophy rates. As the goal of this study is to evaluate current practice, rather than the future of more personalized decision-making, our model focused on assessing the time needed to detect disease progression or activity while on therapy under different decision-making strategies. DMT allocation and patient response to DMTs were simulated by assigning a DMT efficacy profile to each patient and it was assumed that the relative risk of EDSS transition, the rate ratio for relapse occurrence, the rate ratio for new lesion occurrence, and the annual brain volume loss were constant while the patient stayed on the same therapy, but changed (degraded) if the patient's disease activity remained undetected and (potentially) improved if the patient was switched to another DMT.

The results of this paper indicate that using MRI and assistive software leads to benefits in terms of faster detection of disease activity and better long-term health outcomes due to faster escalation to high efficacy DMTs. Indeed, a clear difference in the detection of true disease activity was observed of 28%, 42%, 60%, and 74% after one year for decisions based on clinical information without MRI, NEDA-3 with visual MRI reading, NEDA-3 with software assistance, and NEDA-4 with software assistance, respectively. The undetected disease activity for these treatment strategies after year 1 is 50%, 36%, 18%, and 4%, respectively. As true disease activity that wasn't picked up after one year is more likely to be picked up with a delay in the years later, and as we simulate that an increasing proportion of patients will be on a higher efficacy DMT throughout the years, the difference between the treatment strategies becomes smaller over time, with 20%, 25%, 35%, and 35% of detected true disease activity and 29%, 18%, 3%, and 1% of undetected disease activity, respectively, after 10 years. As a consequence, a higher proportion of patients would be switched to a higher efficacy DMT earlier when the NEDA-3 and NEDA-4 treatment strategies with assistive software are followed.

In MS, it is known that not being on the optimal treatment early in the disease has a significant health impact in later life and that being on a suboptimal treatment is similar to not being treated at all [11]. In this context, our results indicate that the average time a patient with MS has disease activity or progression while on treatment is 2.8 years, 1.9 years, 1.3 years, and 1.0 years when treatment decisions are based on clinical information without MRI, NEDA-3 with visual MRI reading, NEDA-3 with software assistance, and NEDA-4 with software assistance, respectively.

Regarding costs, the real total costs are composed of the sum of costs over the considered horizon, including costs of pharmaceuticals, medical visits, and indirect costs. Costs of DMT are typically treated separately from other health-related costs in health economics studies. Annual wholesale acquisition costs of individual DMTs in MS (see, e.g., ([17] Table 19)) in the US are high, at around $80,000 per year in 2021, but very similar between low and high efficacy DMTs. In our model, the proportion of patients stopping DMT would play a role in the overall average annual cost over the considered cohort. In this study, we decided to focus only on the costs associated with health states. The estimated costs driven by the patients' health states show potential annual differences over the 10- or 15-year horizon of around $2200 per year on average. One has to take into consideration the cost of acquiring an annual MRI and performing radiological reading (with or without assistive software). Such costs can be in the range of $2000–$4000 in the US.

We aimed at developing our models as similar to clinical reality as possible, but theoretical models always have limitations. For example, therapy discontinuation was only modeled under the condition of reaching EDSS 7, while, in reality, intolerability, adverse effects, patient preference, and convenience play an important role in deciding therapy (dis)continuation. Taking such aspects into account would increase the percentage of patients that stop or switch DMTs, but this wasn't modeled, as it would affect all treatment strategies considered in this study. In addition, our simulated observation model imposed a therapy switch if any of the observed parameters exceeded a predefined threshold, without taking into consideration the disease aggressiveness prior to DMT initiation. In practice, the thresholds for deciding that disease activity or progression occurs would need to be patient-specific rather than generic, to allow therapy continuation if there are potential benefits compared to stopping the DMT. In particular, deciding whether the rate of brain volume change is within normal limits or more pronounced compared to healthy controls should be done using age-specific thresholds and taking the stage of the disease into account, since the rate of brain atrophy is not constant over the life span or the course of MS [32,37].

Another way to refine the proposed microsimulation model is to incorporate additional confounding factors as part of the profile of each hypothetical patient. In particular, the age at MS onset could be included, since previous studies have shown that disability accumulates at a different pace depending on the onset age [38]: young-onset patients attain disability milestones earlier in life, but patients diagnosed later in life progress faster through the lower half of the EDSS scale. To account for such relations, the probabilistic distributions of the patient's hidden state parameters, as well as the thresholds of the decision-making criteria, would require adaptations.

Though this study demonstrates a clear benefit in using assistive MRI software in the follow-up of MS patients, several design choices of the simulated model were not made in favor of using MRI (software). For example, the only parameter for which measurement error was generated was the annualized brain volume change. This led to a potential detection of false disease activity in 3% of the simulated decisions with the NEDA-4 (software) strategy over 10 years. This type of misdiagnosis deserves attention when balancing the advantages and disadvantages of implementing such a strategy in the real world. Furthermore, in this study, the EDSS state is used to measure progression, because it has historically been linked to costs and health outcomes. However, patients may have brain atrophy without changes in EDSS, but with a potentially large long-term impact on EDSS and/or cognition. Hence, more refined models and additional clinical evidence should be considered in future studies. Furthermore, in our model, inter-rater variability and other uncertainties were not modeled for the clinical parameters EDSS and the number of relapses. Nevertheless, it is known that estimating EDSS is prone to significant inter-rater variability and even daily variations.

In conclusion, using assistive MRI software to detect and quantify new lesions and/or brain atrophy has a significant impact on the detection of disease activity, treatment decisions, health outcomes, utilities, and costs in patients with MS.

Author Contributions: Conceptualization, D.M.S., W.V.H. and D.S.; methodology, D.M.S., W.V.H., G.N. and D.S.; software, D.M.S.; formal analysis, D.M.S.; investigation, G.E.; writing—original draft preparation, D.M.S. and W.V.H.; writing—review and editing, G.E., A.R., G.N. and D.S.; supervision, A.R. All authors have read and agreed to the published version of the manuscript.

Funding: This research received no external funding.

Institutional Review Board Statement: Not applicable.

Informed Consent Statement: Not applicable.

Data Availability Statement: Not applicable.

Conflicts of Interest: The following authors are employed by icometrix: Diana M. Sima, Giovanni Esposito, Annemie Ribbens, Dirk Smeets. Guy Nagels is medical director of neurology at icometrix; he or his institution (VUB/UZ Brussel) have received research, educational, and travel grants from Biogen, Roche, Genzyme, Merck, Bayer, and Teva. Wim Van Hecke is CEO, founder, shareholder, and member of the board of icometrix.

Appendix A. Model Inputs

Appendix A Tables A1–A4 present details relevant to the disease progression Markov model, including the considered initial distribution, state transition matrix, and assumed relations between variables.

Table A1. Initial EDSS state distribution of the RRMS population entering the model.

	EDSS 0	EDSS 1	EDSS 2	EDSS 3	EDSS 4	EDSS 5	EDSS 6	EDSS 7	EDSS 8	EDSS 9
Proportion	25	25	25	25	0	0	0	0	0	0

EDSS, Kurtzke Expanded Disability Status Scale.

Table A2. Transition Probability Matrix for 10-State Disability (EDSS) in the British Columbia Multiple Sclerosis Dataset.

Age ≥ 28 y		\multicolumn{10}{c}{EDSS State at End of Year}
		0	1	2	3	4	5	6	7	8	9
EDSS State at Start of Year	0	0.6954	0.2029	0.0725	0.0217	0.0042	0.0014	0.0018	0.0001	0.00003	0.00000
	1	0.0583	0.6950	0.1578	0.0609	0.0164	0.0046	0.0064	0.0005	0.0001	0.00001
	2	0.0159	0.1213	0.6079	0.1680	0.0446	0.0185	0.0216	0.0017	0.0005	0.0000
	3	0.0059	0.0496	0.1201	0.5442	0.0911	0.0584	0.1165	0.0103	0.0035	0.0003
	4	0.0016	0.0221	0.0666	0.1152	0.4893	0.1039	0.1681	0.0258	0.0067	0.0006
	5	0.0005	0.0053	0.0294	0.0587	0.0874	0.4869	0.2731	0.0388	0.0188	0.0010
	6	0.0001	0.0013	0.0044	0.0250	0.0307	0.0408	0.7407	0.1090	0.0438	0.0042
	7	0.00001	0.0002	0.0005	0.0025	0.0073	0.0039	0.1168	0.6927	0.1606	0.0156
	8	0.0000	0.00001	0.0000	0.0003	0.0005	0.0005	0.0188	0.0557	0.9034	0.0207
	9	0.0000	0.0000	0.0000	0.00002	0.00004	0.00003	0.0018	0.0057	0.1741	0.8133

EDSS, Kurtzke Expanded Disability Status Scale. Source: [25].

Table A3. Annual Natural History Relapse Rate by EDSS Health State Used in the Model.

	EDSS 0	EDSS 1	EDSS 2	EDSS 3	EDSS 4	EDSS 5	EDSS 6	EDSS 7	EDSS 8	EDSS 9
Relapse rate *	0.71	0.73	0.68	0.72	0.71	0.59	0.49	0.51	0.51	0.51

EDSS, Kurtzke Expanded Disability Status Scale. * Mean number of relapses per patient per year. Source: ([17] Appendix Table E7).

Table A4. Treatment effect parameters for individual DMTs.

Treatment	Relative Risk EDSS Progression (Range)	Rate Ratio for Relapse Rate (Range)
Alemtuzumab	0.25–0.68	0.22–0.35
Dimethyl Fumarate	0.46–0.84	0.43–0.63
Fingolimod	0.51–0.90	0.39–0.55
Glatiramer acetate 20 mg	0.58–0.94	0.55–0.71
Interferon β-1a 30 mcg	0.63–1.00	0.74–0.94
Interferon β-1a 22 mcg	0.52–1.23	0.55–0.85
Interferon β-1a 44 mcg	0.52–0.99	0.54–0.73
Interferon β-1b 250 mcg	0.46–0.89	0.55–0.77
Natalizumab	0.37–0.84	0.25–0.40
Ocrelizumab	0.28–0.76	0.27–0.44
Peginterferon β-1a	0.37–1.02	0.47–0.86
Teriflunomide 7 mg	0.63–1.14	0.67–0.93
Teriflunomide 14 mg	0.52–0.97	0.56–0.79

Source: adapted from ([17] Appendix Table E7).

Appendix B. Utilities and Costs

Appendix B Tables A5 and A6 give numerical details about the cost-utility data used.

Table A5. Utility by EDSS state.

	EDSS 0	EDSS 1	EDSS 2	EDSS 3	EDSS 4	EDSS 5	EDSS 6	EDSS 7	EDSS 8	EDSS 9
Utility	0.9248	0.7614	0.6741	0.5643	0.5643	0.4906	0.4453	0.2686	0.0076	−0.2304

EDSS, Kurtzke Expanded Disability Status Scale. Source: [25].

Table A6. Annual costs by EDSS state (US$ 2021).

Annual Costs	EDSS 0	EDSS 1	EDSS 2	EDSS 3	EDSS 4	EDSS 5	EDSS 6	EDSS 7	EDSS 8	EDSS 9
Direct	$3221	$5536	$7851	$10,165	$12,481	$14,796	$17,111	$19,427	$21,741	$24,056
Indirect	$12,211	$16,704	$21,198	$25,692	$30,187	$34,681	$39,175	$43,669	$48,164	$52,658

EDSS, Kurtzke Expanded Disability Status Scale. Source: ([17] Table 20); values inflated to US$ 2021.

Appendix C. Model Parameter Distributions

The probabilistic distributions used to simulate aR, aNL, and aPBVC, as well as to perform EDSS state transitions, are illustrated in Appendix C Figure A1 below.

The aR is shown for EDSS = 1 (mean aR is 0.58 for low efficacy DMT and 0.24 for high efficacy DMT), for EDSS = 2 (mean aR is 0.44 for low and 0.31 for high efficacy DMT), and for EDSS 3 (mean aR is 0.56 for low and 0.28 for high efficacy DMT). Mean aNL is 6.0 for low, and 2.3 for high efficacy DMT.

Appendix C Table A7 shows the effect of individual decision parameters on the proportion of simulated patients for which disease activity would be detected after one year, using the decision-making criteria in Table 1. 1000 simulated patients are generated for 3 situations: natural disease course, disease course modulated by low efficacy DMTs (with randomly generated efficacy according to the ranges given in Table 2 for the low efficacy DMTs family) and disease course modulated by high efficacy DMTs (with randomly generated efficacy according to the ranges given in Table 2 for the high efficacy DMTs family). For the number of relapses, the number of lesions, and aPBVC, several thresholds are considered, as listed in Table 1. These proportions do not show when several criteria are met simultaneously.

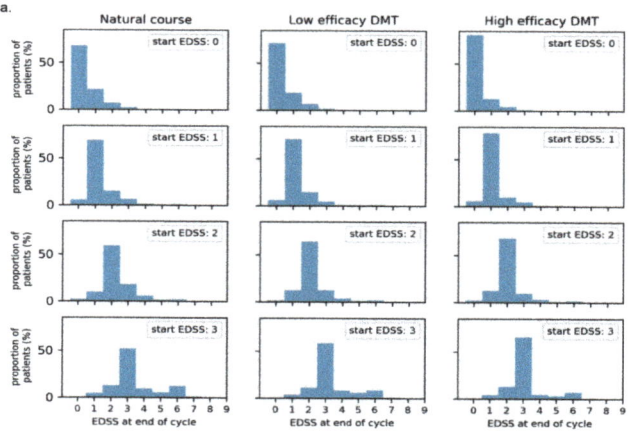

Figure A1. *Cont.*

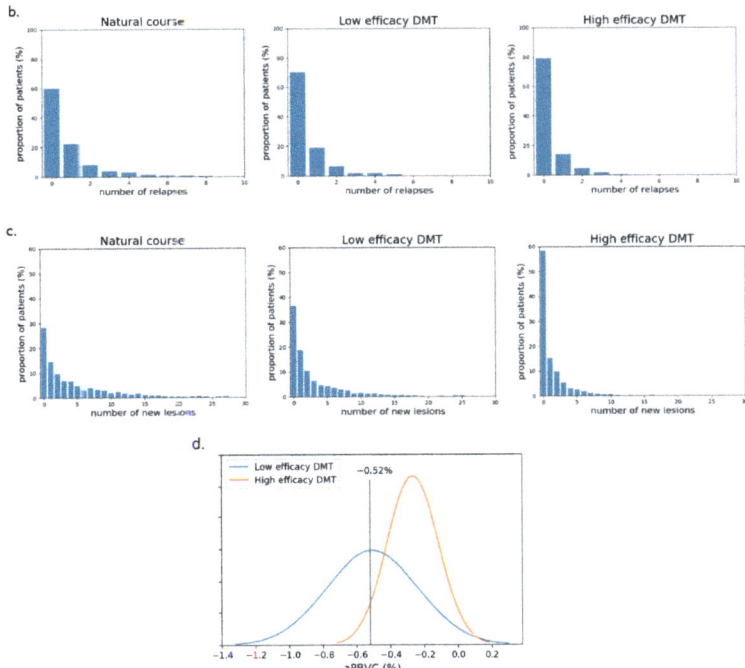

Figure A1. Distribution of simulated disease activity parameters. For comparison purposes, we show the untreated MS (natural course) distributions, together with those modulated by low or high efficacy DMTs. Efficacy rates are randomly generated to be representative for a whole family of DMTs, as specified in Table 2, and are thus not specific for a single DMT. (**a**) EDSS transitions showing the proportion of patients moving to the next EDSS state at the end of a cycle, when the EDSS at the beginning of the cycle was 0, 1, 2, or 3; (**b**) histograms of the number of relapses during one cycle, assuming an EDSS of 1; (**c**) histograms of the number of new lesions during one cycle; (**d**) Gaussian distributions of aPBVC for healthy controls, which is also used as target distribution for high efficacy DMT, and (untreated or on low efficacy DMT) MS patients. The −0.52% threshold giving 5% 'false positives' is illustrated (from [22]). With a mean of the MS distribution at −0.51%, the 'sensitivity' for this threshold is 49%.

Table A7. The proportion of simulated patients where disease activity would be detected based on individual criteria is presented in Table 1, with different threshold choices.

	EDSS Progression	Relapse Progression Using $n^{relapse}$ Threshold of			Lesion Progression Using n^{lesion} Threshold of				PBVC Progression Using α Threshold of		
	-	1 *	2	3	1	2	3 *	4	−0.40	−0.52 *	−0.72
natural course	22%	35%	17%	8%	64%	56%	48%	43%	66%	49%	21%
low efficacy DMT	19%	30%	12%	5%	64%	43%	38%	28%	66%	49%	21%
high efficacy DMT	12%	20%	6%	2%	48%	28%	15%	11%	19%	5%	0%

The * superscript indicates the selected threshold.

References

1. Costello, K.; Halper, J.; Kalb, R.; Skutnik, L.; Rapp, R. *The Use of Disease-Modifying Therapies in Multiple Sclerosis, Principles and Current Evidence—A Consensus Paper by the Multiple Sclerosis Coalition*; The Multiple Sclerosis Coalition: Hackensack, NJ, USA, 2019; Available online: https://ms-coalition.org/the-use-of-disease-modifying-therapies-in-multiple-sclerosis-updated/ (accessed on 10 October 2021).
2. Giovannoni, G.; Butzkueven, H.; Dhib-Jalbut, S.; Hobart, J.; Kobelt, G.; Pepper, G.; Sormani, M.P.; Thalheim, C.; Traboulsee, A.; Vollmer, T. Brain Health: Time Matters in Multiple Sclerosis. *Mult. Scler. Relat. Disord.* **2016**, *9* (Suppl. 1), S5–S48. [CrossRef]
3. University of California, San Francisco MS-EPIC Team; Cree, B.A.C.; Hollenbach, J.A.; Bove, R.; Kirkish, G.; Sacco, S.; Caverzasi, E.; Bischof, A.; Gundel, T.; Zhu, A.H.; et al. Silent Progression in Disease Activity-Free Relapsing Multiple Sclerosis. *Ann. Neurol.* **2019**, *85*, 653–666. [CrossRef] [PubMed]
4. Rosenkrantz, A.B.; Duszak, R.; Babb, J.S.; Glover, M.; Kang, S.K. Discrepancy Rates and Clinical Impact of Imaging Secondary Interpretations: A Systematic Review and Meta-Analysis. *J. Am. Coll. Radiol.* **2018**, *15*. [CrossRef] [PubMed]
5. Van Hecke, W.; Costers, L.; Descamps, A.; Ribbens, A.; Nagels, G.; Smeets, D.; Sima, D.M. A Novel Digital Care Management Platform to Monitor Clinical and Subclinical Disease Activity in Multiple Sclerosis. *Brain Sci.* **2021**, *11*, 1171. [CrossRef] [PubMed]
6. Erbayat Altay, E.; Fisher, E.; Jones, S.E.; Hara-Cleaver, C.; Lee, J.-C.; Rudick, R.A. Reliability of Classifying Multiple Sclerosis Disease Activity Using Magnetic Resonance Imaging in a Multiple Sclerosis Clinic. *JAMA Neurol.* **2013**, *70*, 338–344. [CrossRef]
7. Wang, W.; van Heerden, J.; Tacey, M.A.; Gaillard, F. Neuroradiologists Compared with Non-Neuroradiologists in the Detection of New Multiple Sclerosis Plaques. *AJNR Am. J. Neuroradiol.* **2017**, *38*, 1323–1327. [CrossRef]
8. Adelman, G.; Rane, S.G.; Villa, K.F. The Cost Burden of Multiple Sclerosis in the United States: A Systematic Review of the Literature. *J. Med. Econ.* **2013**, *16*, 639–647. [CrossRef]
9. Chen, A.Y.; Chonghasawat, A.O.; Leadholm, K.L. Multiple Sclerosis: Frequency, Cost, and Economic Burden in the United States. *J. Clin. Neurosci.* **2017**, *45*, 180–186. [CrossRef] [PubMed]
10. Owens, G.M.; Olvey, E.L.; Skrepnek, G.H.; Pill, M.W. Perspectives for Managed Care Organizations on the Burden of Multiple Sclerosis and the Cost-Benefits of Disease-Modifying Therapies. *J. Manag. Care Pharm.* **2013**, *19*, S41–S53. [CrossRef] [PubMed]
11. Hult, K.J. Measuring the Potential Health Impact of Personalized Medicine: Evidence from MS Treatments. In *Economic Dimensions of Personalized and Precision Medicine*; Berndt, E.R., Goldman, D.P., Rowe, J.W., Eds.; National Bureau of Economic Research; University of Chicago Press: Chicago, IL, USA, 2019.
12. Furneri, G.; Santoni, L.; Ricella, C.; Prosperini, L. Cost-Effectiveness Analysis of Escalating to Natalizumab or Switching among Immunomodulators in Relapsing-Remitting Multiple Sclerosis in Italy. *BMC Health Serv. Res.* **2019**, *19*, 436. [CrossRef]
13. Chirikov, V.; Ma, I.; Joshi, N.; Patel, D.; Smith, A.; Giambrone, C.; Cornelio, N.; Hashemi, L. Cost-Effectiveness of Alemtuzumab in the Treatment of Relapsing Forms of Multiple Sclerosis In The United States and Societal Spillover Effects. *Value Health* **2017**, *20*, A722. [CrossRef]
14. Gani, R.; Giovannoni, G.; Bates, D.; Kemball, B.; Hughes, S.; Kerrigan, J. Cost-Effectiveness Analyses of Natalizumab (Tysabri) Compared with Other Disease-Modifying Therapies for People with Highly Active Relapsing-Remitting Multiple Sclerosis in the UK. *Pharmacoeconomics* **2008**, *26*, 617–627. [CrossRef] [PubMed]
15. Kaunzner, U.W.; Gauthier, S.A. MRI in the Assessment and Monitoring of Multiple Sclerosis: An Update on Best Practice. *Ther. Adv. Neurol. Disord.* **2017**, *10*, 247–261. [CrossRef] [PubMed]
16. Tremlett, H.; Zhao, Y.; Rieckmann, P.; Hutchinson, M. New Perspectives in the Natural History of Multiple Sclerosis. *Neurology* **2010**, *74*, 2004–2015. [CrossRef] [PubMed]
17. Institute for Clinical and Economic Review and California Technology Assessment Forum. *Disease-Modifying Therapies for Relapsing-Remitting and Primary-Progressive Multiple Sclerosis: Effectiveness and Value: Final Evidence Report*; Institute for Clinical and Economic Review: Boston, MA, USA, 2017. Available online: http://resource.nlm.nih.gov/101704699 (accessed on 10 October 2021).
18. Dahan, A.; Wang, W.; Gaillard, F. Computer-Aided Detection Can Bridge the Skill Gap in Multiple Sclerosis Monitoring. *J. Am. Coll. Radiol.* **2018**, *15*, 93–96. [CrossRef]
19. Galletto Pregliasco, A.; Collin, A.; Guéguen, A.; Metten, M.A.; Aboab, J.; Deschamps, R.; Gout, O.; Duron, L.; Sadik, J.C.; Savatovsky, J.; et al. Improved Detection of New MS Lesions during Follow-Up Using an Automated MR Coregistration-Fusion Method. *AJNR Am. J. Neuroradiol.* **2018**, *39*, 1226–1232. [CrossRef] [PubMed]
20. van Heerden, J.; Rawlinson, D.; Zhang, A.M.; Chakravorty, R.; Tacey, M.A.; Desmond, P.M.; Gaillard, F. Improving Multiple Sclerosis Plaque Detection Using a Semiautomated Assistive Approach. *AJNR Am. J. Neuroradiol.* **2015**, *36*, 1465–1471. [CrossRef] [PubMed]
21. Zopfs, D.; Laukamp, K.R.; Paquet, S.; Lennartz, S.; Pinto Dos Santos, D.; Kabbasch, C.; Bunck, A.; Schlamann, M.; Borggrefe, J. Follow-up MRI in Multiple Sclerosis Patients: Automated Co-Registration and Lesion Color-Coding Improves Diagnostic Accuracy and Reduces Reading Time. *Eur. Radiol.* **2019**, *29*, 7047–7054. [CrossRef] [PubMed]
22. De Stefano, N.; Stromillo, M.L.; Giorgio, A.; Bartolozzi, M.L.; Battaglini, M.; Baldini, M.; Portaccio, E.; Amato, M.P.; Sormani, M.P. Establishing Pathological Cut-Offs of Brain Atrophy Rates in Multiple Sclerosis. *J. Neurol. Neurosurg. Psychiatry* **2016**, *87*, 93–99. [CrossRef] [PubMed]

23. Smeets, D.; Ribbens, A.; Sima, D.M.; Cambron, M.; Horakova, D.; Jain, S.; Maertens, A.; Van Vlierberghe, E.; Terzopoulos, V.; Van Binst, A.-M.; et al. Reliable Measurements of Brain Atrophy in Individual Patients with Multiple Sclerosis. *Brain Behav.* **2016**, *6*, e00518. [CrossRef]
24. Hettle, R.; Harty, G.; Wong, S.L. Cost-Effectiveness of Cladribine Tablets, Alemtuzumab, and Natalizumab in the Treatment of Relapsing-Remitting Multiple Sclerosis with High Disease Activity in England. *J. Med. Econ.* **2018**, *21*, 676–686. [CrossRef] [PubMed]
25. Palace, J.; Duddy, M.; Bregenzer, T.; Lawton, M.; Zhu, F.; Boggild, M.; Piske, B.; Robertson, N.P.; Oger, J.; Tremlett, H.; et al. Effectiveness and Cost-Effectiveness of Interferon Beta and Glatiramer Acetate in the UK Multiple Sclerosis Risk Sharing Scheme at 6 Years: A Clinical Cohort Study with Natural History Comparator. *Lancet Neurol.* **2015**, *14*, 497–505. [CrossRef]
26. Ribbons, K.A.; McElduff, P.; Boz, C.; Trojano, M.; Izquierdo, G.; Duquette, P.; Girard, M.; Grand'Maison, F.; Hupperts, R.; Grammond, P.; et al. Male Sex Is Independently Associated with Faster Disability Accumulation in Relapse-Onset MS but Not in Primary Progressive MS. *PLoS ONE* **2015**, *10*, e0122686. [CrossRef] [PubMed]
27. Sormani, M.P.; Bruzzi, P.; Miller, D.H. Gasperini, C.; Barkhof, F.; Filippi, M. Modelling MRI Enhancing Lesion Counts in Multiple Sclerosis Using a Negative Binomial Model: Implications for Clinical Trials. *J. Neurol. Sci.* **1999**, *163*, 74–80. [CrossRef]
28. van den Elskamp, I.; Knol, D.; Uitdehaag, B.; Barkhof, F. The Distribution of New Enhancing Lesion Counts in Multiple Sclerosis: Further Explorations. *Mult. Scler.* **2009**, *15*, 42–49. [CrossRef] [PubMed]
29. Aban, I.B.; Cutter, G.R.; Mavinga, N. Inferences and Power Analysis Concerning Two Negative Binomial Distributions with an Application to MRI Lesion Counts Data. *Comput. Stat. Data Anal.* **2008**, *53*, 820–833. [CrossRef] [PubMed]
30. Kalincik, T.; Vivek, V.; Jokubaitis, V.; Lechner-Scott, J.; Trojano, M.; Izquierdo, G.; Lugaresi, A.; Grand'maison, F.; Hupperts, R.; Oreja-Guevara, C.; et al. Sex as a Determinant of Relapse Incidence and Progressive Course of Multiple Sclerosis. *Brain* **2013**, *136*, 3609–3617. [CrossRef]
31. Sormani, M.P.; Bruzzi, P. MRI Lesions as a Surrogate for Relapses in Multiple Sclerosis: A Meta-Analysis of Randomised Trials. *Lancet Neurol.* **2013**, *12*, 669–676. [CrossRef]
32. Azevedo, C.J.; Cen, S.Y.; Jaberzadeh, A.; Zheng, L.; Hauser, S.L.; Pelletier, D. Contribution of Normal Aging to Brain Atrophy in MS. *Neurol. Neuroimmunol. Neuroinflamm.* **2019**, *6*. [CrossRef]
33. Favaretto, A.; Lazzarotto, A.; Margoni, M.; Poggiali, D.; Gallo, P. Effects of Disease Modifying Therapies on Brain and Grey Matter Atrophy in Relapsing Remitting Multiple Sclerosis. *Mult. Scler. Demyelinating Disord.* **2018**, *3*, 1–10. [CrossRef]
34. Ontaneda, D.; Tallantyre, E.C.; Raza, P.C.; Planchon, S.M.; Nakamura, K.; Miller, D.; Hersh, C.; Craner, M.; Bale, C.; Chaudhry, B.; et al. Determining the Effectiveness of Early Intensive versus Escalation Approaches for the Treatment of Relapsing-Remitting Multiple Sclerosis: The DELIVER-MS Study Protocol. *Contemp. Clin. Trials* **2020**, *95*, 106009. [CrossRef] [PubMed]
35. Chirikov, V.; Ma, I.; Joshi, N.; Patel, D.; Smith, A.; Giambrone, C.; Cornelio, N.; Hashemi, L. Cost-Effectiveness of Alemtuzumab in the Treatment of Relapsing Forms of Multiple Sclerosis in the United States. *Value Health* **2019**, *22*, 168–176. [CrossRef] [PubMed]
36. Zimmermann, M.; Brouwer, E.; Tice, J.A.; Seidner, M.; Loos, A.M.; Liu, S.; Chapman, R.H.; Kumar, V.; Carlson, J.J. Disease-Modifying Therapies for Relapsing-Remitting and Primary Progressive Multiple Sclerosis: A Cost-Utility Analysis. *CNS Drugs* **2018**, *32*, 1145–1157. [CrossRef] [PubMed]
37. Ancorra, M.; Nakamura, K.; Lampert, E.J.; Pulido-Valdeolivas, I.; Zubizarreta, I.; Llufriu, S.; Martinez-Heras, E.; Sola-Valls, N.; Sepulveda, M.; Tercero-Uribe, A.; et al. Assessing Biological and Methodological Aspects of Brain Volume Loss in Multiple Sclerosis. *JAMA Neurol.* **2018**, *75*, 1246–1255. [CrossRef] [PubMed]
38. Confavreux, C.; Vukusic, S. Age at Disability Milestones in Multiple Sclerosis. *Brain* **2006**, *129*, 595–605. [CrossRef]

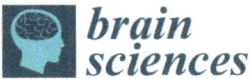

Review

Electronic Health Interventions in the Case of Multiple Sclerosis: From Theory to Practice

Maria Scholz, Rocco Haase, Dirk Schriefer, Isabel Voigt and Tjalf Ziemssen *

Center of Clinical Neuroscience, Department of Neurology, University Hospital Carl-Gustav Carus, Dresden University of Technology, 01307 Dresden, Germany; maria.scholz@uniklinikum-dresden.de (M.S.); Rocco.Haase@uniklinikum-dresden.de (R.H.); Dirk.Schriefer@uniklinikum-dresden.de (D.S.); Isabel.Voigt@uniklinikum-dresden.de (I.V.)
* Correspondence: Tjalf.Ziemssen@uniklinikum-dresden.de; Tel.: +49-351-458-4465

Abstract: (1) Background: eHealth interventions play a growing role in shaping the future healthcare system. The integration of eHealth interventions can enhance the efficiency and quality of patient management and optimize the course of treatment for chronically ill patients. In this integrative review, we discuss different types of interventions, standards and advantages of quality eHealth approaches especially for people with multiple sclerosis (pwMS). (2) Methods: The electronic databases PubMed, Cochrane and Web of Science were searched to identify potential articles for eHealth interventions in pwMS; based on 62 articles, we consider different ways of implementing health information technology with various designs. (3) Results: There already exist some eHealth interventions for single users with a single-use case, interventions with a social setting, as well as eHealth interventions that integrate various single and social interventions and even those that may be used additionally for complex use cases. A key determinant of consumer acceptance is a high-quality user-centric design for healthcare practitioners and pwMS. In pwMS, the different neurological disabilities should be considered, and particular attention must be paid to the course of the treatment and the safety processes of each treatment option. (4) Conclusion: Depending on the field of application and the respective users, interventions are designed for single, social, integrated or complex use. In order to be accepted by their target group, interventions must be beneficial and easy to use.

Keywords: multiple sclerosis; digital health; eHealth; intervention; patient management

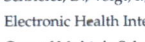

Citation: Scholz, M.; Haase, R.; Schriefer, D.; Voigt, I.; Ziemssen, T. Electronic Health Interventions in the Case of Multiple Sclerosis: From Theory to Practice. *Brain Sci.* 2021, 11, 180. https://doi.org/10.3390/brainsci11020180

Academic Editor: Bruno Brochet
Received: 21 December 2020
Accepted: 28 January 2021
Published: 2 February 2021

Publisher's Note: MDPI stays neutral with regard to jurisdictional claims in published maps and institutional affiliations.

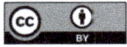

Copyright: © 2021 by the authors. Licensee MDPI, Basel, Switzerland. This article is an open access article distributed under the terms and conditions of the Creative Commons Attribution (CC BY) license (https://creativecommons.org/licenses/by/4.0/).

1. Introduction

In a society of growing digital proficiency, 80 percent of all Internet users go online to seek health information [1]. The use of health information technology (HIT) in healthcare has become increasingly prominent since the late 1980s [2]. Early HIT mainly referred to the digitization of traditional processes in the public health sector. With the development of new technologies, the term has become more general [3]. Focusing on eHealth-assisted patient management, we have also witnessed a steady increase of research interest in the last two decades (Figure 1) [4].

Several approaches exist to defining constructs such as eHealth, telehealth and other HIT terms [5], but we want to provide a common ground for our review: eHealth is defined as "an emerging field in the intersection of medical informatics, public health and business" using information and communication technologies [3]. Such technologies are shown in Figure 2 and may contain personalized health (pHealth), telemedicine and telecare, mobile health (mHealth), clinical information systems (e.g., electronic health record), disease registries and other non-clinical systems, integrated regional and national information networks and Big Data approaches [2,6,7].

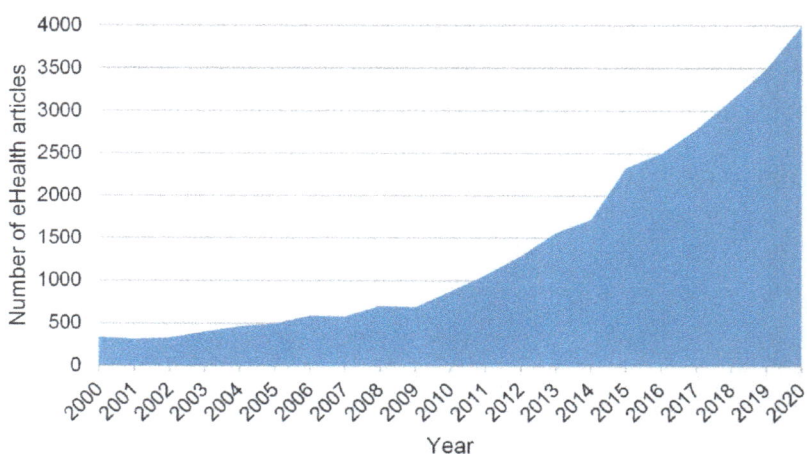

Figure 1. Publication trend: number of publications on the search query of eHealth interventions over the last two decades at PubMed.

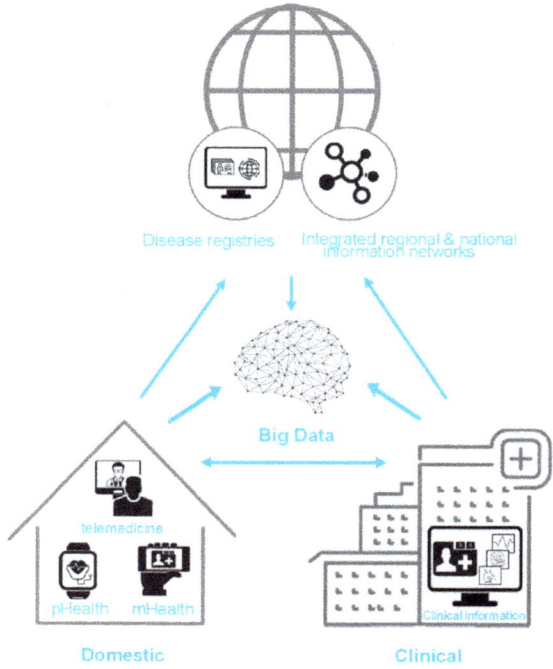

Figure 2. Different eHealth technologies used in domestic settings such as personalized health (pHealth) and mobile health (mHealth), clinical settings or both for collecting or presenting patient data and their interaction possibilities with each other. Clinical information represents all data collected in the clinical environment together yielding the electronic health record.

Good eHealth interventions are easy to use and should enhance efficiency and quality, translate evidence-based knowledge into practice, enable patient empowerment by giving them more control over their health, education and information exchange as well as facilitate specific interventions [8–10]. Especially for people with chronic diseases, adequate treatment and monitoring are difficult to supply [11]. eHealth interventions are an effective way to identify the health needs of people with complex chronic diseases and may meet their long-term care needs because many areas can be addressed and acceptance as well as satisfaction with such interventions is supposed to be high [12].

An important chronic disease is multiple sclerosis (MS), one of the world's most common neurological disorders of young adults that results in central demyelination and neurodegeneration causing multifocal neurological problems [13–16]. Usually, people with MS (pwMS) show their first symptoms at the age of 20 to 40 years; consequently, they live with this chronic disease for the following decades, which is why these patients may be important early adopters of emerging eHealth trends [17]. Additionally, their physical and cognitive impairments complicate traditional face-to-face interventions for pwMS. Such disabilities and the willingness to use digital media for communication with healthcare providers make MS an excellent model for innovative improvements in care delivery, including eHealth interventions [18–20]. In addition to individual disabilities, there are other circumstances that make a face-to-face visit even more challenging. On the one hand, these include geographical barriers. Long distances to specialists, especially in rural areas, mean an enormous effort for patients to obtain the required care. On the other hand, there are special situations such as the recent coronavirus disease (COVID-19) pandemic making smooth patient care problematic. Reducing person-to-person contact in order to stop a rapid spread of the disease is a preventive measure against proliferation [21]. This commandment and the fear of possible infection lead patients to cancel their medical appointments. To enable continuous patient care without a face-to-face visit and to overcome geographical barriers [22], eHealth interventions can serve as a helpful tool. By extending the collection of health data electronically beyond the consultation itself, a continuous recording of all facets of this complex disease may enable a safe and efficient management of the individual disease course. Therefore, HIT serves as a support for medical and health policy practice [11] that reduces costs. Since the quality of care achieved by eHealth interventions may deviate from traditional face-to-face interactions, cost reductions and treatment outcomes need to be balanced. To optimize the specific treatments of pwMS, eHealth interventions can support physicians in long-term documentation and management of treatment steps in any disease-modifying therapy (DMT) [23].

The aim of this integrative review is to offer an overview of eHealth interventions for pwMS grouped into single, social, integrated or complex eHealth interventions. We also provide not only a theoretical description of the benefits of complex interventions but also a practical demonstration. Key factors for a successful development of good patient management are discussed.

2. Materials and Methods

We searched the electronic databases PubMed, Cochrane and Web of Science from 2000 to December 2020 to identify potential articles for eHealth intervention in pwMS. The keywords used in this article were "(eHealth OR telemedicine OR telehealth OR "digital health" OR "mobile Health" OR "personalized Health" OR "electronic health") AND "multiple sclerosis" NOT (Parkinson OR "major depressive disorder" OR epilepsy OR diabetes)". In total, there were 451 articles obtained from the three databases using the keyword searches. After looking for false entries that did not focus on MS and articles that were not written in English or German, 283 articles were determined to be irrelevant to this study and 106 were recognized as duplicates and were therefore removed. The remaining 62 articles were reviewed and discussed. As a taxonomy for eHealth interventions, we consider different ways to implement HIT, for instance, by phone, telehealth, web-based, via remote sensing or virtual technologies [7,24,25], which are designed as an intervention with a single-use case, interventions with a social setting, as well as an eHealth intervention that integrate various single and social interventions and even those that may be used additionally for complex use cases. There are numerous heterogeneous options for classifying eHealth interventions [26,27]. In this integrative review, we applied a classification based on a taxonomy that was developed for the Office for Life Sciences of the UK [28,29]. For some interventions, we provide information for cooperation and funding in brackets. Additionally, we present some success factors of eHealth interventions for pwMS found in the selected literature.

3. Results

3.1. eHealth Interventions for a Single-Use Case

Health technologies for a single-use case focus on a single purpose for an individual user. Typically, single-use interventions are consumer-initiated and record vital measurements, training values, health behavior, medication and food intake [8,11]. In this way, pwMS use applications that focus on their disease. Patients can record their medication intake, subsequent consultations and disease-related vital signs to get an overview of their disease progression. It is also feasible to inform pwMS about the latest results and guidelines for different MS treatments and medications via single-use technologies or to remind them of appointments or medication intake [18,30,31].

The Multiple Sclerosis Centers of Excellence website (Veterans Health Administration; 2003) is such a single-use application for an eHealth intervention. It prepares caregivers for the special needs of MS and empowers patients to care for themselves by asking questions and providing guidelines on the website [32]. Self-managing MS is feasible with MS Energize (AUT Ventures, New Zealand; New Zealand; Kiwinet, New Zealand; MEA Mobile, Stuttgart, Germany; 2019) [33], MSCopilot (AD SCIENTIAM, Paris, France; 2019) [34], MS COMPASS++ (PEARS HEALTH CYBER, Czech Republic; 2015) [35], via digital diary [36], MS Invigor8 [37], Managing Fatigue [38], MS Sherpa (MS sherpa BV, Nijmegen, Netherlands; 2019) [39], MyMS&Me (Irody, Inc., Boston, MA, USA; 2020) [40] and other mobile applications [41]. Especially wireless and wearable devices are useful interventions to enhance rehabilitation in pwMS [26,42]. Functions of the autonomic nervous system, upper and lower limb functions, movement, cognition and other body functions can be permanently recorded with accelerometers, gyroscopes and glove-type monitors and thus provide a more precise overview of the disease [26]. Special offers such as Home-Based Tablet App for Dexterity Training (Swiss Multiple Sclerosis Society, Bayer AG; 2020) [43], the personalized mobile application WalkWithMe [44], the App for Dual-Task Assessment and Training Regarding Cognitive-Motor Interference (Novartis Pharma AG;; Swedisch PROMOBILIA foundation; Flemish MS Liga; 2016) [45] and additional eHealth interventions [46–52] offer exercises to reduce various disabilities.

3.2. Social eHealth Interventions

The availability of supporters can help chronically ill patients to face their daily challenges and improve their self-management in chronic diseases. Social eHealth interventions can provide social support from other users such as experts, physicians or other patients [8]. Social eHealth interventions enable these physically and cognitively impaired people to participate digitally in communities and stay "connected" with friends and family [53]. With the application of gamification, patients are encouraged and motivated to make greater use of eHealth interventions and achieve goals more easily [8]. Gamification is the application of game design elements such as rewards, challenges and competition, teamwork, point scoring and rankings [54].

Social media such as the BartsMS Blog, the SMsocialnetwork [26], PatientsLikeMe [55], the Overcoming Multiple Sclerosis [56] website and telemedicine support such as My Support Plus [57], ECHO [58], CareCall [59], Tele-MIT [60], Multiple Sclerosis at Home Access [61] and *Télé-SEP* [62] try to prevent misinformation, disseminate valid information and improve quality of care. Patients can talk about their illness or ask specialists for advice before their visit. The T-EDSS is a telephone-based Expanded Disability Status Scale) (EDSS) that simplifies communication for physicians and patients by eliminating the need to commute to health centers [63]. YouTube videos created by pwMS are used for communication (e.g., dealing with blindness or chronic illness in daily life) and education between patients [64]. However, patients should be careful as long as all information is not regularly checked for accuracy and correctness. In addition to online offers, gamification is a playful way to train physical and cognitive areas, even if it does not replace telerehabilitation [26]. To improve sensory strategies, pwMS can use gamification intervention such as Nintendo® Wii® Balance Board® (Nintendo, Kyoto, Japan), Xbox 360® (Microsoft, Redmond, WA, USA) and Kinect console (Microsoft, Redmond, WA, USA) [65,66], More Stamina [67] or BrainHQ® tool (PositScience, San Francisco, CA, USA) [68]. Visual feedback exercises can be used to train balance [69]. To improve functional outcomes, home-based physical telerehabilitation [15] or web-based telephone consultations like FACETS [70] have become a useful complement to standard interventions.

3.3. Integrated eHealth Interventions

Integrated eHealth interventions link patients with the healthcare system. Apps and websites are used to provide information exchange between healthcare providers, deliver video and image instructions to patients and encourage them speaking about their experience with the disease and the way they deal with it. This is an optimal way to prepare caregivers for the special requirements of MS [32]. It is also applied to remind participants to take medication and monitor their compliance, eating habits and emotional well-being. Furthermore, integrated eHealth is used to send educational and motivational messages or to provide feedback to patients and to support them in self-managing their chronic condition [8,11,32,53].

The web-based Mellen Center Care On-Line (MCCO) (Cleveland Clinic., Cleveland, OH, USA; 1998) [71] patient portal provides improved patient–physician communication, information about the disease through appropriate links and control over disease progression as well as future clinical visits [18]. Other integrated eHealth interventions that simplify and control clinical procedures or reduces costs and geographical barriers are "GP at Hand" (Babylon GP at Hand, London, UK; 2021), MS Mosaic (Duke Health and Duke University; 2004), Floodlight (Genentech, Inc., Basel, Switzerland; 2021), ElevateMS (Sage Bionetworks, Novartis Pharmaceuticals Corporation, Seattle, WA, USA; 2017), MSmonitor (TEVA Netherlands; 2014), PatientConcept (NeuroSys GmbH, Ulm, Germany; 2015), PatientSite (Beth Israel Deaconess Medical Center, Boston, MA, USA; 2000), [9,17,26,72,73] the Open MS BioScreen [74], MS PATHS (Biogen, Cambridge, UK; 2020) [75], MSProDiscuss (Adelphi Communications Ltd.; Novartis, London, UK; 2020) [76] and Multiple Sclerosis Documentation System (MSDS)^{3D} (MedicalSyn GmbH, Stuttgart, Germany; 2010) [77]. MSDS^{3D} can not only be used for the collection and interpretation of patient data, but also to monitor drug safety as well as for conveying information to the patient and to get a clinical opinion from an expert neurologist or radiologist via the expert advice tool of MSDS^{3D} [78,79].

3.4. Complex eHealth Interventions

Complex eHealth interventions have multiple components for interaction. They focus on the optimal management of a particular disease. Data, collected electronically by patient, physician or nurse, are analyzed by the system and used for the prognosis of the chronic disease. This enables the early recognition of critical events and correlations in social processes. Furthermore, the interpretation of complex data by the system enables a quick prediction of answers to various questions [80]. These systems increase safety and control the efficacy of MS therapies [26,27]. The next step for MSDS^{3D} will be the inclusion of specific management pathways. The implementation of such clinical pathways for disease monitoring or the treatment of symptomatic disabilities will enable data-driven standardized care and make it measurable and verifiable [81]. The quality of care can be assessed implementing guidelines [23] and pharmacoeconomic outcomes can be analyzed as well [82].

The Home Automated Tele management (HAT) system is such an intervention that analyzes patient self-testing results and reviews computer-generated alerts. It implements computerized decision support based on individualized alert setup and real-time monitoring of patient self-testing data. A personalized training plan with written descriptions and a video of the therapist performing the exercise is uploaded to a HAT home unit for each patient [83]. Another intervention is the MS SCDS toolkit that facilitates quality initiatives and ensures that care conforms to best practices. This toolkit supports initial and follow-up visits [84].

The Integrated Care Portal Multiple Sclerosis (IBMS) is an eHealth portal solution that is adapted to the clinical patterns of MS and associated patient needs to improve the overall diagnostic and therapeutic quality of care [85]. Therefore, IBMS is connected to the existing $MSDS^{3D}$ and enables fast and easy networking of all participating healthcare providers. Necessary medical diagnostic services such as magnetic resonance imaging (MRI) or laboratory examinations are accessible more quickly from any location. Therapeutic decisions are supported by experts and implemented efficiently and in accordance with guidelines. Information on examination results, previous illnesses or medication can be read into an electronic patient record that is accessed by different physicians any time so that they can quickly and purposefully consider interdisciplinary patient information for treatment (see Figure 3 for the basic concept of IBMS). Patients with difficult disease progression and complex care requirements can be assigned to the specialized setting of the University Hospital Dresden in order to guarantee the best possible care being tailored to their needs. Patients with less complex care needs can be treated locally by general practitioners or neurologists in private practices for routine presentations or information meetings. This efficient demand-oriented use of health services is intended to reduce the physician workload and treatment costs.

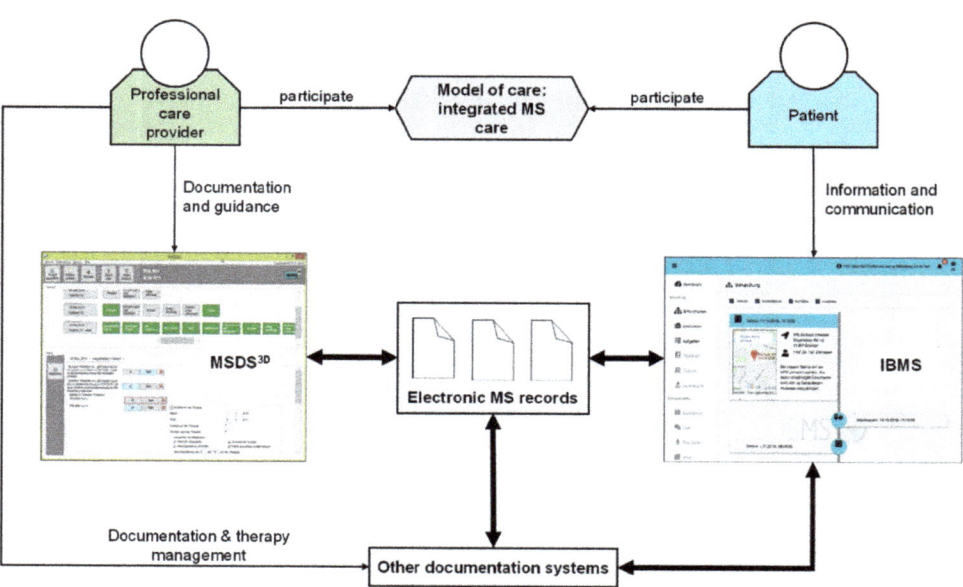

Figure 3. eHealth application of informal care, example of a basic concept, adapted from [85]. Multiple sclerosis (MS); Multiple Sclerosis Documentation System^{3D} (MSDS^{3D}); Integrated Care Portal Multiple Sclerosis (IBMS).

In addition to the integration of professional healthcare providers in the treatment of MS, IBMS has set itself the goal of improving the integration of patients and their families. Patients and their family (if requested by the patients) should also be able to view diagnostic results and other medically relevant data on their treatment in a comprehensible form. Moreover, pwMS and their family can receive recommendations for treatment based on the latest guidelines. In this way, the willingness of the family to participate in the coordination of patient care can be improved and the patients have a stronger involvement in their treatment management. Obstacles in treatment management are distance to healthcare, complex clinical patterns or job constraints. The use of modern information and communication technologies must make treatment as independent of time and place as possible in order to overcome such obstacles. This reduces not only job-related restrictions and the associated costs but also strengthens the mental resources of family members.

3.5. Success Factors of eHealth Interventions for pwMS

After looking through the existing landscape of eHealth interventions for pwMS, we identified general factors of success and failure that can influence the use of eHealth interventions. A key determinant of consumer acceptance and engagement with these programs is a high-quality user-centric design [36]. This includes the accommodation for varying physical and cognitive impairments and providing high-quality information, choice and control as part of overcoming practical challenges [87].

Visual deficits require a large font with large line spacing, low contrast to black letters on a white background, no color and no blinking effects for the interventions. Because of possible motor impairment, there must be an alternative for control beyond mouse or keyboard. One possibility would be the linguistic control or using only a few keyboard buttons. Cognitive limitations can be bypassed by creating an intuitive user interface [18]. To improve walking impairments and avoid comorbidities such as cardiovascular disease, eHealth interventions should enhance the physical activity [88].

In order to provide pervasive and patient-centered care, the design of interventions should be appropriate and tailored both for healthcare practitioner and for patients [10,11]. Individual counselling, group contacts and self-management also increase the use of eHealth applications [7,8,10].

Social support can increase empowerment and self-management skills and motivate chronically ill people like pwMS to search for health information online [7,8,89,90]. Furthermore, gaming-based systems such as the Nintendo® Wii® Fit console or Kinect motion sensor motivate patients to use eHealth applications [1,9]. The adaptation of digital self-monitoring tools to a patient's personal situation, guidance to increase the value of the data and integration of digital self-monitoring into treatment plans are features that can increase user acceptance [91]. The design of eHealth interventions must be tailored to different users and consider a wide range of aspects. Therefore, it is necessary to design flexible interfaces. Especially chronically ill patients like pwMS need an adaptive design for various symptoms. EHealth interventions are not only used for rehabilitation but also for preventing risk behaviors [1,4,8,9,53]. To meet all needs and demands of pwMS, healthcare professionals, researchers and industry partners must work together to develop effective eHealth solutions [92].

In addition to the design requirements and the consideration of different user perspectives, application support plays an important role in the uncomplicated implementation of interventions. A lack of knowledge about new technologies and programs by patients and even professional nurses makes it harder to use the applications without errors. Therefore, training on such technologies and programs for caregivers and patients is required in order to provide easy access and act in accordance with predefined protocols. Continuous data recording and user acceptance of an intervention can only be achieved if device and system errors as well as technical difficulties in uploading self-monitored data are avoided or promptly remedied. In order to ensure a legally secure consultation between patient and healthcare professional as well as sound patient management, an appropriate standard of care must be achieved [93–95]. This means, on the one hand, protecting electronic data from misuse and manipulation and, on the other hand, interconnecting different systems and making data transparent [24,96]. A major challenge remains to ensure interoperability between different types of systems and data sources [2]. The basis for successful data exchange between participating individuals is the assurance of standards for data protection and data security. Informations critical to the individual should only be collected, stored or disseminated following their guidelines. In this context, it must be transparently defined what kind of data are collected and how they are stored, who ultimately owns them, how the patient can access them, and who gets (partial) access to them [97]. Especially in industry-funded projects, different interests clash when it comes to who gets access to study data, as well as when and how. Significant progress has been made in this area in recent years, not the least due to the European General Data Protection Regulation. However, the more complex the scope and the larger the group of the addressed audience, the higher the requirements are for establishing a (multinational) eHealth project as well as those for monitoring compliance with existing regulations. In principle, integrated and complex eHealth interventions offer a more promising approach here as opposed to a plethora of individual apps, as a smaller number of bundled data protection processes enables a more careful examination of the respective conditions through the patient. Likewise, longer support times and more easily reachable responsible entities can be expected for data protection inquiries in larger projects [98].

4. Discussion

EHealth interventions are helpful tools to close the supply shortfall in the healthcare system and to improve the care of chronically ill patients because they can present the course of illness more comprehensively and more accurately than face-to-face visits. They are designed for various use cases and different users. On the one hand, individual health parameters of patients can be entered and interactions with physicians or other patients can take place. On the other hand, health systems are interconnected to exchange data, give feedback and receive optimal disease management. For the implementation of eHealth interventions, a number of requirements for various deficits in relation to different diseases must be considered. Well-designed interventions can provide relief to the patient and all other persons involved in the recovery process if the digital divide in chronic care can be minimized [24].

PwMS may be an ideal, trend-adopting group of eHealth users. There are already several eHealth interventions on the market for MS, specifically targeted to the impairments of the disease. One example is the MSDS^{3D}. A special feature of MSDS^{3D} is the focus on the management of individual DMTs, which ensures a comprehensive and safe treatment of the patient. The system also includes a module focusing on treatment satisfaction. Treatment satisfaction is an important factor for patient compliance and an indication of comorbidity; therefore, it should be added to any eHealth intervention directly [36]. Being connected to MSDS^{3D} via the IBMS portal, both physicians and patients are able to follow the course of disease exactly. In addition, patients and their family can exchange information with healtcare professionals via the platform and obtain the latest information.

Our research is not without limitations. In the present review, only those papers published in English or German in PubMed, Cochrane or Web of Science were included. This may have resulted in the omission of eHealth interventions from other databases, in other languages, without a product name or not (freely accessible) published commercial interventions of private companies. Our definition of eHealth has also led us not to include domains such as robotics. In this paper, we only presented various interventions and mentioned their positive aspects. However, we did focus only on the effect of eHealth interventions on treatment or patient management. It is to be determined whether eHealth interventions help to provide a better picture of disease status than standard interventions and whether these technologies are associated with improvements in long-term patient outcomes. It is important to know how effective the individual interventions are and to identify the most useful and cost-effective technology. This could increase acceptance of the use of eHealth interventions. However, the comparison of the interventions is difficult due to the differently used methods. In addition, long-term studies are necessary to determine the long-term effect of an intervention, but for cost reasons, this is rarely done. It would also be informative to know how interventions can assist the paradigm shift of healthcare from disease-focused to patient-centered and facilitate conducting pragmatic clinical trials.

Future research should focus on patients' self-monitoring to empower them in viewing and understanding their disease progression independently of the physician and in making self-determined decisions regarding treatment. For this, interventions should not only be able to display data and results in an easy-to-understand manner but should also enable specific treatment options for each outcome (e.g., specific exercises for foot drop; different medication options). An option to make appointments with specialists would complement the intervention. This all leads us to a system that combines all health-related aspects in a patient-centered eHealth approach.

Author Contributions: Conceptualization, M.S., R.H. and T.Z.; methodology, M.S.; writing—review and editing, M.S.; visualization, I.V.; supervision, D.S., R.H. and T.Z.; project administration, T.Z. All authors have read and agreed to the published version of the manuscript.

Funding This research received no external funding.

Acknowledgments: The MSDS^{3D} module development was supported by the Hertie Foundation, Novartis, Teva, Roche, Sanofi, Biogen and Merck. The BMS portal was supported by the University Hospital Carl Gustav Carus Dresden, the Technical University of Dresden, the MedicalSyn GmbH and the Carus Consilium GmbH, which cooperated in the project Integrated Care Portal Multiple Sclerosis. The implementation of the project is made possible by funding from the European Regional Development Fund (ERDF) and the Free State of Saxony.

Conflicts of Interest: T.Z. received personal compensation from Biogen, Bayer, Celgene, Novartis, Roche, Sanofi and Teva for consulting services and additional financial support for the research activities from Bayer, BAT, Biogen, Novartis, Teva and Sanofi. R.H. received personal compensation by Sanofi and travel grants by Celgene and Sanofi.

References

1. Ploeg, J.; Markle-Reid, M.; Valaitis, R.; McAiney, C.; Duggleby, W.; Bartholomew A.; Sherifali, D. Web-based interventions to improve mental health, general caregiving outcomes, and general health for informal caregivers of adults with chronic conditions living in the community: Rapid evidence review. *J. Med. Internet Res.* **2017**, *19*, e263. [CrossRef] [PubMed]
2. Gray, C.S.; Mercer, S.; Palen, T.; McKinstry, B.; Hendry, A. EHealth advances in support of people with complex care needs: Case examples from Canada, Scotland and the US. *Healthc. Q.* **2016**, *19*, 29–37. [CrossRef] [PubMed]
3. Eysenbach, G. What is e-health? *J. Med. Internet Res.* **2001**, *3*, E20. [CrossRef] [PubMed]
4. Barello, S.; Triberti, S.; Graffigna, G.; Libreri, C.; Serino, S.; Hibbard, J.; Riva, G. EHealth for patient engagement: A systematic review. *Front. Psychol.* **2015**, *6*, 2013. [CrossRef] [PubMed]
5. Oh, H.; Rizo, C.; Enkin, M.; Jadad, A. What is eHealth, (3): A systematic review of published definitions. *J. Med. Internet Res.* **2005**, *7*, e1. [CrossRef]
6. Saner, H.; van der Velde, E. eHealth in cardiovascular medicine: A clinical update. *Eur. J. Prev. Cardiol.* **2016**, *23*, 5–12. [CrossRef]
7. Vorderstrasse, A.; Lewinski, A.; Melkus, G.D.; Johnson, C. social support for diabetes self-management via eHealth interventions. *Curr. Diabetes Rep.* **2016**, *16*, 56. [CrossRef]
8. Allam, A.; Kostova, Z.; Nakamoto K.; Schulz, P.J. The effect of social support features and gamification on a Web-based intervention for rheumatoid arthritis patients: Randomized controlled trial. *J. Med. Internet Res.* **2015**, *17*, e14. [CrossRef]
9. Marziniak, M.; Brichetto, G.; Feys, P.; Meyding-Lamade, U.; Vernon, K.; Meuth, S.G. The use of digital and remote communication technologies as a tool for multiple sclerosis management: Narrative review. *JMIR Rehabil. Assist. Technol.* **2018**, *5*, e5. [CrossRef]
10. Conway, N.; Webster, C.; Smith, B.; Wake, D. eHealth and the use of individually tailored information: A systematic review. *Health Inform. J.* **2017**, *23*, 218–233.
11. Abaza, H.; Marschollek, M. mHealth application areas and technology combinations *. A comparison of literature from high and low/middle income countries. *Methods Inf. Med.* **2017**, *56*, e105–e122. [PubMed]
12. Wallin, E.E.; Mattsson, S.; Olsson, E.M. The preference for internet-based psychological interventions by individuals without past or current use of mental health treatment delivered online: A survey study with mixed-methods analysis. *JMIR Ment. Health* **2016**, *3*, e25. [CrossRef] [PubMed]
13. Browne, P.; Chandraratna, D.; Angood, C.; Tremlett, H.; Baker, C.; Taylor, B.V.; Thompson, A.J. Atlas of multiple sclerosis 2013 A growing global problem with widespread inequity. *Neurology* **2014**, *83*, 1022–1024. [CrossRef]
14. Goldenberg, M.M. Multiple sclerosis review. *P T Peer Rev. J. Formul. Manag.* **2012**, *37*, 175–184.

15. Khan, F.; Amatya, B.; Kesselring, J.; Galea, M. Telerehabilitation for persons with multiple sclerosis. *Cochrane Database Syst. Rev.* **2015**, *4*, CD010508. [CrossRef]
16. Vickrey, B.G.; Hays, R.D.; Harooni, R.; Myers, L.W.; Ellison, G.W. A health-related quality of life measure for multiple sclerosis. *Qual. Life Res. Int. J. Qual. Life Asp. Treat. Care Rehabil.* **1995**, *4*, 187–206. [CrossRef]
17. Nielsen, A.S.; Halamka, J.D.; Kinkel, R.P. Internet portal use in an academic multiple sclerosis center. *J. Am. Med. Inform. Assoc. JAMIA* **2012**, *19*, 128–133. [CrossRef]
18. Atreja, A.; Mehta, N.; Miller, D.; Moore, S.; Nichols, K.; Miller, H.; Harris, C.M. One size does not fit all: Using qualitative methods to inform the development of an Internet portal for multiple sclerosis patients. *AMIA Annu. Symp. Proc. AMIA Symp.* **2005**, *2005*, 16–20.
19. Haase, R.; Schultheiss, T.; Kempcke, R.; Thomas, K.; Ziemssen, T. Use and acceptance of electronic communication by patients with multiple sclerosis: A multicenter questionnaire study. *J. Med. Internet Res.* **2012**, *14*, e135. [CrossRef]
20. Leavitt, V.M.; Riley, C.S.; de Jager, P.L.; Bloom, S. eSupport: Feasibility trial of telehealth support group participation to reduce loneliness in multiple sclerosis. *Mult. Scler.* **2019**, *26*, 1797–1800. [CrossRef]
21. Prem, K.; Liu, Y.; Russell, T.W.; Kucharski, A.J.; Eggo, R.M.; Davies, N.; Jit, M.; Klepac, P. The effect of control strategies to reduce social mixing on outcomes of the COVID-19 epidemic in Wuhan, China: A modelling study. *Lancet Public Health* **2020**, *5*, e261–e270. [CrossRef]
22. Marrie, R.A.; Leung, S.; Tyry, T.; Cutter, G.R.; Fox, R.; Salter, A. Use of eHealth and mHealth technology by persons with multiple sclerosis. *Mult. Scler. Relat. Disord.* **2019**, *27*, 13–19. [CrossRef] [PubMed]
23. Hobart, J.; Bowen, A.; Pepper, G.; Crofts, H.; Eberhard, L.; Berger, T.; Boyko, A.; Boz, C.; Butzkueven, H.; Celius, E.G.; et al. International consensus on quality standards for brain health-focused care in multiple sclerosis. *Mult. Scler.* **2018**, *25*, 1809–1818. [CrossRef] [PubMed]
24. Gammon, D.; Berntsen, G.K.; Koricho, A.T.; Sygna, K.; Ruland, C. The chronic care model and technological research and innovation: A scoping review at the crossroads. *J. Med. Internet Res.* **2015**, *17*, e25. [CrossRef] [PubMed]
25. Weidemann, M.L.; Trentzsch, K.; Torp, C.; Ziemssen, T. Enhancing monitoring of disease progression-remote sensing in multiple sclerosis. *Nervenarzt* **2019**, *90*, 1239–1244. [CrossRef]
26. Lavorgna, L.; Brigo, F.; Moccia, M.; Leocani, L.; Lanzillo, R.; Clerico, M.; Abbadessa, G.; Schmierer, K.; Solaro, C.; Prosperini, L.; et al. e-Health and multiple sclerosis: An update. *Mult. Scler.* **2018**, *24*, 1657–1664. [CrossRef]
27. Matthews, P.M.; Block, V.J.; Leocani, L. E-health and multiple sclerosis. *Curr. Opin. Neurol.* **2020**, *33*, 271–276. [CrossRef]
28. Taylor, K. *Connected Health: How Digital Technology is Transforming Health and Social Care*; Deloitte Center for Health Solutions: London, UK, 2015.
29. Deloitte UK Center for Health Solutions. *Digital Health in the UK: An Industry Study for the Office of Life Sciences*; Deloitte Center for Health Solutions: London, UK, 2015.
30. Goodwin, R.A.; Lincoln, N.B.; das Nair, R.; Bateman, A. Evaluation of NeuroPage as a memory aid for people with multiple sclerosis: A randomised controlled trial. *Neuropsychol. Rehabil.* **2020**, *30*, 15–31. [CrossRef]
31. Settle, J.R.; Maloni, H.W.; Bedra, M.; Finkelstein, J.; Zhan, M.; Wallin, M.T. Monitoring medication adherence in multiple sclerosis using a novel web-based tool: A pilot study. *J. Telemed. Telecare* **2016**, *22*, 225–233. [CrossRef]
32. Hatzakis, M.J., Jr.; Allen, C.; Haselkorn, M.; Anderson, S.M.; Nichol, P.; Lai, C.; Haselkorn, J.K. Use of medical informatics for management of multiple sclerosis using a chronic-care model. *J. Rehabil. Res. Dev.* **2006**, *43*, 1–16. [CrossRef]
33. Babbage, D.R.; van Kessel, K.; Drown, J.; Thomas, S.; Sezier, A.; Thomas, P.; Kersten, P. MS energize: Field trial of an app for self-management of fatigue for people with multiple sclerosis. *Internet Interv.* **2019**, *18*, 100291. [CrossRef] [PubMed]
34. Maillart, E.; Labauge, P.; Cohen, M.; Maarouf, A.; Vukusic, S.; Donzé, C.; Gallien, P.; de Sèze, J.; Bourre, B.; Moreau, T.; et al. MSCopilot, a new multiple sclerosis self-assessment digital solution: Results of a comparative study versus standard tests. *Eur. J. Neurol.* **2020**, *27*, 429–436. [CrossRef] [PubMed]
35. MS COMPASS+, Pears Health Cyber's MS Compass+, Mobile Application at the Eyeforpharma Barcelona Awards. Available online: http://www.pearshealthcyber.com/wp-content/rskompas/index2.html (accessed on 21 December 2020).
36. Zettl, U.K.; Bauer-Steinhusen, U.; Glaser, T.; Hechenbichler, K.; Limmroth, V. Evaluation of an electronic diary for improvement of adherence to interferon beta-1b in patients with multiple sclerosis: Design and baseline results of an observational cohort study. *BMC Neurol.* **2013**, *13*, 117.
37. Moss-Morris, R.; McCrone, P.; Yardley, L.; van Kessel, K.; Wills, G.; Dennison, L. A pilot randomised controlled trial of an Internet-based cognitive behavioural therapy self-management programme, (MS Invigor8) for multiple sclerosis fatigue. *Behav. Res. Ther.* **2012**, *50*, 415–421. [CrossRef] [PubMed]
38. Plow, M.; Packer, T.; Mathiowetz, V.G.; Preissner, K.; Ghahari, S.; Sattar, A.; Bethoux, F.; Finlayson, M. REFRESH protocol: A non-inferiority randomised clinical trial comparing internet and teleconference to in-person 'Managing Fatigue' interventions on the impact of fatigue among persons with multiple sclerosis. *BMJ Open* **2020**, *10*, e035470.
39. Van Oirschot, P.; Heerings, M.; Wendrich, K.; den Teuling, B.; Martens, M.B.; Jongen, P.J. Symbol digit modalities test variant in a smartphone app for persons with multiple sclerosis: Validation study. *JMIR mHealth uHealth* **2020**, *8*, e18160. [CrossRef]
40. Golan, D.; Sagiv, S.; Glass-Marmor, L.; Miller, A. Mobile phone-based e-diary for assessment and enhancement of medications adherence among patients with multiple sclerosis. *Mult. Scler. J. Exp. Transl. Clin.* **2020**, *6*. [CrossRef]

41. Salimzadeh, Z.; Damanabi, S.; Kalankesh, L.R. Ferdousi, R. Mobile applications for multiple sclerosis: A Focus on self-management. *Acta Inform. Med.* **2019**, *27*, 12–18. [CrossRef]
42. Block, V.J.; Lizée, A.; Crabtree-Hartman, E.; Bevan, C.J.; Graves, J.S.; Bove, R.; Green, A.J.; Nourbakhsh, B.; Tremblay, M.; Gourraud, P.A.; et al. Continuous daily assessment of multiple sclerosis disability using remote step count monitoring. *J. Neurol.* **2017**, *264*, 316–326. [CrossRef]
43. Van Beek, J.J.W.; van Wegen, E.E.H.; Rietberg, M.B.; Nyffeler, T.; Bohlhalter, S.; Kamm, C.P.; Nef, T.; Vanbellingen, T. Feasibility of a home-based tablet app for dexterity training in multiple sclerosis: Usability study. *JMIR mHealth uHealth* **2020**, *8*, e18204. [CrossRef]
44. Van Geel, F.; Geurts, E.; Abasıyanık, Z.; Coninx, K.; Feys, P. Feasibility study of a 10-week community-based program using the WalkWithMe application on physical activity, walking, fatigue and cognition in persons with Multiple Sclerosis. *Mult. Scler. Relat. Disord.* **2020**, *42*, 102067. [CrossRef] [PubMed]
45. Tacchino, A.; Veldkamp, R.; Coninx, K.; Brulmans, J.; Palmaers, S.; Hämäläinen, P.; D'Hooge, M.; Vanzeir, E.; Kalron, A.; Brichetto, G.; et al. Design, development, and testing of an app for dual-task assessment and training regarding cognitive-motor interference, (CMI-APP) in people with multiple sclerosis: Multicenter pilot study. *JMIR mHealth uHealth* **2020**, *8*, e15344. [CrossRef] [PubMed]
46. Tallner, A.; Pfeifer, K.; Maurer, M. Web-based interventions in multiple sclerosis: The potential of tele-rehabilitation. *Ther. Adv. Neurol. Disord.* **2016**, *9*, 327–335. [CrossRef] [PubMed]
47. Fuchs, T.A.; Ziccardi, S.; Dwyer, M.G.; Charvet, L.E.; Bartnik, A.; Campbell, R.; Escobar, J.; Hojnacki, D.; Kolb, C.; Oship, D.; et al. Response heterogeneity to home-based restorative cognitive rehabilitation in multiple sclerosis: An exploratory study. *Mult. Scler. Relat. Disord.* **2019**, *34*, 103–111. [CrossRef] [PubMed]
48. Thirumalai, M.; Rimmer, J.H.; Johnson, G.; Wilroy, J.; Young, H.J.; Mehta, T.; Lai, B. TEAMS, (Tele-Exercise and Multiple Sclerosis), a tailored telerehabilitation mhealth app: Participant-centered development and usability study. *JMIR mHealth uHealth* **2018**, *6*, e10181. [CrossRef]
49. Casey, B.; Coote, S.; Byrne, M. Activity matters: A web-based resource to enable people with multiple sclerosis to become more active. *Transl. Behav. Med.* **2019**, *9*, 120–128. [CrossRef]
50. Tacchino, A.; Pedullà, L.; Bonzano, L.; Vassallo, C.; Battaglia, M.A.; Mancardi, G.; Bove, M.; Brichetto, G. A new app for at-home cognitive training: Description and pilot testing on patients with multiple sclerosis. *JMIR mHealth uHealth* **2015**, *3*, e85. [CrossRef]
51. Silveira, S.L.; McCroskey, J.; Wingo, B.C.; Motl, R.W. eHealth-based behavioral intervention for increasing physical activity in persons with multiple sclerosis: Fidelity protocol for a randomized controlled trial *JMIR Res. Protoc.* **2019**, *8*, e12319. [CrossRef]
52. D'Hooghe, M.; van Gassen, G.; Kos, D.; Bouquiaux, O.; Cambron, M.; Decoo, D.; Lysandropoulos, A.; van Wijmeersch, B.; Willekens, B.; Penner, I.K.; et al. Improving fatigue in multiple sclerosis by smartphone-supported energy management: The MS TeleCoach feasibility study. *Mult. Scler. Relat. Disord.* **2018**, *22*, 90–96. [CrossRef]
53. Agbakoba, R.; McGee-Lennon, M.; Bouamrane, M.M.; Watson, N.; Mair, F. Implementing a national scottish digital health & wellbeing service at scale: A qualitative study of stakeholders' views. *Stud. Health Technol. Inform.* **2015**, *216*, 487–491.
54. Edney, S.; Plotnikoff, R.; Vandelanotte, C.; Olds, T.; De Bourdeaudhuij, I.; Ryan, J.; Maher, C. "Active Team" a social and gamified app-based physical activity intervention: Randomised controlled trial study protocol. *BMC Public Health* **2017**, *17*, 859. [CrossRef] [PubMed]
55. Chiauzzi, E.; Hekler, E.B.; Lee, J.; Towner, A.; DasMahapatra, P.; Fitz-Randolph, M. In search of a daily physical activity "sweet spot": Piloting a digital tracking intervention for people with multiple sclerosis. *Digit. Health* **2019**, *5*. [CrossRef] [PubMed]
56. O'Donnell, J.M.; Jelinek, G.A.; Gray, K.M.; de Livera, A.; Brown, C.R.; Neate, S.L.; O'Kearney, E.L.; Taylor, K.L.; Bevens, W.; Weiland, T.J. Therapeutic utilization of meditation resources by people with multiple sclerosis: Insights from an online patient discussion forum. *Inform. Health Soc Care* **2020**, *45*, 374–384. [CrossRef] [PubMed]
57. Landtblom, A.M.; Guala, D.; Martin, C.; Olsson-Hau, S.; Haghighi, S.; Jansson, L. Fredrikson, S. RebiQoL: A randomized trial of telemedicine patient support program for health-related quality of life and adherence in people with MS treated with Rebif. *PLoS ONE* **2019**, *14*, e0218453. [CrossRef]
58. Johnson, K.L.; Hertz, D.; Stobbe, G.; Alschuler, K.; Kalb, R.; Alexander, K.S.; Kraft, G.H.; Scott, J.D. Project extension for community healthcare outcomes, (ECHO) in multiple sclerosis: Increasing clinician capacity. *Int. J. MS Care* **2017**, *19*, 283–289. [CrossRef]
59. Mercier, H.W.; Ni, P.; Houlihan, B.V.; Jette, A.M. Differential impact and use of a telehealth intervention by persons with MS or SCI. *Am. J. Phys. Med. Rehabil.* **2015**, *94*, 987–999. [CrossRef]
60. Kahraman, T.; Savci, S.; Ozdogar, A.T.; Gedik, Z.; Idiman, E. Physical, cognitive and psychosocial effects of telerehabilitation-based motor imagery training in people with multiple sclerosis: A randomized controlled pilot trial. *J. Telemed. Telecare* **2020**, *26*, 251–260. [CrossRef]
61. Healey, K.; Zabad, R.; Young, L.; Lindner, A.; Lenz, N.; Stewart, R.; Charlton, M. Multiple sclerosis at home access, (MAHA): An initiative to improve care in the community. *Int. J. MS Care* **2019**, *21*, 101–112. [CrossRef]
62. Derache, N.; Hauchard, K.; Seguin, F.; Ohannessian, R.; Defer, G. Retrospective evaluation of regional telemedicine team meetings for multiple sclerosis, (MS) patients: Experience from the Caen MS expert center in Normandy, France. *Rev. Neurol.* **2020**. [CrossRef]
63. Syed, M.J.; Shah, Z.; Awan, S.; Wasay, M.; Fredrikson, S. Telephone validation of an Urdu translated version of the extended disability severity scale in multiple sclerosis patients. *Mult. Scler. Relat. Disord.* **2020**, *48*, 102684.

64. Fernandez-Luque, L.; Elahi, N.; Grajales, F.J., 3rd. An analysis of personal medical information disclosed in YouTube videos created by patients with multiple sclerosis. *Stud. Health Technol. Inform.* **2009**, *150*, 292–296. [PubMed]
65. Ortiz-Gutiérrez, R.; Cano-de-la-Cuerda, R.; Galán-del-Río, F.; Alguacil-Diego, I.M.; Palacios-Ceña, D.; Miangolarra-Page, J.C. A telerehabilitation program improves postural control in multiple sclerosis patients: A Spanish preliminary study. *Int. J. Environ. Res. Public Health* **2013**, *10*, 5697–5710. [CrossRef] [PubMed]
66. Gutiérrez, R.O.; del Río, F.G.; de la Cuerda, R.C.; Diego, I.M.A.; González, R.A.; Page, J.C. A telerehabilitation program by virtual reality-video games improves balance and postural control in multiple sclerosis patients. *NeuroRehabilitation* **2013**, *33*, 545–554. [CrossRef] [PubMed]
67. Giunti, G.; Rivera-Romero, O.; Kool, J.; Bansi, J.; Sevillano, J.L.; Granja-Dominguez, A.; Izquierdo-Ayuso, G.; Giunta, D. Evaluation of more stamina, a mobile app for fatigue management in persons with multiple sclerosis: Protocol for a feasibility, acceptability, and usability study. *JMIR Res. Protoc.* **2020**, *9*, e18196. [CrossRef]
68. Bove, R.M.; Rush, G.; Zhao, C.; Rowles, W.; Garcha, P.; Morrissey, J.; Schembri, A.; Alailima, T.; Langdon, D.; Possin, K.; et al. A videogame-based digital therapeutic to improve processing speed in people with multiple sclerosis: A feasibility study. *Neurol. Ther.* **2019**, *8*, 135–145. [CrossRef]
69. Brichetto, G.; Spallarossa, P.; de Carvalho, M.L.; Battaglia, M.A. The effect of Nintendo(R) Wii(R) on balance in people with multiple sclerosis: A pilot randomized control study. *Mult. Scler.* **2013**, *19*, 1219–1221. [CrossRef]
70. Thomas, S.; Pulman, A.; Thomas, P.; Collard, S.; Jiang, N.; Dogan, H.; Smith, A.D.; Hourihan, S.; Roberts, F.; Kersten, P.; et al. Digitizing a face-to-face group fatigue management program: Exploring the views of people with multiple sclerosis and health care professionals via consultation groups and interviews. *JMIR Form. Res.* **2019**, *3*, e10951. [CrossRef]
71. Miller, D.M.; Moore, S.M.; Fox, R.J.; Atreja, A.; Fu, A.Z.; Lee, J.C.; Saupe, W.; Stadtler, M.; Chakraborty, S.; Harris, C.M.; et al. Web-based self-management for patients with multiple sclerosis: A practical, randomized trial. *Telemed. J. E-health Off. J. Am. Telemed. Assoc.* **2011**, *17*, 5–13. [CrossRef]
72. Jongen, P.J.; Sinnige, L.G.; van Geel, B.M.; Verheul, F.; Verhagen, W.I.; van der Kruijk, R.A.; Haverkamp, R.; Schrijver, H.M.; Baart, J.C.; Visser, L.H.; et al. The interactive web-based program MSmonitor for self-management and multidisciplinary care in multiple sclerosis: Concept, content, and pilot results. *Patient Prefer. Adherence* **2015**, *9*, 1741–1750. [CrossRef]
73. Lang, M.; Mayr, M.; Ringbauer, S.; Cepek, L. PatientConcept app: Key characteristics, implementation, and its potential benefit. *Neurol. Ther.* **2019**, *8*, 147–154. [CrossRef]
74. Schleimer, E.; Pearce, J.; Barnecut, A.; Rowles, W.; Lizee, A.; Klein, A.; Block, V.J.; Santaniello, A.; Renschen, A.; Gomez, R.; et al. A precision medicine tool for patients with multiple sclerosis, (the open MS BioScreen): Human-centered design and development. *J. Med. Internet Res.* **2020**, *22*, e15605. [CrossRef] [PubMed]
75. Mowry, E.M.; Bermel, R.A.; Williams, J.R.; Benzinger, T.L.S.; de Moor, C.; Fisher, E.; Hersh, C.M.; Hyland, M.H.; Izbudak, I.; Jones, S.E.; et al. Harnessing real-world data to inform decision-making: Multiple sclerosis partners advancing technology and health solutions, (MS PATHS). *Front. Neurol.* **2020**, *11*, 632. [CrossRef] [PubMed]
76. Ziemssen, T.; Piani-Meier, D.; Bennett, B.; Johnson, C.; Tinsley, K.; Trigg, A.; Hach, T.; Dahlke, F.; Tomic, D.; Tolley, C.; et al. A physician-completed digital tool for evaluating disease progression, (multiple sclerosis progression discussion tool): Validation study. *J. Med. Internet Res.* **2020**, *22*, e16932. [CrossRef] [PubMed]
77. Ziemssen, T.; Kempcke, R.; Eulitz, M.; Grossmann, L.; Suhrbier, A.; Thomas, K.; Schultheiss, T. Multiple sclerosis documentation system, (MSDS): Moving from documentation to management of MS patients. *J. Neural Transm.* **2013**, *120*, S61–S66. [CrossRef] [PubMed]
78. Haase, R.; Wunderlich, M.; Dillenseger, A.; Kern, R.; Akgun, K.; Ziemssen, T. Improving multiple sclerosis management and collecting safety information in the real world: The MSDS3D software approach. *Expert Opin. Drug Saf.* **2018**, *17*, 369–378. [CrossRef]
79. Chang, C.H. Patient-reported outcomes measurement and management with innovative methodologies and technologies. *Qual. Life Res.* **2007**, *16*, 157–166. [CrossRef]
80. Coorey, G.M.; Neubeck, L.; Usherwood, T.; Peiris, D.; Parker, S.; Lau, A.Y.; Chow, C.; Panaretto, K.; Harris, M.; Zwar, N.; et al. Implementation of a consumer-focused eHealth intervention for people with moderate-to-high cardiovascular disease risk: Protocol for a mixed-methods process evaluation. *BMJ Open* **2017**, *7*, e014353. [CrossRef]
81. Ziemssen, T.; Kern, R.; Voigt, I.; Haase, R. Data collection in multiple sclerosis: The MSDS approach. *Front. Neurol.* **2020**, *11*, 445. [CrossRef]
82. Ness, N.-H.; Haase, R.; Kern, R.; Schriefer, D.; Ettle, B.; Cornelissen, C.; Akguen, K.; Ziemssen, T. The multiple sclerosis health resource utilization survey, (MS-HRS): Development and validation study. *J. Med. Internet Res.* **2020**, *22*, e17921. [CrossRef]
83. Finkelstein, J.; Lapshin, O.; Castro, H.; Cha, E.; Provance, P.G. Home-based physical telerehabilitation in patients with multiple sclerosis: A pilot study. *J. Rehabil. Res. Dev.* **2008**, *45*, 1361–1373. [CrossRef]
84. Claire Simon, K.; Hentati, A.; Rubin, S.; Franada, T.; Maurer, D.; Hillman, L.; Tideman, S.; Szela, M.; Meyers, S.; Frigerio, R.; et al. Successful utilization of the EMR in a multiple sclerosis clinic to support quality improvement and research initiatives at the point of care. *Mult. Scler. J. Exp. Transl. Clin.* **2018**, *4*. [CrossRef] [PubMed]
85. Voigt, I.; Benedict, M.; Susky, M.; Scheplitz, T.; Frankowitz, S.; Kern, R.; Müller, O.; Schlieter, H.; Ziemssen, T. A digital patient portal for patients with multiple sclerosis. *Front. Neurol.* **2020**, *11*, 400. [CrossRef] [PubMed]

86. De Vito Dabbs, A.; Myers, B.A.; Mc Curry, K.R.; Dunbar-Jacob, J.; Hawkins, R.P.; Begey, A.; Dew, M.A. User-centered design and interactive health technologies for patients. *Comput. Inform. Nurs.* **2009**, *27*, 175–183. [CrossRef] [PubMed]
87. Giunti, G.; Kool, J.; Rivera Romero, O.; Dorronzoro Zubiete, E. Exploring the specific needs of persons with multiple sclerosis for mhealth solutions for physical activity: Mixed-methods study. *JMIR mHealth uHealth* **2018**, *6*, e37. [CrossRef]
88. Dlugonski, D.; Motl, R.W.; Mohr, D.C.; Sandroff, B.M. Internet-delivered behavioral intervention to increase physical activity in persons with multiple sclerosis: Sustainability and secondary outcomes. *Psychol. Health Med.* **2012**, *17*, 636–651. [CrossRef]
89. Lee, K.; Hoti, K.; Hughes, J.D.; Emmerton, L. Dr Google and the consumer: A qualitative study exploring the navigational needs and online health information-seeking behaviors of consumers with chronic health conditions. *J. Med. Internet Res.* **2014**, *16*, e262. [CrossRef]
90. Tonheim, A.N.; Babic, A. Assessing information needs for a personal multiple sclerosis application. *Stud. Health Technol. Inform.* **2018**, *247*, 486–490.
91. Wendrich, K.; van Oirschot, P.; Martens, M.B.; Heerings, M.; Jongen, P.J.; Krabbenborg, L. Toward digital self-monitoring of multiple sclerosis: Investigating first experiences, needs, and wishes of people with MS. *Int. J. MS Care* **2019**, *21*, 282–291. [CrossRef]
92. Giunti, G.; Fernández, E.G.; Zubiete, E.D.; Romero, O.R. Supply and demand in mhealth apps for persons with multiple sclerosis: Systematic search in app stores and scoping literature review. *JMIR mHealth uHealth* **2018**, *6*, e10512. [CrossRef]
93. Frielitz, F.S.; Storm, N.; Hiort, O.; Katalinic, A.; von Sengbusch, S. The creation of a data protection policy: A guide to telemedicine healthcare projects. *Bundesgesundheitsblatt Gesundh. Gesundh.* **2019**, *62*, 479–485. [CrossRef]
94. Garska, H. Data protection in telemedicine. *Hautarzt Z. Dermatol. Venerol. Verwandte Geb.* **2019**, *70*, 343–345. [CrossRef] [PubMed]
95. Alaqra, A.S.; Fischer-Hubner, S.; Framner, E. Enhancing privacy controls for patients via a selective authentic electronic health record exchange service: Qualitative study of perspectives by medical professionals and patients. *J. Med. Internet Res.* **2018**, *20*, e10954. [CrossRef] [PubMed]
96. McGillion, M.; Yost, J.; Turner, A.; Bender, D.; Scott, T.; Carroll, S.; Ritvo, P.; Peter, E.; Lamy, A.; Furze, G.; et al. Technology-enabled remote monitoring and self-management—Vision for patient empowerment following cardiac and vascular surgery: User testing and randomized controlled trial protocol. *JMIR Res. Protoc.* **2016**, *5*, e149. [CrossRef] [PubMed]
97. Meingast, M.; Roosta, T.; Sastry, S. Security and privacy issues with health care information technology. *Conf. Proc. IEEE Eng. Med. Biol. Soc.* **2006**, *2006*, 5453–5458.
98. Kern, R.; Haase, R.; Eisele, J.C.; Thomas, K.; Ziemssen, T. Designing an electronic patient management system for multiple sclerosis: Building a next generation multiple sclerosis documentation system. *Interact. J. Med. Res.* **2016**, *5*, e2. [CrossRef]

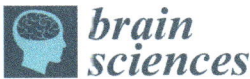

Systematic Review

Is mHealth a Useful Tool for Self-Assessment and Rehabilitation of People with Multiple Sclerosis? A Systematic Review

Bruno Bonnechère [1,*], Aki Rintala [2], Annemie Spooren [1], Ilse Lamers [1,3] and Peter Feys [1,3]

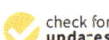

Citation: Bonnechère, B.; Rintala, A.; Spooren, A.; Lamers, I.; Feys, P. Is mHealth a Useful Tool for Self-Assessment and Rehabilitation of People with Multiple Sclerosis? A Systematic Review. *Brain Sci.* 2021, *11*, 1187. https://doi.org/10.3390/brainsci11091187

Academic Editor: Lorenzo Priano

Received: 28 July 2021
Accepted: 2 September 2021
Published: 9 September 2021

Publisher's Note: MDPI stays neutral with regard to jurisdictional claims in published maps and institutional affiliations.

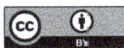

Copyright: © 2021 by the authors. Licensee MDPI, Basel, Switzerland. This article is an open access article distributed under the terms and conditions of the Creative Commons Attribution (CC BY) license (https://creativecommons.org/licenses/by/4.0/).

1. REVAL-Rehabilitation Research Center, Faculty of Rehabilitation Sciences, Hasselt University, B-3590 Diepenbeek, Belgium; annemie.spooren@uhasselt.be (A.S.); ilse.lamers@uhasselt.be (I.L.); peter.feys@uhasselt.be (P.F.)
2. Faculty of Social Services and Health Care, LAB University of Applied Sciences, FI-15210 Lahti, Finland; aki.rintala@lab.fi
3. University MS Center Hasselt-Pelt, B-3500 Hasselt, Belgium
*   Correspondence: bruno.bonnechere@uhasselt.be

Abstract: The development of mobile technology and mobile Internet offers new possibilities in rehabilitation and clinical assessment in a longitudinal perspective for multiple sclerosis management. However, because the mobile health applications (mHealth) have only been developed recently, the level of evidence supporting the use of mHealth in people with multiple sclerosis (pwMS) is currently unclear. Therefore, this review aims to list and describe the different mHealth available for rehabilitation and self-assessment of pwMS and to define the level of evidence supporting these interventions for functioning problems categorized within the International Classification of Functioning, Disability and Health (ICF). In total, 36 studies, performed with 22 different mHealth, were included in this review, 30 about rehabilitation and six for self-assessment, representing 3091 patients. For rehabilitation, most of the studies were focusing on cognitive function and fatigue. Concerning the efficacy, we found a small but significant effect of the use of mHealth for cognitive training (Standardized Mean Difference (SMD) = 0.28 [0.12; 0.45]) and moderate effect for fatigue (SMD = 0.61 [0.47; 0.76]). mHealth is a promising tool in pwMS but more studies are needed to validate these solutions in the other ICF categories. More replications studies are also needed as most of the mHealth have only been assessed in one single study.

Keywords: mHealth; multiple sclerosis; telemonitoring; longitudinal assessment; rehabilitation; fatigue; walking; cognition

1. Introduction

People with Multiple Sclerosis (pwMS) may manifest heterogeneous symptoms and functioning problems that require continuous and long-term rehabilitation programs in clinical and community settings across the disability spectrum. In high-income countries, the pressure on healthcare systems is increasing [1] and the continuity of high-level care is threatened due to lack of reimbursement, while in some countries access to the specialized MS centers has always been poor [2]. Furthermore, a vast majority of pwMS often present fatigue, emotional or cognitive dysfunction, or restricted physical mobility or a combination of those which limits access to rehabilitation centers. In this context, the WHO stated that lack of access to specialized centers or healthcare professionals is one of the most important limitations for the rehabilitation process [3]. The use of mobile technologies and electronic health (eHealth) could be an alternative to tackle the above-mentioned limitations (i.e., lack of access to centers) of rehabilitation of pwMS or complement current rehabilitation services. eHealth is also expected to facilitate the monitoring of functioning of pwMS between medical consultations, which is informative to define whether to continue or adapt medical treatment.

The number of healthcare interventions delivered via personal mobile devices (mHealth) has increased exponentially thanks to the availability of mobile technology (the number of smartphone subscriptions worldwide today surpasses six billion and is forecast to further grow by several hundred million in the next few years [4]). The development and implementation of mHealth open new perspectives and opportunities in the healthcare sector. Previous studies highlighted that mHealth has already been accepted by patients. Amongst the most important benefits identified by the patients are easy access to personalized information, convenience, better information on their health, and the ability to communicate more easily with healthcare professionals [5,6]. So far, most studies have focused on patients with cancer [7–9], patients with cardiovascular diseases [10,11], or older adults with [12] or without cognitive impairment [13].

Concerning pwMS, a meta-analysis showed that technology-based distance physical rehabilitation intervention has a positive effect on physical activity and walking ability when compared to usual care or no intervention [14]. Another review synthesized the different eHealth technologies that are available for the management of pwMS [15]. eHealth is a broader term than mHealth; eHealth is composed of the electronic records, self-remote disease monitoring (i.e., blood markers, vital signs), mobile and wired communication for advice and education, and tools to facilitate self-management (i.e., physical activity tracker, rehabilitation exercises reminder or calendar). This previous review was published in 2018 and given the important development of technology-supported rehabilitation tools a lot of new solutions have been developed. Furthermore, there is currently a lack of information about the different mHealth currently available, and the level of evidence supporting them, in pwMS.

Therefore, the aim of this paper is first to describe the different mHealth applications currently available to assist the rehabilitation of pwMS and the tools that exist to perform longitudinal self-assessment of the patients. The second aim of this review is to determine the level of evidence supporting the use of mHealth in pwMS on their functioning according to the International Classification of Functioning, Disability, and Health (ICF).

2. Methods

2.1. Search Strategy and Selection Criteria

Records were searched on three databases (Pubmed, Biber, and Scopus) to identify eligible studies published between 2011 (after the release of the first generation of iPad, which was an important step in the development of mobile applications) and June 2021. MeSH terms and free words referring to e-health intervention in pwMS ('multiple sclerosis', 'ms', 'ehealth', 'mhealth', 'mobile apps, smartphone intervention', 'apps', 'self-monitoring', 'self-assessment', 'functioning', 'intervention', 'rehabilitation') were used as keywords. The complete search strategy is presented in Table S1.

2.2. Eligibility Criteria

A PICOs approach was used as inclusion and exclusion criteria, which were assessed by the study team [16].

- **Population**: pwMS performing training (rehabilitation exercises) or self-assessment in home-environment, studies with inpatient treatment or assisted-rehabilitation were not included.
- **Intervention**: mHealth rehabilitation intervention (planned and supervised interventions), or self-assessment studies with repeated measurements over time, using any type of support (e.g., smartphones, phones, apps, web applications). Studies using non-specific games, virtual reality or active video games (e.g., Nintendo Wii, Microsoft Xbox Kinect), or computer-supported therapy were not included.
- **Control**: usual care or no intervention.
- **Outcome measures**: any type of outcome measure related to the International Classification of Functioning, Disability and Health (ICF).
- **Study design**: RCTs, explorative studies.

A flow diagram of the study selection with the screened articles and the selection process is presented in Figure 1.

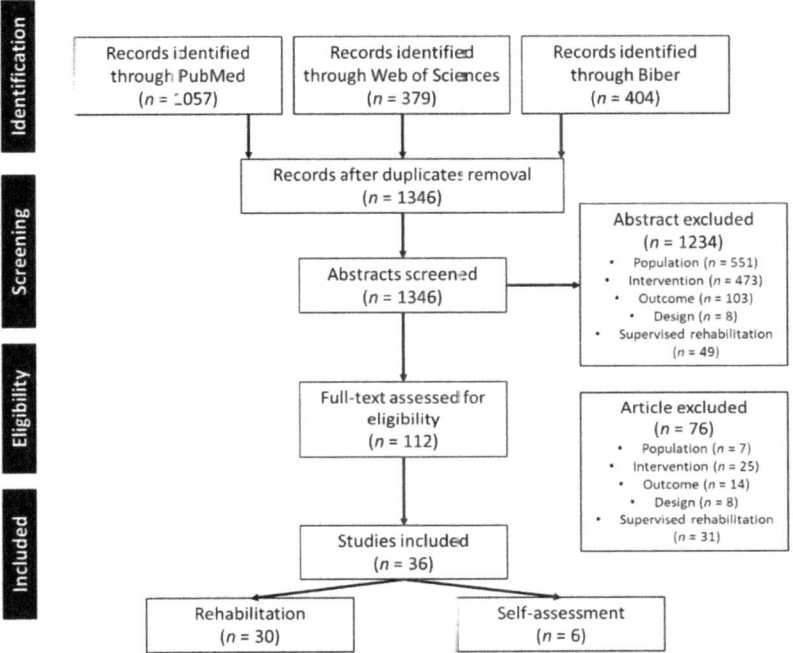

Figure 1. Flowchart of study selection.

2.3. Quality Assessment

Since we included different types of articles, the critical appraisal of the methodological quality was based on the Downs and Black checklist [17], as this checklist is the best option to assess the quality and risk of bias for both RCT and non-RCT [18].

2.4. Data Extraction

The following information was extracted from the included studies: characteristics of the patients (age, sex ratio, type of MS and severity), type and duration of the mHealth intervention, study design, main outcomes, and ICF domains evaluated.

2.5. Statistical Analysis

For studies assessing the efficacy of a rehabilitation program, we performed a meta-analysis. The measure of treatment effect was the standardized mean difference effect size (standardized mean difference (SMD)), defined as the between-group difference in mean values divided by the pooled SD computed using the Hedge's g method ($Hedges'g = \frac{M_1 - M_2}{SD_{pooled}}$). If different tests were used to assess the same ICF domains in the same study, the different results were pooled to have one unique SMD as recommended by Cochrane's group [19]. A positive SMD implies better therapeutic effects in the intervention group compared to the control. We assessed the heterogeneity in stratified analyses by type of ICF domains. We calculated the variance estimate tau^2 as a measure of between-trial heterogeneity. We prespecified a tau^2 of 0.0 to represent no heterogeneity, 0.0–0.2 to represent low heterogeneity, 0.2–0.4 to represent moderate heterogeneity, and above 0.4 to represent high heterogeneity between trials [20]. To deal with high or moderate heterogeneity we used random-effect models and presented forest plots for the different ICF domains. We checked for publication bias using funnel plot [21] and Egger's test for the intercept was applied to check the asymmetry [22].

2.6. Ethical Approval

This systematic review was reported following the Preferred Reporting Items for Systematic Reviews and Meta-Analyses (PRISMA) recommendations [23]. For the present study, no ethics committee approval was necessary.

3. Results

For the sake of clarity, this section has been divided into three different parts; first, we will present the characteristics of the included studies and the patients; then we will describe the different mHealth used in these studies and finally, we will present the clinical efficacy for the different domains in the ICF.

3.1. Search Results

In total, 1346 articles were found with the systematic review. A total of 112 full-text articles were assessed and 36 papers were included in the analysis. The PRISMA flowchart on the study selection is presented in Figure 1.

3.2. Characteristics of the Included Studies

Thirty studies about the use of mHealth for rehabilitation interventions of pwMS were included in this review, representing a total of 1962 patients [24–53]. The majority of these studies ($n = 25; 3\%$) were RCTs. Concerning the patients, the majority of the patients were female ($76 \pm 10\%$); concerning the type of MS the majority of the included patients (79%) have relapsing-remitting multiple sclerosis (RRMS), 16% have secondary progressive multiple sclerosis (SPMS) and 5% primary progressive multiple sclerosis (PPMS), and the average EDSS is 3.5 ± 1.1. The median duration of the intervention was 9 weeks [p25 = 8 weeks, p75 = 12 weeks] for a median time of 18 h [p25 = 13.25 h, p75 = 27 h]. Finally, for the ICF, 16 (53%) of the studies reported outcomes related to cognition, 11 (37%) to fatigue, 10 (33%) to quality of life, 7 (23%) on motor function, and 6 (20%) on activity level; we observed that most of the studies are assessing different primary outcomes (ICF domains). The complete description of the included studies is presented in Table 1. Amongst the 30 studies, 16 different mHealth apps have been tested.

Concerning the self-assessment tools six studies, using six different mHealth applications, were included in the review, representing 1129 participants (955 pwMS [88% with RRMS, 5% with SPMS and 7% with PPMS, average EDSS 2.5 ± 0.5] and 174 healthy participants) [54–59]. The median duration of the follow-up was 12 weeks [p25 = 6 weeks, p75 = 24 weeks].

The characteristics of the studies and participants are summarized in Table 2.

Table 1. Characteristics of the included studies (study design, mean duration on the intervention, targeted ICF function) on mHealth for rehabilitation and description of the participants.

Study	D&B (/28)	Study Design	Intervention	Duration	Participants	Type of MS and Disability Level	ICF Motor Function	Activity Level	Cognition	Fatigue	Quality of Life
Cerasa et al., 2013 [24]	23	RCT	RehaCom	6 weeks of training (2 × 60 min/week)	17 MS patients 33 (4) years old 85% female	RRMS: 17 EDSS: 3 (0; 4.0)			X	X	
Amato et al., 2014 [25]	21	RCT	Attention Processing Training Program (APT)	12 weeks of training (2 × 60 min/week)	88 MS patients 41 (11) years old 78% female	Type not available EDSS: 2.7 (1.5)			X		
Charvet et al., 2015 [26]	24	RCT	Luminosity	12 weeks of training (5 × 30 min/week)	20 MS patients 40 (8) years old 70% female	RRMS: 20 EDSS: 2 (0; 3.5)			X		
Hancock et al., 2015 [27]	22	RCT	Posit Science inSight (now BrainHQ)	6 weeks of training (6 × 30 min/week)	40 MS patients 50 (6) years old	Type and EDSS not available			X		
Hubacher et al., 2015 [28]	24	RCT	BrainStim	4 weeks of training (4 × 45 min/week)	10 MS patients 46 (7) years old 50% female	RRMS: 10 EDSS: 2 (1.0; 3.5)			X		
Fischer et al., 2015 [29]	23	RCT	Deprexis	9 weeks of training	90 MS patients 45 (12) years old 78% female	RRMS: 40, SPMS: 21, PPMS: 14, unclear: 18					X
Campbell et al., 2016 [30]	22	RCT	RehaCom	6 weeks of training (3 × 45 min/week)	35 MS patients 47 (8) years old 71% female	RRMS: 27, SPMS: 11 EDSS: 5.0 (3.5; 6.0)			X		
Pedulla et al., 2016 [31]	24	RCT	COGNI-TRAcK	8 weeks of training (5 × 30 min/week)	28 MS patients 47 (6) years old 71% female	RRMS: 17, SPMS: 11 EDSS: 3.8 (1.9)			X		
Charvet et al., 2017 [32]	23	RCT	BrainHQ	12 weeks of training (5 × 60 min/week)	135 MS patients 51 (13) years old 77% female	RRMS: 89, SPMS: 35, PPMS: 7, EDSS: 3.5 (2.5; 4.5)			X		

Table 1. Cont.

Study	D&B (/28)	Study Design	Intervention	Duration	Participants	Type of MS and Disability Level	ICF Motor Function	ICF Activity Level	ICF Cognition	ICF Fatigue	Quality of Life
Messinis et al., 2017 [33]	23	RCT	RehaCom	10 weeks of training (2 × 60 min/week)	58 MS patients 46 (10) years old 69% female	RRMS: 58 EDSS: 3.2 (1.0; 5.5)			X	X	
Conroy et al., 2018 [34]	23	RCT	MS HAT system	6 months of intervention Self-paced rehabilitation	54 MS patients 50 (12) years old 77% female	RRMS: 14, SPMS: 35, PPMS: 2 PDSS: 4.1 (1.5)	X	X			
Stuifbergen et al., 2018 [35]	22	RCT	MAPSS-MS	8 weeks of training 2 h/week group session + 3 × 45 min/week home-based training program	183 MS patients 50 (8) years old 87% female	RRMS: 124 EDSS 5.2 (1.6)			X		X
Fjeldstad-Pardo et al., 2018 [36]	21	RCT	CG: exercise sheet tIG: telerehabilitation aIG: in-person rehabilitation + exercise sheet	8 weeks -CG: 5 × week -tIG: 2 × week -aIG: 2 × week	30 MS patients 55 (12) years old 68% female	RRMS: 18, SPMS: 8, PPMS: 4 EDSS: 4.3 (1.1)	X	X	X	X	X
Pöttgen et al., 2018 [37]	23	RCT	ELEVIDA	12 weeks of intervention Self-paced rehabilitation	275 MS patients 41 (11) years old 81% female	RRMS: 200, SPMS: 40, PPMS: 11, unclear: 24				X	X
Cavalera et al., 2019 [38]	24	RCT	MBSR program (mindfulness)-MBI (intervention group) or online psychoeducation (active control group)	8 weeks of training 1 weekly session	121 MS patients 42 (8) years old 34% female	RRMS: 113; SPMS: 8 EDSS: median 3					X

Table 1. Cont.

Study	D&B (/28)	Study Design	Intervention	Duration	Participants	Type of MS and Disability Level	Motor Function	Activity Level	ICF Cognition	ICF Fatigue	Quality of Life
Chiaravalloti et al., 2018 [39]	23	RCT	Processing speed apps (similar to BrainHQ)	5 weeks of training 2/week	21 MS patients 48 (8) years old 75% female	RRMS: 21			X		
Plow et al., 2019 [40]	22	RCT	Contact-control social support intervention Fasting-mimicking diet physical activity plus fatigue self-management intervention PA-only physical activity only intervention	12 week intervention 12 week follow-up Mix between group phone calls and individualized phone calls	208 MS patients 52 (8) years old 85% female	RRMS: 176, SPMS: 11, PPMS: 6, PRMS: 1, unknown: 14		X		X	
Fuchs et al., 2019 [41]	20	Experimental study	BrainHQ	/	51 MS patients 56 years old	RRMS: 35, SPMS: 12, PPMS: 4 EDSS: 4 [2.0; 6.0]			X		
Vilou et al., 2020 [42]	22	Explorative study	BrainHQ	6 weeks of training (2 × 20 min/week) -weekly contact + 2 weeks scheduled visit (semi-assisted)	47 MS patients 35 (16) years old 85% female	RRMS: 47 EDSS: 3.2 (2.0)			X		
Jeong et al., 2020 [43]	23	Retrospective analysis	MS-HAT	6 months of follow-up 2.5 h/week	17 MS patients 60 (11) years old	Type and EDSS not available	X	X	X		X
Kratz et al., 2020 [44]	24	RCT (pilot)	Web-based and telephone delivered exercises therapy	-Home: 30 min endurance 2× week; 3× week strength training lower extremity + 2 functional exercises per week -in-person: 30 endurance-tr + 30 resistance + home exercise for 8 weeks	20 MS patients 48 (8) years old 90% of female	RRMS: 16, SPMS: 1, PPMS: 1				X	

Table 1. Cont.

Study	D&B (/28)	Study Design	Intervention	Duration	Participants	Type of MS and Disability Level	ICF Motor Function	Activity Level	Cognition	Fatigue	Quality of Life
Flachenecker et al., 2020 [45]	23	RCT	Behavior-oriented exercise and physical activity promotion program via web and telephone-based program	12 weeks on intervention -Strength training (1–2 times per week) -Endurance training (10–60 min/1–2 times per week)	64 MS patients 47 (9) years old 62% of female	RRMS: 39, SPMS: 25 EDSS: 4.3 (3.5; 5.0)	X			X	X
Manns et al., 2020 [46]	22	Pre-post intervention (single group)	SitLess+ MoveMore FitBit on (tracking instrument-self monitoring tool) ActivPAL3 (tracking for activity level during 7 days after each time point)	15 weeks of training -7 weeks with SitLess -7 weeks with MoveMore	41 MS patients (39 post intervention and 36 complete follow-up) 50 (10) years old 90% of female	RRMS: 26, SPMS: 11, PPMS: 4 EDSS: 5.5 (3.7)		X		X	
Donkers et al., 2020 [47]	24	RCT (pilot)	Web-based exercise webbasedphysio.com	26 weeks of training Adaptation of the exercises every two weeks	48 MS patients 54 (12) years old 65% of female	Type and EDSS not available	X				X
Messinis et al., 2020 [48]	24	RCT	RehaCom	8 weeks of training (3 × 45 min/week)	36 MS patients 46 (4) years old 66% of female	SPMS: 36 EDSS: 5.5 (4.5; 7.0)			X	X	X
Minen et al., 2020 [49]	23	RCT	RELAXaHEAD	90 days Self-paced training	62 MS patients 40 (10) years old 89% female	Type and EDSS not available			X	X	X
Van Geel et al., 2020 [50]	25	Cohort study	Walk-With-Me app	10 weeks of training	12 participants 43 (38.5; 50) years old 100% female	RRMS: 11, SPMS: 1 EDSS not available		X	X	X	X

Table 1. Cont.

Study	D&B (/28)	Study Design	Intervention	Duration	Participants	Type of MS and Disability Level	ICF Motor Function	ICF Activity Level	ICF Cognition	ICF Fatigue	ICF Quality of Life
Bove et al., 2020 [51]	26	RCT	AKL-T03 (web-based)	6 weeks of training (5 × 25 min/week)	44 MS patients 51 (13) years old 80% female	RRMS: 33, SPMS: 7, PPMS: 2, CIS: 1, undetermined: 1 EDSS: 3.5 (2.5; 4.5)			X	X	
Tarakci et al., 2021 [52]	24	RCT	Web-based and telphone delivered exercises therapy	12 weeks program (3 × 60 min/week)	30 MS patients 41 (11) years old 77% of female	RRMS: 30 EDSS: 3.4 (1.5)		X		X	X
Williams et al., 2021 [53]	23	RCT	Phone instruction and illustrated training booklet and activity diary	8 weeks of training (2 × 60 min/week)	50 MS patients 51 (10) years old 76% females	RRMS: 31, SPMS: 6, PPMS: 7, undetermined: 6 EDSS not available	X				

The X indicate the main ICF domains assessed. D&B: Downs and Black checklist, RCT: Randomized Controlled Trial, MS: Multiple Sclerosis, RRMS: Relapsing Remitting Multiple Sclerosis, SPMS: Secondary Progressive Multiple Sclerosis, PPMS: Primary Progressive Multiple Sclerosis, CIS: Clinically Isolated Syndrome, EDSS: Expanded Disability Status Scales, PDSS: Patient Determined Disease Steps. MS-HAT: MS Home Automated Telehealth, MAPSS-MS: Memory, Attention, and Problem Solving Skills for Persons with Multiple Sclerosis, MBSR: Mindfulness Based Stress Reduction, PA: Physical Activity.

Table 2. Characteristics of the included studies (study design, mean duration on the intervention, targeted ICF function) on mHealth for self-assessment and description of the participants.

Study	D&B (/28)	Study Design	Intervention	Duration	Participants	Type of MS and Disability Level	ICF Motor Function	ICF Activity Level	ICF Cognition	ICF Fatigue	ICF Quality of Life
Miller et al., 2011 [54]	24	RCT	MCCO-enhanced (Web-Based)	12 months: self-monitoring functioning at any moment, comparing MCCO-original with MCCO-enhanced	206 MS patients	Not available					X
Greiner et al., 2015 [55]	18	Pilot study	MSdialog (Web-Based and App)	6-week study, following stages: 5-min online survey, training teleconference, weekly health reports, 5-min usability survey at weeks 3 and 6, follow-up call interview with selected patients	76 MS patients 68% female	Not available			X	X	

Table 2. Cont.

Study	D&B (/28)	Study Design	Intervention	Duration	Participants	Type of MS and Disability Level	Motor Function	Activity Level	ICF Cognition	Fatigue	Quality of Life
D'Hooghe et al., 2018 [56]	21	Cohort study	MS TeleCoach (Web-Based)	2-week run-in period: assess baseline activity level per patient 12-week period: target number of activity counts gradually increased through telecoaching	75 MS patients 67% female	RRMS: 75 EDSS: 2				X	
Midaglia et al., 2019 [57]	20	Observational study	Floodlight (App)	Active monitoring for 24 weeks: Daily Mood Question: daily, MSIS-29: fortnightly, SDMT: weekly, pinching test: weekly, Draw a Shape Test: daily, 5UTT: daily, 2MWT: daily Passive monitoring; gait behavior: continuous, mobility pattern: continuous	101 participants (76 MS patients) 40 years old 70% female	RRMS: 69, SPMS: 4, PPMS: 3 EDSS: 2.4 (1.4)		X	X		
Newland et al., 2019 [58]	18	Pilot study	FatigueApp.com (App)	FatigueApp.com: collect data for 5 weeks on Patient-Reported Outcomes Measurement Information System (PROMIS)	32 MS patients 49 (11) years old 81% female	RRMS: 30, SPMS: 2 EDSS: 3 (2; 4.8)				X	
Pratap et al., 2020 [59]	21	Observational pilot study	ElevateMS (App)	12 weeks Completed baseline assessments, including self-reported physical ability and longitudinal assessments of quality of life and daily health Completed functional tests as an independent assessment of MS-related motor activity	629 participants (490 MS patients) 47 (11) years old 50% female	RRMS: 423, SPMS: 30, PPMS: 42, undetermined: 2		X			X

The X indicate the main ICF domains assessed. D&B: Downs and Black checklist, RCT: Randomized Controlled Trial, MS: Multiple Sclerosis, RRMS: Relapsing Remitting Multiple Sclerosis, SPMS: Secondary Progressive Multiple Sclerosis, PPMS: Primary Progressive Multiple Sclerosis, EDSS: Expanded Disability Status Scales. MCCO-enhanced: The Mellen Center Care Online, MSIS-29: Multiple Sclerosis Impact Scale, SDMT: Symbol Digital Modalities Test, 5UTT: 5 U-Turn Test, 2MWT: 2-Minute Walk Test.

3.3. Quality Assessment

The quality of the included papers was checked using the Downs and Black checklist Overall, the average score for the included studies is 21.9 out of 28 (22.2 for studies on rehabilitation, 20.3 for studies assessing self-assessment). The average results for the different questions and sub-analysis of the Downs and Black checklist are presented in Figure 2.

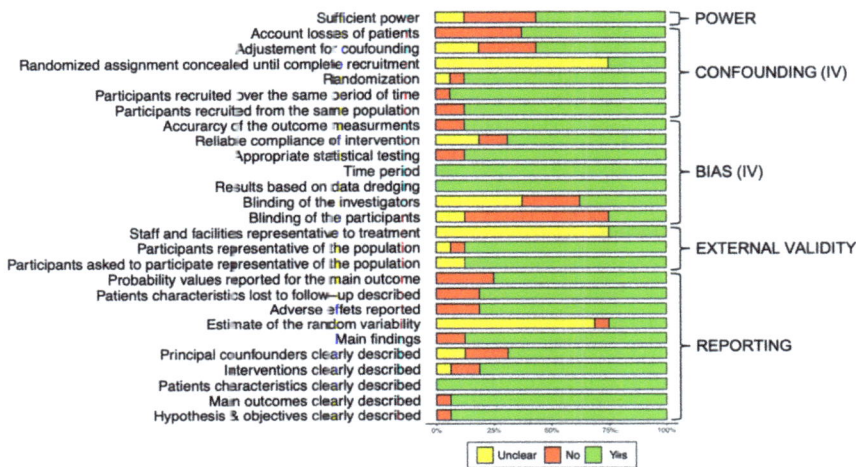

Figure 2. Quality of the study, author's judgment broken down for each question of the Downs and Black checklist across all included studies (IV): internal validity, for the question about the data dredging the green color indicates that there is no problem and data were acquired directly and have not been imputed.

When analyzing individual items, we observed that, due to the nature of the training, the blinding of the participants was not possible, on the other hand, the blinding of the investigators was not guaranteed either. Another potential source of bias is the uncertainty about the randomization assignment until the complete recruitment. The last important point is that a high number of studies do not take into consideration the patients that did not complete the intervention (loss in follow-up) so leading to uncertainty on reasons of non-adherence. Only a few studies used intention-to-treat analysis. On average 90.6% of the included patients completed the entire protocol and were included in the final analysis.

3.4. Description of the Available mHealth Solutions

First, we present the mHealth solutions that are mainly used for rehabilitation purposes. Most of the proposed mHealth solutions have been studied for cognition, QoL, and fatigue and were limited to one single ICF domain. We later discuss the applications for the respective domains, although some overlap occurred.

RehaCom [24,30,33,48] is a comprehensive and sophisticated system of software for computer-assisted cognitive rehabilitation. It proposes different solutions for screening and training cognitive functions and offers apps for home training.

BrainHQ [32,41,42] is a platform providing a set of more than 30 mini brain training exercises designed to challenge different cognitive functions (processing speed, attention, working memory, and executive function through visual and auditory domains). The initial level of challenge is low and the difficulty is adapted on an individual basis as learning and abilities improve over time. The company was previously known as Posit Sciences [27].

Luminosity [25] is a platform providing cognitive training exercises embedded in games. As for BrainHQ different cognitive functions can be challenged in a set of different mini-games.

The Memory, Attention, and Problem Solving Skills for Persons with Multiple Sclerosis (MAPSS-MS) intervention [35] aims to help pwMS acquire the highest level of cognitive functioning and functional independence. It includes problems solving and lifestyle adjustments (sleep, stress management, physical activity) that support cognitive functioning and will support persons with MS in the use of compensatory cognitive strategies and cognitive skills. The cognitive training is done with Luminosity app.

BrainStim [28] is a computerized training tool based on the working memory (WM) model of Baddeley [60]. It consists of three different modules targeting both, verbal and visual-spatial aspects of WM.

COGNI-TRAcK [31] implements three different types of exercises which were shown to be effective in improving the cognitive status of healthy subjects. The exercises consisted of (i) a visuospatial WM task; (ii) an "operation" N-back task; (iii) a "dual" N-back task [61].

The Attention Processing training (APT) program [25] is a cognitive rehabilitation intervention that targets focused, sustained, selective, alternating, and divided attention. The aim is to increase the ability to respond to specific stimuli [62].

ELEVEDIA [37] content is based on cognitive behavioral therapy strategies and is conveyed chiefly via the technique of a 'simulated dialogue'. Program modules are composed of an introduction and a summary and include homework tasks. Patients are advised to access the program once to twice per week.

The MS Home Automated Telehealth (MS HAT) system [34,43] is supporting patient-centered care, self-management and allows easier patient–provider communication. Three interfaces are available: patient unit, server, and clinical unit. The patient unit had interactive options for data collection, educational content, exercise information, and therapist–patient communication, access to exercises, response to exercise-specific assessments, and documenting exercise data from home. Exercises consist of task-oriented training such as digitized writing tracking or manipulating light bulbs or keys. Exercise adherence feedback was via diary entries, calendars, and graphs [63].

AKL-TO3 [51] is engaging the patients in simultaneous sensory and motor tasks and is designed to engage the frontal neural network. It enabled real-time monitoring of progress and continuously challenges patients so that the training is never too easy or difficult encouraging patients to improve performance.

RELAXaHEAD [49] is designed for pain management and in particular migraine and neck pain. It contained a headache diary, which includes features for tracking headache characteristics, headache medications and sleep, and tracking medication side effects and menstrual cycles. The app also contains a serious game module to ease muscle relaxation.

WalkWithMe [50] has been developed to motivate and stimulate patients to walk more and farther. It allows to track the walking activities and follow up on progress. The app detects the walking speed and gives feedback during walking with verbal feedback (i.e., pace) by the virtual coach.

Webbasedphysio.com [47] is an internet-delivered therapeutic exercise program. The web-based physio allows people the flexibility to do their own, individualized exercise program at a time and location which is convenient to them, thus enhancing the individual's ability to self-manage their condition on a long-term basis.

Deprexis [29] is an online program based on principles of cognitive-behavioral therapy. It consists of 10 sequential modules—psycho-education, behavioral activation, cognitive modification, mindfulness and acceptance, interpersonal skills, relaxation, physical exercise and lifestyle modification, problem-solving, expressive writing and forgiveness, positive psychology, and emotion-focus interventions.

The Mindfulness Based Stress Reduction (MBSR) [38] deals with stress management, relaxation training, sleep hygiene, fatigue, and social relationships. The course materials were developed using existing informative MS videos, created by the Italian MS Association, recording new interviews and generating new exercises.

Concerning the mHealth apps that are mainly used for self-assessment:

MSdialog [55] is a web and mobile (i.e., cell phone and tablet) based software application that combines information from RebiSmart (with health information recorded by patients via their personal computer or smartphone to collect and store real-time data regarding administration of Rebif (interferon β-1a), clinical outcomes, and patient reported outcomes). MSdialog offers a practical means by which patients record and exchange information with their healthcare specialists intending to support the patient–physician relationship and offering patients a method of engaging in the pharmaceutical management of their MS and patients' self-reported outcomes [64].

MS Telecoach [56] provides a combination of monitoring, self-management, and motivational messages, focusing on energy management of physical activity to improve fatigue levels. It has two components: telemonitoring (physical activity through accelerometers and self-reported fatigue impact levels) and tele-coaching (motivational messages and advice).

Floodlight [57] is a combination of continuous sensor data capture and standard clinical outcome measures. It involves performing a set of daily active tests to evaluate cognition, upper extremity function, gait, and balance domains and contribute sensor data via passive monitoring, also including self-reported patient outcomes.

The Mellen Center Care Online (MCCO-enhanced) [54] is an electronic messaging system between clinician and patient. It contains a self-monitoring and self-management system to assess MS symptoms and the pwMS receives graphical feedback to evaluate symptom changes

FatigueApp.com [58] is collecting data to correlate fatigue measures with other symptoms and quality of life. Fatigue questionnaires are completed every morning for 6 consecutive days and again 4 weeks later.

ElevateMS [59] allows collecting different data in the real-world environment of the patients such as self-reported measures of symptoms and health via 'check-in'-surveys Independent assessments of motor function occur via sensor-based active functional tests, participants are encouraged to complete surveys daily, and notifications to perform more comprehensive functional tests are provided once a week.

3.5. Outcome Data Related to ICF

3.5.1. Rehabilitation

Amongst the included RCTs, 20 were included in the meta-analysis assessing the efficacy of mHeath for rehabilitation [24,26–31,33–37,39,40,44,45,47–49,51,65], representing 1393 pwMS. When considering all the studies and ICF domains together, the heterogeneity between the studies was moderate (tau^2 = 0.30, 95%CI [0.26; 0.62]), therefore we decided to use random-effect model. The funnel plot did not show significant asymmetry (Egger's intercept = 0.45, p = 0.91) (Figure S1). The sensitivity analysis did not show any outlier (Figure S2).

The overall effect of mHealth intervention in pwMS is moderate (SMD = 0.50 [0.35; 0.66]) and statistically significant ($p < 0.0001$). Since different studies evaluated human functioning at different aspects according to the ICF, we then performed subgroup analysis to assess the efficacy across the different ICF. The forest plot is presented in Figure 3.

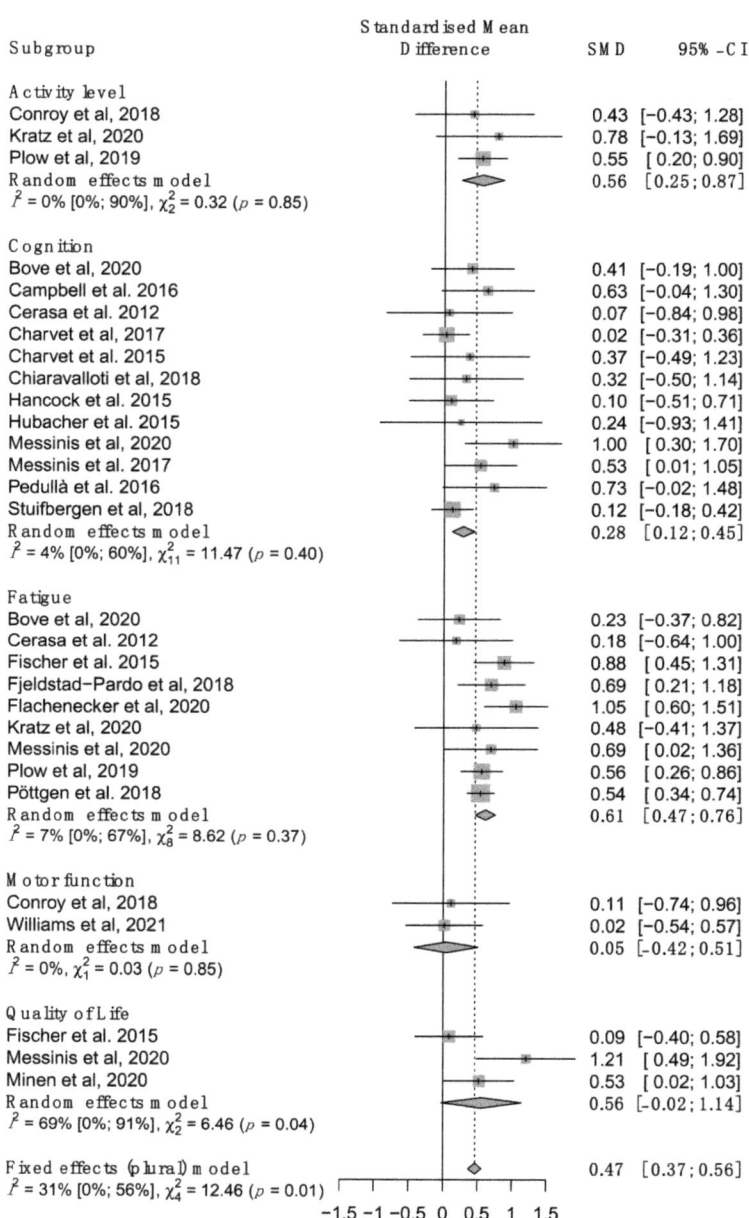

Figure 3. Stratified meta-analysis according to ICF domains, results are indicated with 95% confidence intervals Positive Standardized Mean Differences (SMD) indicates superior efficacy of the mHealth intervention compared to control group [24,26–31,33–37,39,40,44,45,47–49,51,65].

At the ICF domains level, we observed the biggest effect for fatigue (SMD = 0.61 [0.47; 0.76]), followed by outcome measures at the activity level (SMD = 0.56 [0.25; 0.87]) and cognitive impairment (SMD = 0.28 [0.12; 0.45]). Note that for activity level these results must be interpreted carefully due to the small number of included studies ($n = 3$). For the domains of motor function and quality of life the results were not significant but only included two and three studies, respectively. Using a fixed-effect model to summarize the overall ICF functioning we found an overall moderate effect (SMD 0.47 [0.37; 0.56], $p < 0.0001$).

We then summarized the main results and conclusions of the studies that were not included in the meta-analysis.

Concerning cognitive function, Fuchs et al., 2019 investigated the clinical characteristics predicting response to a home-based restorative cognitive training. Significant improvements were observed after training [41]. Villou et al., 2020 is an explorative study that reported statistical improvement of various cognitive functions after training such as visuospatial memory, visual attention, task-switching, reading speed and response inhibition, and verbal learning [42].

For fatigue, Stuifenbergen et al., 2018 analyzed the acceptability and effect of MAPSS-MS on cognitive function and fatigue. The authors find similar results as with usual care; interestingly, the improvements were maintained during the follow-up at 3 and 6 months and were superior in the intervention group [35].

For the quality of life, Cavalera et al., 2013 showed an improvement of QoL after 8 weeks of intervention using a mindfulness program but the progress was not maintained over time (6-month follow-up after the end of the intervention) [38]. Tarakci et al., 2021 compared an in-person rehabilitation program with a telerehabilitation program. After 12 weeks of training, the results were similar in the two groups for fatigue and activity level [52]. Manns et al., 2020 demonstrated a reduction of fatigue after a combined intervention (SitLess and MoveMore) but the difference was not significant compared to usual care [46]. Interestingly the total sedentary time decreased in the intervention group and these results are maintained over time.

Van Geel et al. reported that using the WalkWithMe app induced a significant improvement in quality of life, walking, and leisure, 36-Item Short-Form Health Survey (SF-36) quality of life, cognition, cognitive fatigability, lower limb strength, and dominant hand function. However, it was an observational study without a control group [50].

3.5.2. Self-Assessment

Concerning the efficacy of self-assessment and monitoring, only six studies were included in this review.

Miller et al. highlighted group differences between the MCCO-original and MCCO-enhanced groups. MCCO-original had a higher European Quality of Life level after 12 months of regularly self-monitoring their quality of life [54].

Greiner et al. performed a 6-week longitudinal observation and showed that MSdialog was adapted to monitor patient-reported outcomes. Amongst the different functions evaluated by the pwMS, fatigue (99%), physical health (96%), cognitive deficits (93%), pain (91%) and sleep quality (91%) were the most important. These numbers represent the weight given by the patients for these different functions that scored the MS quality-of-life questionnaire using a visual analogical scale [55].

D'Hooghe et al. showed that it is feasible to use the MS TeleCoach at home without supervision. The authors observed a significant decrease in fatigue and an increase in cognitive function after 12 weeks of use [56].

Midaglia et al. assessed the usability and acceptability of the Floodlight for active monitoring and passive monitoring intervention. After 24 weeks of intervention, mHealth had an acceptable impact on daily activities including cognition and physical activity for 80% of the pwMS [57].

Newland et al. reported that the FatigueApp could collect self-reported symptoms including fatigue, self-reported EDSS (EDSS-SR), pain, and cognition [58]. Participants were asked to complete the questionnaires for 7 consecutive days and then again 4 weeks later.

Pratap et al. in a large study including more than 500 pwMS described that ElevateMS can be used to longitudinally (12 weeks period) to collect information about the most common symptoms of MS. During this follow-up, they observed that the most frequent complaints are fatigue (63%), memory issues (42%) and difficulty with walking (41%). After the intervention, there were significantly increased functional performances and QoL [59].

3.6. Summary

To summarize the findings of this study we listed the different mHealth according to the targeted ICF domain for both rehabilitation and self-assessment in Table 3.

Table 3. Overview of the different mHealth solutions for rehabilitation and self-assessment according to the mean ICF targeted.

Functioning (ICF)	mHealth	
	Rehabilitation	Self-Assessment
Cognition	BrainHQ [27,32,39,41,42] Lumosity [26] RehaCom [24,30,33] BrainStim [28] COGNI-TRAcK [31] MAPPS-MS * [35] APT [25] MS-HAT [43] Walk-With-Me [50] AKL-T03 [51]	MSdialog [55] Floodlight [57]
Fatigue	RehaCom [24,33] ELEVEDIA [37] MAPPS-MS [35] SitLess and MoveMore [46] Walk-With-Me [50] AKL-T03 [51]	MSdialog [55] MS TeleCoach [56] FatigueApp.com [58]
Quality of Life	ELEVEDIA [37] MBSR [38] MS-HAT [43] webbasedphysio.com [47] RehaCom [48] RELAXaHEAD [49] Walk-With-Me [50]	MCCO-enhanced [54] ElevateMS [59]
Activity Level	MS-HAT system [34] SitLess and MoveMore [46] Walk-With-Me [50]	Floodlight [57] ElevateMS [59]
Motor Function	MS-HAT system [34,43] webbasedphysio.com [47]	/

* The cognitive training module of MAPPS-MS is done with Luminosity.

4. Discussion

The main result of this review is the high number of solutions (applications) currently being tested with pwMS for rehabilitation (n = 16), despite the relatively recent development and use of these new apps in rehabilitation. On another side, the development of mHealth for self-assessment and home-monitoring is still limited (six apps found). Consequently, one of the downsides is that there are only very few studies performed with the same mHealth which makes it more difficult to compare the studies and thus to determine the level of evidence. Therefore, rather than comparing the efficacy of each particular mHealth, we performed the analysis at the ICF domain level. The most studied ICF domain is cognition: we found a small but significant effect of the training using mHealth (SMD = 0.28 [0.12; 0.45]) which is consistent with other meta-analyses summarizing the effect of computerized cognitive training, including computer solutions and supervised training (SMD = 0.30 [0.18; 0.43]) [66]. It is important to note here that there is currently a lack of information about the transfer of the benefits gained in the mHealth solution in the activity of daily living as most of the studies only assess direct or near transfer effects. The second most studied function is fatigue, with a moderate effect (SMD = 0.61 [0.47; 0.76]). The effect of mHealth is a bit lower than the effect of pharmacological treatment (i.e., amantadine): SMD = 1.09 [0.87; 1.30] [67], but similar to the effect of exercise therapy (SMD = 0.53 [0.33; 0.73]) [68].

For the motor function and quality of life, there are, currently, not enough studies available, but the few studies available also seem to indicate a favorable effect. The paucity of studies investigating the effects of mHealth applications to train motor functions is somehow surprising. However, we excluded studies including wearables and thus the number of interventions done to increase physical activity based on step count (i.e., [69]). The low numbers of studies investigating the effects of mHealth interventions on quality of life may be expected as the quality of life is often thought to be the result of improving specific ICF domains.

Another major finding of this systematic review regarding self-assessment is the fact that mHealth can be used directly by the patients to continuously monitor several different functions in their living environment. The solutions are not only well accepted by the patients, but several studies also show that using this type of mHealth is directly beneficial for the patients. This positive effect may be mediated by a better knowledge of the diseases and symptoms (education) [70] but also by the more active participation of the patient in his treatment (patients' engagement) [71].

There are several limitations to this review. The first one is the lack of standardization in the nomenclature used to describe the different mHealth currently tested in research. Therefore, due to the small numbers of studies published, we ended up including studies assessing different types of applications and intervention modalities or duration. The heterogeneity between the studies, and the patients, makes it more difficult to compare studies and especially to generalize the results. There is also a huge heterogeneity in the duration of the intervention for both the duration of the intervention (ranging from minimum 4 to maximal 26 weeks) and the total amount of training (ranging from 4 to 65 h). Unfortunately, due to the small number of studies included in the different ICF levels, we could not perform meta-regression to determine if there is a dose–response relationship between the amount of training using the mHealth and the clinical outcome.

A third important limitation is that most of the included studies on the rehabilitation aspects (except [32,35,38,40,45]) have relatively small sample sizes and the results are likely to be underpowered [72]. Furthermore, the percentage of participants that were included in the final analysis is 90% and information about the adherence to the intervention was missing (usually a threshold of 80% is applied to determine if the participants do a sufficient amount of exercises [73]). Concerning the meta-analysis, due to the relatively small number of included studies, the results must also be interpreted carefully, especially for the ICF motor function and quality of life. Concerning motor functions, most of the current solutions are focusing on walking while patients may also experience severe disability in upper limbs functions and dexterity, efforts must be made to develop solutions that focus on these problems. Concerning the external validity of this review and the translation to the clinic, it is important to note that the vast majority of the applications were tested in pwMS with mild disability (EDSS = 3.5 ± 1.1) with RRMS (79%), and thus not guaranteed to be applicable to the same extent in more disabled patients with restricted mobility. Further studies must therefore focus on more disabled patients to determine the feasibility of mHealth with these patients if the efficacy is similar.

Finally, most of presented solutions are still at the research project stage and applications are not yet widely available to patients or their treating clinicians.

Despite these limitations, this review highlights interesting and promising results for patients. However, there are still a few points that should be addressed before these solutions can be used in daily practice. The first, and probably most important is the recognition of the m- and eHealth apps as medical devices. In June 2020, the US Food and Drug Administration (FDA) permitted the marketing of the first game-based digital therapeutic device to improve attention function in children with attention deficit hyperactivity disorder (ADHD). The mHeath, EndeavorRx, is indicated to improve attention function as measured by computer-based testing and is the first digital therapeutic intended to improve symptoms associated with ADHD, as well as the first game-based therapeutic granted marketing authorization by the FDA for any type of condition. The device is intended for use as part of a therapeutic program that may include clinician-directed therapy, medication, and/or educational programs, which further address symptoms of the disorder [74]. Interestingly this solution is developed by Akili, the company that has developed AKL-T03 which also shows significant results in pwMS [51]. The COVID-19 pandemic has not only disrupted healthcare systems but has also allowed for a very significant acceleration in the development, implementation, and recognition of mHealth in the clinics [75]. It is important to note, however, that most of the measures taken during the crisis may be temporary and it is hoped that efforts will continue in this direction once the crisis is over. For example, it will be important to adapt the nomenclature of interventions, as mobile solutions are currently placed in the same categories as drugs, which poses problems for the validation and reimbursement of these interventions [76]. Another limitation is that, for the moment, the majority of the analyzed mHealth is being developed during research projects and is therefore not easily accessible for patients, except for BrainHQ and Luminosity that are two commercial (gaming) companies. As an indication, the price of an annual subscription to these companies is less than USD 100 per year for a full premium account. RehaCom is also already widely used by clinical centers but mostly for research purposes.

This brings us to the second biggest current limitation which is the lack of reimbursement by the social security system. The organization and involvement of healthcare systems in the revalidation process is country-specific and we will not discuss reimbursement specifically here. However, we know that two of the most important barriers to the implementation of telemedicine and telehealth for the patients, regardless of the pathologies or the specialties, are the financial issues and the lack of knowledge and familiarity with the use of (new) technology [77,78]. The pwMS being relatively young, most of them are familiar with smartphones, apps, and mobile technology, therefore the familiarity with the technology should not be an issue for most of the patients [79], but this can be a real barrier for other diseases or patient groups (e.g., older adults with dementia) [80]. Efforts must also be directed to the education of healthcare professionals as they need to be perfectly aware of the technology and its limitations to motivate the patients to use it.

As a result of all the above limitations, in practice, the solutions described in this article are only used by a small fraction of the pwMS. A recent survey performed in the US found that only 3.1% of the pwMS who took part in the survey ($n = 786$) are using mHealth solutions regularly [81].

We will now discuss some ideas for consideration to facilitate the implementation of these solutions in the rehabilitation process.

The first point would be to integrate the mHealth solutions into the healthcare system, with reimbursement for the patients, providing education of the mHealth solutions for healthcare professionals, and the integration of the data collected with the apps (see [54–59]) in patients' medical records. This could speed up and ease the implementation of mHealth in the daily management and rehabilitation of pwMS. This would not only save time but also allow for a more accurate and regular assessment of patients [65]. Furthermore, these assessments could be carried out in the patients' homes. This fits in perfectly with telemonitoring [82] and the use of real-world data [83]. This would therefore allow the development (by increasing the number of potential users, companies may be more inclined to invest in such solutions) and wider use of these solutions.

A last important point is the sustainability of the studied solutions [84]. The speed of the development of mobile technology (hardware and software) is one of the most important considerations, and the technology becomes quickly obsolete (for example there is a new version of the operating systems [Andoid© or iOS©] on average every 6 months). Thus, the apps that have been developed with the previous version are not supported anymore with the more recent one. This is not much of an issue with the commercial solutions, but it is more problematic with the solutions being developed during research projects.

5. Conclusions

This review highlights an important potential of mHealth for pwMS with evidence of a small but significant effect on fatigue and cognition. Although we have seen that current mHealth is, at the moment, not a perfect solution given the high prevalence of fatigue and cognitive impairment in pwMS and the lack of low-cost tools to assist and stimulate the patients at home, the use of apps could be greatly beneficial.

To develop innovative, effective solutions adapted for pwMS whose cognition, quality of life, functionality, and wellbeing are impaired, researchers, clinicians, policy makers, and app developers will need to further collaborate.

Supplementary Materials: The following are available online at https://www.mdpi.com/article/10.3390/brainsci11091187/s1, Table S1: Search strategy for PubMed Figure S1: Funnel plot of the included studies in the meta-analysis; Figure S2: Sensitivity analysis of the included studies in the meta-analysis.

Author Contributions: Systematic review, B.B., A.R. and P.F.; formal analysis, B.B. and P.F.; writing—original draft preparation, B.B.; writing—review and editing, B.B., A.R., A.S., I.L. and P.F.; visualization, B.B.; supervision, P.F., A.R. and I.L.; project administration, P.F. All authors have read and agreed to the published version of the manuscript.

Funding: This research received no external funding.

Institutional Review Board Statement: Not applicable.

Informed Consent Statement: Not applicable.

Data Availability Statement: Not applicable.

Acknowledgments: The authors would like to thank Deschryvere Charlotte, Noels Maite, and Roesner Marianna for their precious help in the search and inclusion of articles.

Conflicts of Interest: The authors declare no conflict of interest.

References

1. Papanicolas, I.; Mossialos, E.; Gundersen, A.; Woskie, L.; Jha, A.K. Performance of UK National Health Service Compared with Other High Income Countries: Observational Study. *BMJ* **2019**, *367*, l6326. [CrossRef]
2. Flachenecker, P.; Buckow, K.; Pugliatti, M.; Kes, V.B.; Battaglia, M.A.; Boyko, A.; Confavreux, C.; Ellenberger, D.; Eskic, D.; Ford, D.; et al. Multiple Sclerosis Registries in Europe—Results of a Systematic Survey. *Mult. Scler.* **2014**, *20*, 1523–1532. [CrossRef]
3. WHO. Fact Sheets: Rehabilitation. 2020. Available online: https://www.who.int/news-room/fact-sheets/detail/rehabilitation (accessed on 1 July 2021).
4. Statista. Number of Smartphone Users Worldwide from 2016 to 2026. Available online: https://www.statista.com/statistics/330695/number-of-smartphone-users-worldwide/ (accessed on 6 July 2021).
5. Anderson, K.; Burford, O.; Emmerton, L. Mobile Health Apps to Facilitate Self-Care: A Qualitative Study of User Experiences. *PLoS ONE* **2016**, *11*, e0156164. [CrossRef]
6. Birkhoff, S.D.; Smeltzer, S.C. Perceptions of Smartphone User-Centered Mobile Health Tracking Apps Across Various Chronic Illness Populations: An Integrative Review. *J. Nurs. Sch.* **2017**, *49*, 371–378. [CrossRef]
7. Hernandez Silva, E.; Lawler, S.; Langbecker, D. The Effectiveness of MHealth for Self-Management in Improving Pain, Psychological Distress, Fatigue, and Sleep in Cancer Survivors: A Systematic Review. *J. Cancer Surviv.* **2019**, *13*, 97–107. [CrossRef] [PubMed]
8. Zheng, C.; Chen, X.; Weng, L.; Guo, L.; Xu, H.; Lin, M.; Xue, Y.; Lin, X.; Yang, A.; Yu, L.; et al. Benefits of Mobile Apps for Cancer Pain Management: Systematic Review. *JMIR Mhealth Uhealth* **2020**, *8*, e17055. [CrossRef] [PubMed]

9. Kapoor, A.; Nambisan, P.; Baker, E. Mobile Applications for Breast Cancer Survivorship and Self-Management: A Systematic Review. *Health Inform. J.* **2020**, *26*, 2892–2905. [CrossRef] [PubMed]
10. Xu, H.; Long, H. The Effect of Smartphone App-Based Interventions for Patients With Hypertension: Systematic Review and Meta-Analysis. *JMIR Mhealth Uhealth* **2020**, *8*, e21759. [CrossRef] [PubMed]
11. Giebel, G.D.; Gissel, C. Accuracy of MHealth Devices for Atrial Fibrillation Screening: Systematic Review. *JMIR Mhealth Uhealth* **2019**, *7*, e13641. [CrossRef] [PubMed]
12. Bateman, D.R.; Srinivas, B.; Emmett, T.W.; Schleyer, T.K.; Holden, R.J.; Hendrie, H.C.; Callahan, C.M. Categorizing Health Outcomes and Efficacy of MHealth Apps for Persons With Cognitive Impairment: A Systematic Review. *J. Med. Internet Res.* **2017**, *19*, e301. [CrossRef] [PubMed]
13. Elavsky, S.; Knapova, L.; Klocek, A.; Smahel, D. Mobile Health Interventions for Physical Activity, Sedentary Behavior, and Sleep in Adults Aged 50 Years and Older: A Systematic Literature Review. *J. Aging Phys. Act.* **2019**, *27*, 565–593. [CrossRef] [PubMed]
14. Rintala, A.; Hakala, S.; Paltamaa, J.; Heinonen, A.; Karvanen, J.; Sjögren, T. Effectiveness of Technology-Based Distance Physical Rehabilitation Interventions on Physical Activity and Walking in Multiple Sclerosis: A Systematic Review and Meta-Analysis of Randomized Controlled Trials. *Disabil. Rehabil.* **2018**, *40*, 373–387. [CrossRef]
15. Marziniak, M.; Brichetto, G.; Feys, P.; Meyding-Lamadé, U.; Vernon, K.; Meuth, S.G. The Use of Digital and Remote Communication Technologies as a Tool for Multiple Sclerosis Management: Narrative Review. *JMIR Rehabil. Assist. Technol.* **2018**, *5*, e5. [CrossRef] [PubMed]
16. Moher, D.; Liberati, A.; Tetzlaff, J.; Altman, D.G. Preferred Reporting Items for Systematic Reviews and Meta-Analyses: The PRISMA Statement. *J. Clin. Epidemiol.* **2009**, *62*, 1006–1012. [CrossRef] [PubMed]
17. Downs, S.H.; Black, N. The Feasibility of Creating a Checklist for the Assessment of the Methodological Quality Both of Randomised and Non-Randomised Studies of Health Care Interventions. *J. Epidemiol. Community Health* **1998**, *52*, 377–384. [CrossRef] [PubMed]
18. Deeks, J.J.; Dinnes, J.; D'Amico, R.; Sowden, A.J.; Sakarovitch, C.; Song, F.; Petticrew, M.; Altman, D.G.; International Stroke Trial Collaborative Group; European Carotid Surgery Trial Collaborative Group. Evaluating Non-Randomised Intervention Studies. *Health Technol. Assess.* **2003**, *7*, 1–173. [CrossRef]
19. Higgins, J.P.T.; Thomas, J.; Chandler, J.; Cumpston, M.; Li, T.; Page, M.; Welch, V. *Cochrane Handbook for Systematic Reviews of Interventions*, 2nd ed.; Wiley-Blackwell: Hoboken, NJ, USA, 2019; ISBN 978-1-119-53662-8.
20. Carter, E.C.; Schönbrodt, F.D.; Gervais, W.M.; Hilgard, J. Correcting for Bias in Psychology: A Comparison of Meta-Analytic Methods. *Adv. Methods Pract. Psychol. Sci.* **2019**, *2*, 115–144. [CrossRef]
21. Sterne, J.A.C.; Sutton, A.J.; Ioannidis, J.P.A.; Terrin, N.; Jones, D.R.; Lau, J.; Carpenter, J.; Rücker, G.; Harbord, R.M.; Schmid, C.H.; et al. Recommendations for Examining and Interpreting Funnel Plot Asymmetry in Meta-Analyses of Randomised Controlled Trials. *BMJ* **2011**, *343*, d4002. [CrossRef]
22. Pustejovsky, J.E.; Rodgers, M.A. Testing for Funnel Plot Asymmetry of Standardized Mean Differences. *Res. Synth. Methods* **2019**, *10*, 57–71. [CrossRef]
23. Liberati, A.; Altman, D.G.; Tetzlaff, J.; Mulrow, C.; Gøtzsche, P.C.; Ioannidis, J.P.A.; Clarke, M.; Devereaux, P.J.; Kleijnen, J.; Moher, D. The PRISMA Statement for Reporting Systematic Reviews and Meta-Analyses of Studies That Evaluate Health Care Interventions: Explanation and Elaboration. *PLOS Med.* **2009**, *6*, e1000100. [CrossRef]
24. Cerasa, A.; Gioia, M.C.; Valentino, P.; Nisticò, R.; Chiriaco, C.; Pirritano, D.; Tomaiuolo, F.; Mangone, G.; Trotta, M.; Talarico, T.; et al. Computer-Assisted Cognitive Rehabilitation of Attention Deficits for Multiple Sclerosis: A Randomized Trial with FMRI Correlates. *Neurorehabil. Neural Repair* **2013**, *27*, 284–295. [CrossRef]
25. Amato, M.; Goretti, B.; Viterbo, R.; Portaccio, E.; Niccolai, C.; Hakiki, B.; Iaffaldano, P.; Trojano, M. Computer-Assisted Rehabilitation of Attention in Patients with Multiple Sclerosis: Results of a Randomized, Double-Blind Trial. *Mult. Scler.* **2014**, *20*, 91–98. [CrossRef]
26. Charvet, L.; Shaw, M.; Haider, L.; Melville, P.; Krupp, L. Remotely-Delivered Cognitive Remediation in Multiple Sclerosis (MS): Protocol and Results from a Pilot Study. *Mult. Scler. J.—Exp. Transl. Clin.* **2015**, *1*, 205521731560962. [CrossRef]
27. Hancock, L.M.; Bruce, J.M.; Bruce, A.S.; Lynch, S.G. Processing Speed and Working Memory Training in Multiple Sclerosis: A Double-Blind Randomized Controlled Pilot Study. *J. Clin. Exp. Neuropsychol.* **2015**, *37*, 113–127. [CrossRef]
28. Hubacher, M.; Kappos, L.; Weier, K.; Stöcklin, M.; Opwis, K.; Penner, I.-K. Case-Based FMRI Analysis after Cognitive Rehabilitation in MS: A Novel Approach. *Front. Neurol.* **2015**, *6*, 78. [CrossRef]
29. Fischer, A.; Schröder, J.; Vettorazzi, E.; Wolf, O.T.; Pöttgen, J.; Lau, S.; Heesen, C.; Moritz, S.; Gold, S.M. An Online Programme to Reduce Depression in Patients with Multiple Sclerosis: A Randomised Controlled Trial. *Lancet Psychiatry* **2015**, *2*, 217–223. [CrossRef]
30. Campbell, J.; Langdon, D.; Cercignani, M.; Rashid, W. A Randomised Controlled Trial of Efficacy of Cognitive Rehabilitation in Multiple Sclerosis: A Cognitive, Behavioural, and MRI Study. *Neural Plast.* **2016**, *2016*, 1–9. [CrossRef] [PubMed]
31. Pedullà, L.; Brichetto, G.; Tacchino, A.; Vassallo, C.; Zaratin, P.; Battaglia, M.A.; Bonzano, L.; Bove, M. Adaptive vs. Non-Adaptive Cognitive Training by Means of a Personalized App: A Randomized Trial in People with Multiple Sclerosis. *J. Neuroeng. Rehabil.* **2016**, *13*, 88. [CrossRef] [PubMed]
32. Charvet, L.E.; Yang, J.; Shaw, M.T.; Sherman, K.; Haider, L.; Xu, J.; Krupp, L.B. Cognitive Function in Multiple Sclerosis Improves with Telerehabilitation: Results from a Randomized Controlled Trial. *PLoS ONE* **2017**, *12*, e0177177. [CrossRef]

33. Messinis, L.; Nasios, G.; Kosmidis, M.H.; Zampakis, P.; Malefaki, S.; Ntoskou, K.; Nousia, A.; Bakirtzis, C.; Grigoriadis, N.; Gourzis, P.; et al. Efficacy of a Computer-Assisted Cognitive Rehabilitation Intervention in Relapsing-Remitting Multiple Sclerosis Patients: A Multicenter Randomized Controlled Trial. *Behav. Neurol.* 2017, 2017, 1–17. [CrossRef] [PubMed]
34. Conroy, S.S.; Zhan, M.; Culpepper, W.J.; Royal, W.; Wallin, M.T. Self-Directed Exercise in Multiple Sclerosis: Evaluation of a Home Automated Tele-Management System. *J. Telemed. Telecare* 2018, 24, 410–419. [CrossRef]
35. Stuifbergen, A.K.; Becker, H.; Perez, F.; Morrison, J.; Brown, A.; Kullberg, V.; Zhang, W. Computer-Assisted Cognitive Rehabilitation in Persons with Multiple Sclerosis: Results of a Multi-Site Randomized Controlled Trial with Six Month Follow-Up. *Disabil. Health J.* 2018, 11, 427–434. [CrossRef]
36. Fjeldstad-Pardo, C.; Thiessen, A.; Pardo, G. Telerehabilitation in Multiple Sclerosis: Results of a Randomized Feasibility and Efficacy Pilot Study. *Int. J. Telerehabil.* 2018, 10, 55–64. [CrossRef] [PubMed]
37. Pöttgen, J.; Moss-Morris, R.; Wendebourg, J.-M.; Feddersen, L.; Lau, S.; Köpke, S.; Meyer, B.; Friede, T.; Penner, I.-K.; Heesen, C.; et al. Randomised Controlled Trial of a Self-Guided Online Fatigue Intervention in Multiple Sclerosis. *J. Neurol. Neurosurg. Psychiatry* 2018, 89, 970–976. [CrossRef] [PubMed]
38. Cavalera, C.; Rovaris, M.; Mendozzi, L.; Pugnetti, L.; Garegnani, M.; Castelnuovo, G.; Molinari, E.; Pagnini, F. Online Meditation Training for People with Multiple Sclerosis: A Randomized Controlled Trial. *Mult. Scler.* 2019, 25, 610–617. [CrossRef]
39. Chiaravalloti, N.D.; Goverover, Y.; Costa, S.L.; DeLuca, J. A Pilot Study Examining Speed of Processing Training (SPT) to Improve Processing Speed in Persons With Multiple Sclerosis. *Front. Neurol.* 2018, 9, 685. [CrossRef]
40. Plow, M.; Finlayson, M.; Liu, J.; Motl, R.W.; Bethoux, F.; Sattar, A. Randomized Controlled Trial of a Telephone-Delivered Physical Activity and Fatigue Self-Management Interventions in Adults With Multiple Sclerosis. *Arch. Phys. Med. Rehabil.* 2019, 100, 2006–2014. [CrossRef] [PubMed]
41. Fuchs, T.A.; Ziccardi, S.; Dwyer, M.G.; Charvet, L.E.; Bartnik, A.; Campbell, R.; Escobar, J.; Hojnacki, D.; Kolb, C.; Oship, D.; et al. Response Heterogeneity to Home-Based Restorative Cognitive Rehabilitation in Multiple Sclerosis: An Exploratory Study. *Mult. Scler. Relat. Disord.* 2019, 34, 103–111. [CrossRef]
42. Vilou, I.; Bakirtzis, C.; Artemiadis, A.; Ioannidis, P.; Papadimitriou, M.; Konstantinopoulou, E.; Aretouli, E.; Messinis, L.; Nasios, G.; Dardiotis, E.; et al. Computerized Cognitive Rehabilitation for Treatment of Cognitive Impairment in Multiple Sclerosis: An Explorative Study. *J. Integr. Neurosci* 2020, 19, 341–347. [CrossRef]
43. Jeong, I.C.; Liu, J.; Finkelstein, J. Association Between System Usage Pattern and Impact of Web-Based Telerehabilitation in Patients with Multiple Sclerosis. *Stud. Health Technol. Inform.* 2020, 272, 346–349. [CrossRef]
44. Kratz, A.L.; Atalla, M.; Whibley, D.; Myles, A.; Thurston, T.; Fritz, N.E. Calling Out MS Fatigue: Feasibility and Preliminary Effects of a Pilot Randomized Telephone-Delivered Exercise Intervention for Multiple Sclerosis Fatigue. *J. Neurol. Phys. Ther.* 2020, 44, 23–31. [CrossRef]
45. Flachenecker, P.; Bures, A.K.; Gawlik, A.; Weiland, A.-C.; Kuld, S.; Gusowski, K.; Streber, R.; Pfeifer, K.; Tallner, A. Efficacy of an Internet-Based Program to Promote Physical Activity and Exercise after Inpatient Rehabilitation in Persons with Multiple Sclerosis: A Randomized, Single-Blind, Controlled Study. *Int. J. Environ. Res. Public Health* 2020, 17, 4544. [CrossRef]
46. Manns, P.J.; Mehrabani, G.; Norton, S.; Aminian, S.; Motl, R.W. The SitLess With MS Program: Intervention Feasibility and Change in Sedentary Behavior. *Arch. Rehabil. Res. Clin. Transl.* 2020, 2, 100083. [CrossRef] [PubMed]
47. Donkers, S.J.; Nickel, D.; Paul, L.; Wegers, S.R.; Knox, K.B. Adherence to Physiotherapy-Guided Web-Based Exercise for Persons with Moderate-to-Severe Multiple Sclerosis: A Randomized Controlled Pilot Study. *Int. J. MS Care* 2020, 22, 208–214. [CrossRef]
48. Messinis, L.; Kosmidis, M.H.; Nasios, G.; Konitsiotis, S.; Ntoskou, A.; Bakirtzis, C.; Grigoriadis, N.; Patrikelis, P.; Panagiotopoulos, E.; Gourzis, P.; et al. Do Secondary Progressive Multiple Sclerosis Patients Benefit from Computer- Based Cognitive Neurorehabilitation? A Randomized Sham Controlled Trial. *Mult. Scler. Relat. Disord.* 2020, 39, 101932. [CrossRef] [PubMed]
49. Minen, M.T.; Schaubhut, K.B.; Morio, K. Smartphone Based Behavioral Therapy for Pain in Multiple Sclerosis (MS) Patients: A Feasibility Acceptability Randomized Controlled Study for the Treatment of Comorbid Migraine and Ms Pain. *Mult. Scler. Relat. Disord.* 2020, 46, 102489. [CrossRef] [PubMed]
50. Van Geel, F.; Geurts, E.; Abasıyanık, Z.; Coninx, K.; Feys, P. Feasibility Study of a 10-Week Community-Based Program Using the WalkWithMe Application on Physical Activity, Walking, Fatigue and Cognition in Persons with Multiple Sclerosis. *Mult. Scler. Relat. Disord.* 2020, 42, 102067. [CrossRef] [PubMed]
51. Bove, R.; Rowles, W.; Zhao, C.; Anderson, A.; Friedman, S.; Langdon, D.; Alexander, A.; Sacco, S.; Henry, R.; Gazzaley, A.; et al. A Novel In-Home Digital Treatment to Improve Processing Speed in People with Multiple Sclerosis: A Pilot Study. *Mult. Scler.* 2021 27, 778–789. [CrossRef] [PubMed]
52. Tarakci, E.; Tarakci, D.; Hajebrahimi, F.; Budak, M. Supervised Exercises versus Telerehabilitation. Benefits for Persons with Multiple Sclerosis. *Acta. Neurol. Scand.* 2021. [CrossRef] [PubMed]
53. Williams, K.L.; Low Choy, N.L.; Brauer, S.G. Center-Based Group and Home-Based Individual Exercise Programs Have Similar Impacts on Gait and Balance in People With Multiple Sclerosis: A Randomized Trial. *PM R* 2021, 13, 9–18. [CrossRef] [PubMed]
54. Miller, D.M.; Moore, S.M.; Fox, R.J.; Atreja, A.; Fu, A.Z.; Lee, J.-C.; Saupe, W.; Stadtler, M.; Chakraborty, S.; Harris, C.M.; et al. Web-Based Self-Management for Patients with Multiple Sclerosis: A Practical, Randomized Trial. *Telemed. e-Health* 2011, 17, 5–13. [CrossRef] [PubMed]
55. Greiner, P.; Sawka, A.; Imison, E. Patient and Physician Perspectives on MSdialog, an Electronic PRO Diary in Multiple Sclerosis. *Patient* 2015, 8, 541–550. [CrossRef] [PubMed]

56. D'hooghe, M.; Van Gassen, G.; Kos, D.; Bouquiaux, O.; Cambron, M.; Decoo, D.; Lysandropoulos, A.; Van Wijmeersch, B.; Willekens, B.; Penner, I.-K.; et al. Improving Fatigue in Multiple Sclerosis by Smartphone-Supported Energy Management: The MS TeleCoach Feasibility Study. *Mult. Scler. Relat. Disord.* **2018**, *22*, 90–96. [CrossRef]
57. Midaglia, L.; Mulero, P.; Montalban, X.; Graves, J.; Hauser, S.L.; Julian, L.; Baker, M.; Schadrack, J.; Gossens, C.; Scotland, A.; et al. Adherence and Satisfaction of Smartphone- and Smartwatch-Based Remote Active Testing and Passive Monitoring in People With Multiple Sclerosis: Nonrandomized Interventional Feasibility Study. *J. Med. Internet Res.* **2019**, *21*, e14863. [CrossRef]
58. Newland, P.; Oliver, B.; Newland, J.M.; Thomas, F.P. Testing Feasibility of a Mobile Application to Monitor Fatigue in People With Multiple Sclerosis. *J. Neurosci. Nurs.* **2019**, *51*, 331–334. [CrossRef]
59. Pratap, A.; Grant, D.; Vegesna, A.; Tummalacherla, M.; Cohan, S.; Deshpande, C.; Mangravite, L.; Omberg, L. Evaluating the Utility of Smartphone-Based Sensor Assessments in Persons With Multiple Sclerosis in the Real-World Using an App (ElevateMS): Observational, Prospective Pilot Digital Health Study. *JMIR Mhealth Uhealth* **2020**, *8*, e22108. [CrossRef] [PubMed]
60. Baddeley, A. *Working Memory*; Clarendon Press: Oxford, UK; Oxford University Press: Oxford, UK, 1986.
61. Tacchino, A.; Pedullà, L.; Bonzano, L.; Vassallo, C.; Battaglia, M.A.; Mancardi, G.; Bove, M.; Brichetto, G. A New App for At-Home Cognitive Training: Description and Pilot Testing on Patients with Multiple Sclerosis. *JMIR Mhealth Uhealth* **2015**, *3*, e85. [CrossRef]
62. Sohlberg, M.M.; Mateer, C.A. Effectiveness of an Attention-Training Program. *J. Clin. Exp. Neuropsychol.* **1987**, *9*, 117–130. [CrossRef]
63. Finkelstein, J.; Wood, J.; Shan, Y. Implementing Physical Telerehabilitation System for Patients with Multiple Sclerosis. In Proceedings of the 2011 4th International Conference on Biomedical Engineering and Informatics (BMEI), Shanghai, China, 15–17 October 2011; pp. 1883–1886.
64. Exell, S.; Thristan, M.; Dangond, F.; Marhardt, K.; St Charles-Krohe, M.; Turner-Bowker, D.M. A Novel Electronic Application of Patient-Reported Outcomes in Multiple Sclerosis—Meeting the Necessary Challenge of Assessing Quality of Life and Outcomes in Daily Clinical Practice. *Eur. Neurol. Rev.* **2014**, *9*, 49. [CrossRef]
65. Williams, A.; Fossey, E.; Farhall, J.; Foley, F.; Thomas, N. Impact of Jointly Using an E-Mental Health Resource (Self-Management And Recovery Technology) on Interactions Between Service Users Experiencing Severe Mental Illness and Community Mental Health Workers: Grounded Theory Study. *JMIR Ment. Health* **2021**, *8*, e25998. [CrossRef]
66. Lampit, A.; Heine, J.; Finke, C.; Barnett, M.H.; Valenzuela, M.; Wolf, A.; Leung, I.H.K.; Hill, N.T.M. Computerized Cognitive Training in Multiple Sclerosis: A Systematic Review and Meta-Analysis. *Neurorehabil. Neural. Repair* **2019**, *33*, 695–706. [CrossRef] [PubMed]
67. Yang, T.-T.; Wang, L.; Deng, X.-Y.; Yu, G. Pharmacological Treatments for Fatigue in Patients with Multiple Sclerosis: A Systematic Review and Meta-Analysis. *J. Neurol. Sci.* **2017**, *380*, 256–261. [CrossRef]
68. Heine, M.; van de Port, I.; Rietberg, M.B.; van Wegen, E.E.H.; Kwakkel, G. Exercise Therapy for Fatigue in Multiple Sclerosis. *Cochrane Database Syst. Rev.* **2015**, CD009956. [CrossRef]
69. Tramontano, M.; Morone, G.; De Angelis, S.; Casagrande Conti, L.; Galeoto, G.; Grasso, M.G. Sensor-Based Technology for Upper Limb Rehabilitation in Patients with Multiple Sclerosis: A Randomized Controlled Trial. *Restor. Neurol. Neurosci.* **2020**, *38*, 333–341. [CrossRef] [PubMed]
70. Wendebourg, M.J.; Heesen, C.; Finlayson, M.; Meyer, B.; Pöttgen, J.; Köpke, S. Patient Education for People with Multiple Sclerosis-Associated Fatigue: A Systematic Review. *PLoS ONE* **2017**, *12*, e0173025. [CrossRef]
71. Rieckmann, P.; Centonze, D.; Elovaara, I.; Giovannoni, G.; Havrdová, E.; Kesselring, J.; Kobelt, G.; Langdon, D.; Morrow, S.A.; Oreja-Guevara, C.; et al. Unmet Needs, Burden of Treatment, and Patient Engagement in Multiple Sclerosis: A Combined Perspective from the MS in the 21st Century Steering Group. *Mult. Scler. Relat. Disord.* **2018**, *19*, 153–160. [CrossRef] [PubMed]
72. Brydges, C.R. Effect Size Guidelines, Sample Size Calculations, and Statistical Power in Gerontology. *Innov. Aging* **2019**, *3*, igz036. [CrossRef]
73. Bonnechère, B.; Langley, C.; Sahakian, B.J. The Use of Commercial Computerised Cognitive Games in Older Adults: A Meta-Analysis. *Sci. Rep.* **2020**, *10*, 15276. [CrossRef]
74. US Food & Drug Administration. FDA Permits Marketing of First Game-Based Digital Therapeutic to Improve Attention Function in Children with ADHD. Available online: https://www.fda.gov/news-events/press-announcements/fda-permits-marketing-first-game-based-digital-therapeutic-improve-attention-function-children-adhd (accessed on 28 June 2021).
75. Marra, C.; Gordon, W.J.; Stern, A.D. Use of Connected Digital Products in Clinical Research Following the COVID-19 Pandemic: A Comprehensive Analysis of Clinical Trials. *BMJ Open* **2021**, *11*, e047341. [CrossRef]
76. Carl, J.R.; Jones, D.J.; Lindhiem, O.J.; Doss, B.D.; Weingardt, K.R.; Timmons, A.C.; Comer, J.S. Regulating Digital Therapeutics for Mental Health: Opportunities, Challenges, and the Essential Role of Psychologists. *Br. J. Clin. Psychol.* **2021**. [CrossRef]
77. Scott Kruse, C.; Karem, P.; Shifflett, K.; Vegi, L.; Ravi, K.; Brooks, M. Evaluating Barriers to Adopting Telemedicine Worldwide: A Systematic Review. *J. Telemed. Telecare.* **2018**, *24*, 4–12. [CrossRef] [PubMed]
78. Rangachari, P.; Mushiana, S.S.; Herbert, K. A Narrative Review of Factors Historically Influencing Telehealth Use across Six Medical Specialties in the United States. *Int. J. Environ. Res. Public Health* **2021**, *18*, 4995. [CrossRef] [PubMed]
79. Almathami, H.K.Y.; Win, K.T.; Vlahu-Gjorgievska, E. Barriers and Facilitators That Influence Telemedicine-Based, Real-Time, Online Consultation at Patients' Homes: Systematic Literature Review. *J. Med. Internet Res.* **2020**, *22*, e16407. [CrossRef]

80. Engelsma, T.; Jaspers, M.W.M.; Peute, L.W. Considerate MHealth Design for Older Adults with Alzheimer's Disease and Related Dementias (ADRD): A Scoping Review on Usability Barriers and Design Suggestions. *Int. J. Med. Inform.* **2021**, *152*, 104494. [CrossRef] [PubMed]
81. Bevens, W.; Gray, K.; Neate, S.L.; Nag, N.; Weiland, T.J.; Jelinek, G.A.; Simpson-Yap S. Characteristics of MHealth App Use in an International Sample of People with Multiple Sclerosis. *Mult. Scler. Relat. Disord.* **2021**, *54*, 103092. [CrossRef]
82. Spina, E.; Trojsi, F.; Tozza, S.; Iovino, A.; Iodice, R.; Passaniti, C.; Abbadessa, G.; Bonavita, S.; Leocani, L.; Tedeschi, G.; et al. How to Manage with Telemedicine People with Neuromuscular Diseases? *Neurol. Sci.* **2021**. [CrossRef]
83. Bergier, H.; Duron, L.; Sordet, C.; Kawka, L.; Schlencker, A.; Chasset, F.; Arnaud, L. Digital Health, Big Data and Smart Technologies for the Care of Patients with Systemic Autoimmune Diseases: Where Do We Stand? *Autoimmun. Rev.* **2021**, *20*, 102864. [CrossRef]
84. Bornechère, B.; Omelina, L.; Kostkova, K.; Van Sint Jan, S.; Jansen, B. The End of Active Video Games and the Consequences for Rehabilitation. *Physiother. Res. Int.* **2018**, *23*, e1752. [CrossRef]

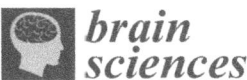

Communication

An ID-Associated Application to Facilitate Patient-Tailored Management of Multiple Sclerosis

Michael Lang [1,*], Daniela Rau [1], Lukas Cepek [1], Fia Cürten [2], Stefan Ringbauer [2] and Martin Mayr [2]

1. NeuroPoint Patientenakademie, 89073 Ulm, Germany; rau@neuropoint.de (D.R.); cepek@neuropoint.de (L.C.)
2. NeuroSys GmbH, 89081 Ulm, Germany; fia.cuerten@neurosys.de (F.C.); stefan.ringbauer@neurosys.de (S.R.); martin.mayr@neurosys.de (M.M.)
* Correspondence: lang@neuropoint.de; Tel.: +49-731-15979794

Abstract: Despite improvements in diagnosis and treatment, multiple sclerosis (MS) is the leading neurological cause of disability in young adults. As a chronic disease, MS requires complex and challenging management. In this context, eHealth has gained an increasing relevance. Here, we aim to summarize beneficial features of a mobile app recently implemented in clinical MS routine as well as beyond MS. PatientConcept is a CE-certified, ID-associated multilingual software application allowing patients to record relevant health data without disclosing any identifying data. Patients can voluntarily share their health data with selected physicians. Since its implementation in 2018, about 3000 MS patients have used PatientConcept. Initially developed as a physician–patient communication platform, the app maps risk management plans of all current disease modifying therapies and thereby facilitates adherence to specified monitoring appointments. It also allows continuous monitoring of various PROs (Patient Reported Outcomes), enabling a broad overview of the disease course. In addition, various studies/projects currently assess monitoring, follow-up, diagnostics and telemetric evaluations of patients with other diseases beyond MS. Altogether, PatientConcept offers a broad range of possibilities to support physician–patient communication, implementation of risk management plans and assessment of PROs. It is a promising tool to facilitate patient-tailored management of MS and other chronic diseases.

Keywords: multiple sclerosis; chronic disease; disease management; Patient Reported Outcomes; e-health; app; communication; digital tools

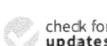

Citation: Lang, M.; Rau, D.; Cepek, L.; Cürten, F.; Ringbauer, S.; Mayr, M. An ID-Associated Application to Facilitate Patient-Tailored Management of Multiple Sclerosis. *Brain Sci.* **2021**, *11*, 1061. https://doi.org/10.3390/brainsci11081061

Academic Editors: Stephen D. Meriney and Cristoforo Comi

Received: 15 July 2021
Accepted: 11 August 2021
Published: 12 August 2021

Publisher's Note: MDPI stays neutral with regard to jurisdictional claims in published maps and institutional affiliations.

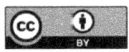

Copyright: © 2021 by the authors. Licensee MDPI, Basel, Switzerland. This article is an open access article distributed under the terms and conditions of the Creative Commons Attribution (CC BY) license (https://creativecommons.org/licenses/by/4.0/).

1. Introduction

"Every 5 min, someone, somewhere in the world is diagnosed with MS" [1]. As the leading neurological cause of disability in young adults [1], MS is considered a growing global problem [2,3]. Disease symptoms are highly individual, ranging from fatigue, visual and bladder disorders, spasticity and mobility restriction to psychological disorders such as depression [4,5] which have a severe impact on the patient's life.

Despite improvements in the diagnosis of MS and a major expansion of effective treatment options [2], disease management remains complex and challenging. As with other chronic diseases, it usually requires long periods of supervision, including regular monitoring and routine visits to observe disease progress or complications [6]. Therefore there is a high demand for individually tailored concepts that facilitate patients' access to healthcare and support the treating physicians in the provision of healthcare services.

During recent years, the development of digital healthcare technologies including mobile phone apps has gained an increasing relevance in disease management [7–10]. In particular for complex and unpredictable diseases such as MS, eHealth can improve monitoring and individual treatment [11], and furthermore promises to expand the possibilities for patients to manage their own care [12]. The relevance of eHealth is also underlined by the German Digital Healthcare Act, a recently passed law to support the future use of apps and other digital applications in the health system [13].

We successfully implemented an ID-associated application to facilitate patient-tailored management of MS [14]. Here, we aim to summarize its features in clinical routine with MS patients as well as its use in projects beyond MS, demonstrating the broad spectrum of possible applications and thus its adaptability to different diseases and individual patient needs.

2. Materials

The PatientConcept app is a CE (Conformité Européenne) certified mobile health software application that was developed in 2016 by a multidisciplinary team of physicians (neurologists, psychiatrists, experts on diabetes) and statisticians in cooperation with an IT company. Development was conducted in compliance with essential health and safety requirements of Directive 93/42/EEC and the product-related harmonized standards and specifications DIN EN ISO 14971, DIN EN ISO 62304, IEC 62366 and DIN EN ISO 13485 [14]. To ensure data safety, the app employs a secure ID associated data management, in which each patient receives their own, worldwide explicit ID for the patient's mobile device. This approach allows distinguishing between medical data (e.g., blood values, disease history) and optional patient identifying data (optional details exclusively stored locally on the smartphone: name, phone number and date of birth). Thus, patients can record relevant health data without disclosing any identifying data. In case patients voluntarily decide to share their health data with selected physicians, practices and/or pharmacies by providing their personal ID, physicians can access health data and bidirectional communication is enabled.

The PatientConcept app is available for free download via the German app store (for both iOS and android smartphones or tablets). It can be used in a multilingual manner (German, English, Italian, French, Portuguese) [14].

3. Results

3.1. Application in the Field of MS

The app was initially developed as a doctor–patient communication platform with the aim of improving patient education, facilitating and thereby strengthening the communication between patients and their physicians, and to ease the daily routine of chronically ill patients. For example, the app provides a medication timer and simplifies requesting follow-up prescriptions for drugs and non-pharmacological therapies (physiotherapy, ergotherapy) from the treating physician with minimal effort.

The app enables bidirectional structured communication: Not only can patients contact their treating physician, but the physician can also communicate specifically with the patient. The patient can thereby receive regular information from the treatment center via push-news, e.g., on current seminars and disease-related updates and useful tips.

Since its implementation in 2018, about 3000 MS patients are/have been using the application. Meanwhile, many additional functions were added to the application. Risk management plans for all current disease modifying therapies have been integrated into the app to accompany the patient in adhering to the specified monitoring. In addition to reminding the patient of monitoring appointments (imaging, laboratory or consultative examinations) according to the guidelines of the respective therapy, the app also controls compliance. ToDo messages that have not been carried out or limit values that have been exceeded automatically result in specific information being sent to the responsible treatment practitioner (Figure 1).

The app offers the possibility of entering various monitoring parameters, which are also checked by the system through an implemented red-flag warning system that can automatically inform the physician via red-flag email in case of critical data (e.g., aberrant blood values). In addition to the parameters specified in the risk management plan, the daily step count and important patient-reported outcome (PRO) measurements can be monitored (Figure 2) in PatientConcept and the upcoming MS-DiGA Emendia (described below). Examples include the assessment of cognition, pinching and drawing tests. Tests/questionnaires can be completed by the patients on a regular basis. Physicians receive supplementary information on the individual disease course via features such as the MS diary. Overall, physicians are provided with a broad treatment overview, e.g., on therapy history and disease progression (Figure 3).

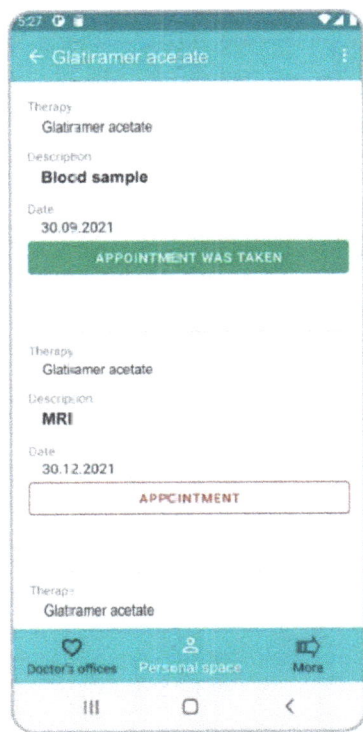

Figure 1. Risk Management Plan. PatientConcept currently maps all risk management plans in MS therapy. Control appointments are specified and checked by the system.

Importantly, the app allows safe use across all indications. Through its anonymous ID-based data management system anonymous disease- and therapy-associated patient data can be collected over a prolonged period of time for research into therapy benefits and patient care.

Beyond the indication MS, the APP is used by about 1000 migraine patients and is currently also used in the indication of dizziness and gastroenterology, and furthermore for the follow-up of breast cancer patients in Germany and COVID patients in Luxembourg. In the meantime, the APP has been in sustained use in the indication of MS since its first publication 4 years ago, and there are more than 2 year data sets used in everyday clinical practice.

A new development for digital support of MS-therapy is the mobile health application Emendia (Latin: "emendare"—to improve), which is planned for market launch in Germany as a Digital Health Application (DiGA) in 2022. According to the German Digital Care Act, DiGAs can be prescribed by a physician at the expense of the statutory health insurance companies. To be approved as a DiGA, such an app has to comply with the strict medical guidelines of the Federal Institute for Drugs and Medical Devices. Emendia MS can provide opportunities for improved self-assessment of the patient's disease status. This is accomplished by a combined collection of subjective parameters of the patient's perceived well-being (e.g., self-perceived overall health) on the one hand and objective patient data (e.g., on motor function via sensors in the smartphone) on the other hand. In addition, Emendia MS aims to strengthen the health literacy of patients by providing valid, understandable information to help them better cope with their disease in everyday life. In contrast to the previously described system PatientConcept, which has been designed as a system for patient–physician communication, Emendia MS has been primarily created for individual use by the patient. Nevertheless, patients receive the opportunity to transmit their health data to the attending physician. In the case that the practice treats patients using either the PatientConcept or Emendia MS system, the backends of both systems are connected enabling interoperability. Patient searches across both systems via patient ID are made possible by this seamless connection without the need for an additional log-in (Figure 4).

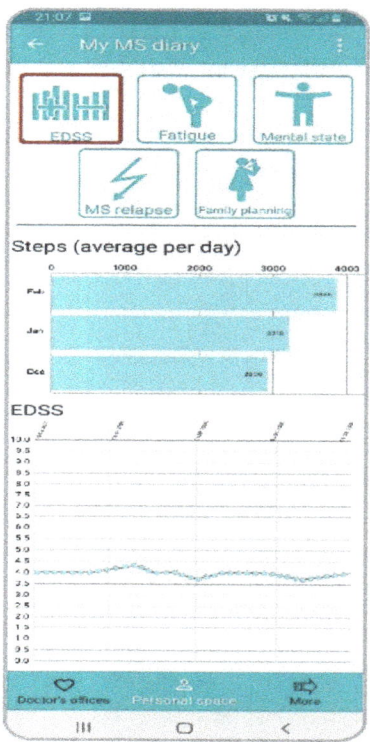

Figure 2. Monitoring of PROs. Patients complete tests/questionnaires on a regular basis, allowing monitoring of various patient reported outcomes.

3.2. Further Applications beyond MS

Besides MS, other chronic diseases also require permanent and continuous medical care. Therefore, we investigated whether the app is suitable for the management of patients with hereditary transthyretin-amyloidosis in an interdisciplinary setting (neurology/cardiology/gastroenterology, etc.) and according to GDPR (general data protection regulation). Time required for the consultation can be optimized, conversations are more specific and targeted, and the exchange between treating colleagues intensified [15].

Patients require monitoring not only during a disease, but also afterwards. The app is currently being used in a nationwide project in 40 cancer centres for continuous tumor follow-up of breast cancer patients (PRO B (Charite, Berlin); https://pro-b-projekt.de

(accessed on 12 August 2021)). Corresponding projects are also planned for the follow-up care of patients with prostate carcinomas and testicular tumors.

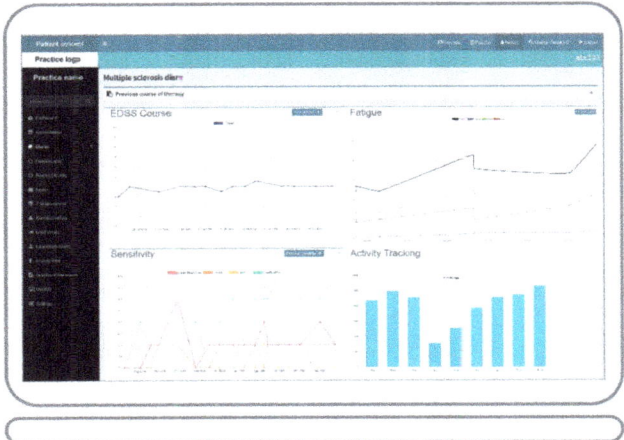

Figure 3. Treatment overview: Using a browser-supported portal for therapy monitoring, no additional software installation is necessary. The attending physician receives a comprehensive overview of the therapy course.

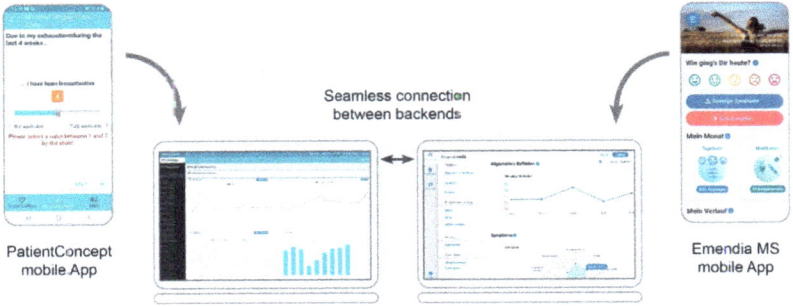

Figure 4. DiGA. Illustration of the interoperability of the PatientConcept and Emendia MS systems. A switch button enables seamless connection without additional log-in between the systems.

In addition, the Luxemburg based CON-VINCE study (https://researchluxembourg.lu/covid-19-taskforce/con-vince, (accessed on 12 August 2021)) currently investigates the use of the app (available in five languages) in monitoring COVID patients across Luxembourg [16].

Beyond the aspect of monitoring, possibilities and limitations of the app as a diagnosis-supporting tool for the differentiation of selected neurological clinical pictures and disease groups were tested [17]. Diagnosis of rare neurological diseases is often difficult. Therefore, the aim was to use diagnosis-supporting procedures that recognise patterns in vast amounts of raw data via artificial intelligence (AI) and generate diagnostic suggestions based on these patterns. By means of specifically generated questionnaires, the app was able to support diagnostics through implemented differential diagnoses and could be used supportively for telemedical solutions (ARTIS Project— www.patientconcept.de/artis (accessed on 12 August 2021)).

As possibilities in the telemetric evaluation of examinations are increasing, we recently tested the transmission of high-resolution images from the peripheral consultation to the ophthalmological specialist via PatientConcept. Analysis of 150 patients in five neurological practices demonstrated the basic feasibility of a telemetric assessment of ocular fundus images using the app [18].

For patients with Parkinson's disease we also plan to launch a digital health application by the end of 2021/beginning of 2022. This results from further development of a project in which sensor data and diary entries from Parkinson's patients were joint. The aim of the DiGA is to record the status of Parkinson's disease and optimise therapeutic decisions.

4. Discussion

"The disease with a thousand faces" [19]—this well-known term for the chronic disease multiple sclerosis already implies the high and complex demands on disease management. One of the central aspects of disease management should be continuous and regular monitoring of safety [20]. Risk management plans define specific examinations for each drug; compliance with these is tedious as well as time- and cost-consuming and thus a major challenge for both patients and physicians. Nevertheless, implementation of risk management plans is indispensable to reduce or avoid serious side effects. To facilitate continuous monitoring, digital applications such as mobile apps have proven useful. In recent years, their development has advanced rapidly and can be of profound benefit [8,9]. mHealth (mobile Health) potentially may deliver healthcare regardless of time and place or geographical constraints [21,22]. Particularly for MS with its long and unpredictable disease course, long-term monitoring preferably with digital applications is a necessity [11,23]. Examples of apps supporting monitoring include the Novartis SymTrac app, My MS manager and MS dialog app [8]. The PatientConcept app and the integrated risk management plan can better help to comply with predefined and monitored requirements by reminding patients of their regular imaging, laboratory or consultation examinations and controlling for documented aberrant values.

Monitoring should not only contain safety aspects, but also clinical and subclinical disease activity to evaluate treatment effectiveness, supporting individualized treatment [20]. In addition to clinical and radiological monitoring, the patients themselves can contribute to evaluating the efficacy of their medication by documenting PRO measurements. These are provided directly by the patient and include symptoms, activity limitations, cognitive and health status, level of fatigue or quality of life [20,24]. Besides their relevance in clinical trials that increasingly define PROs as secondary or tertiary outcomes, PROs are playing an important role also in clinical practice in order to better understand the impact of MS and its therapy on the patient's life under real world conditions [24,25].

Continuous assessment of PROs via the PatientConcept app enables the physician to follow the progression of the disease based on various parameters over time compared to the limited possibilities of a "snapshot" during the personal visit to the practice. It also saves valuable time that physicians could use more sensibly for their patients. In addition, continuous PRO monitoring facilitates the physician in discussing past processes and events with the patient more clearly. The immediate check of patient entries by the system, which informs of any aberrant values, allows the physician to intervene earlier and to make necessary treatment adjustments, resulting in a more patient-tailored therapy approach. The integrated walking assessment via step counts (by the smartphone) could be beneficial for evaluating the severity of the disease, as it facilitates a meaningful assessment of patient mobility [26]. PROs are one example of giving patients a voice. PREMs (patient-reported experience measures) should also be monitored long-term and integrated as a standard in order to identify and prevent problems at an early stage [26].

Patients should also be well informed and involved in treatment decisions to achieve patient engagement. Recognizing that each patient with their different needs is individual displays a core aspect of patient engagement [27], that results in better outcomes and treatment adherence [28–31]. Poor adherence displays a major challenge in MS management [32,33]. Adherence to prescribed disease-modifying treatments (DMTs) can be further improved by a better general connectivity of the patient to the practice or patient portal. Intensified support of MS patients via patient support programs (through patient portal, MS nurse or physicians) has been shown to be beneficial for improving quality of care, patients' quality of life, patient participation and adherence in earlier studies [34–39]. Therefore, the app was initially developed to intensify bidirectional patient–physician communication and to increase patients' commitment to the practice, thereby providing continuous support for chronically ill patients without burdening the physician's time budget.

Since the Digital Health Care Act was introduced in December 2019, DiGAs are receiving growing attention. While a survey revealed that physicians perceive digital health applications as an opportunity, measures to increase acceptance particular among general practitioners appear sensible [40]. The presented DiGA Emendia is unique in allowing the patient to share health data with the treating physician, offering the advantage that a long-term use of Emendia for medical consultation and optimized therapy decisions could be ensured. Currently, 17 DIGAs are listed with others under review [41], aiming at further supporting patients in coping with their disease.

To reduce the patient's burden, disease management should not only be tailored to the individual patient but should also include multidisciplinary assessment [42]. This aspect is of high relevance because a multimodal, interdisciplinary approach is indispensable for an effective management of multisymptomatic diseases such as MS and involves close and continuous collaboration between various specialists [43]. Applying such an interdisciplinary approach for MS patients has been shown to be difficult [44]. Since the parallel use of different apps is not expedient, a consolidated approach is desirable. While most devices are developed for use in the context of one specific disease, the PatientConcept platform (various complementary APPs but only one portal for the physician) can be employed across indications and thus allows easier interdisciplinary exchange and potentially improves the flow of information on medical content for the benefit of patients. This enables specific requests to a specialised centre even in structurally weak regions. Thus, the app might offer an opportunity to improve the quality of care and treatment and to increase the effectiveness of therapeutic measures in MS care. Particularly in times of a pandemic, continuous monitoring could be carried out with the help of the app, potentially supplying profound benefit.

Even though various mHealth (mobile Health) tools have been developed to ease disease management, monitoring, rehabilitation and education of MS patients [8], the usage of available medical software applications remains comparably low. Reasons include concerns about privacy and security [45]. To our knowledge, PatientConcept App was one of the first CE-certified apps and is utilizing a worldwide explicit ID used by the patient to allow safe and structured data management and transfer while ensuring the highest security standards and data privacy. This ID-based data management system could also provide large real-world data sets of anonymous disease-related and therapy-associated patient data over a prolonged period of time to evaluate therapy benefits and patient care outside of clinical trials.

5. Conclusions

The ID-associated CE-certified PatientConcept app is widely used, not only by MS patients, and offers a broad range of possibilities for enhancing bidirectional physician–patient communication, aiming at improving treatment adherence. The use of automated routines can facilitate the indispensable implementation of risk management plans. With its various adaptable features including the assessment of PROs and its possible implementation also in interdisciplinary approaches, the application is a promising tool to facilitate patient-tailored management of multiple sclerosis and other chronic diseases. The usage of PatientConcept with its secure data storage in daily patient care could also provide relevant data on the efficacy of medical measures in the real world.

Author Contributions: Conceptualization, M.L., M.M., F.C., D.R. and L.C.; methodology, M.L. and M.M.; software, S.R.; validation, M.L. and M.M.; formal analysis, S.R.; investigation, M.L. and M.M.; data curation, S.R.; writing—original draft preparation, M.L., F.C. and M.M.; writing—review and editing, M.L. and M.M.; visualization, M.M. and F.C.; supervision, M.L.; project administration, M.L. and M.M.; funding acquisition, M.L. and M.M. All authors have read and agreed to the published version of the manuscript.

Funding: PatientConcept system has received financial support from the Bavarian state, Neuropoint Patient Academy and Systemhaus Ulm, Almirall, Alnylam, Bayer, Biogen, Novartis, Roche, Sanofi Genzyme and Teva.

Institutional Review Board Statement: Cited studies were approved by the Ethics Committee of the LÄK Stuttgart (F-2018-038, F-2018-061, F-2019-099; F-2016-013).

Informed Consent Statement: Informed consent was obtained from all subjects involved in the study.

Acknowledgments: Editorial support (writing assistance, based on authors' detailed directions) was provided by Katrin Blumbach (med:unit GmbH).

Conflicts of Interest: M. Lang, D. Rau, L. Cepek and M. Mayr have received travel grants, speaker's honoraria, financial research support, consultancy fees from Almirall, Alnylam, Bayer, Biogen, Bristol-Myers Squibb, Lilly, Merck, Novartis, Roche, Sanofi Genzyme and Teva. F. Cürten and S. Ringbauer have nothing to declare.

References

1. Multiple Sclerosis International Federation. Atlas of MS 2020, 3rd edition. Part 1: Mapping Multiple Sclerosis around the World. Available online: https://www.msif.org/wp-content/uploads/2020/10/Atlas-3rd-Edition-Epidemiology-report-EN-updated-30-9-20.pdf (accessed on 19 May 2021).
2. Coetzee, T.; Thompson, A.J. Atlas of MS 2020: Informing global policy change. *Mult. Scler.* **2020**, *26*, 1807–1808. [CrossRef] [PubMed]
3. Walton, C.; King, R.; Rechtman, L.; Kaye, W.; Leray, E.; Marrie, R.A.; Robertson, N.; La Rocca, N.; Uitdehaag, B.; van der Mei, I.; et al. Rising prevalence of multiple sclerosis worldwide: Insights from the Atlas of MS, third edition. *Mult. Scler.* **2020**, *26*, 1816–1821. [CrossRef]
4. Ziemssen, T. Multiple sclerosis beyond EDSS: Depression and fatigue. *J. Neurol. Sci.* **2009**, *277*, S37–S41. [CrossRef]
5. Kip, M.; Zimmermann, A. *Krankheitsbild Multiple Sklerose. Weißbuch Multiple Sklerose*; Springer: Berlin/Heidelberg, Germany, 2016.
6. Reynolds, R.; Dennis, S.; Hasan, I.; Slewa, J.; Chen, W.; Tian, D.; Bobba, S.; Zwar, N. A systematic review of chronic disease management interventions in primary care. *BMC Fam. Pract.* **2018**, *19*, 11. [CrossRef]
7. WHO: mHealth. New Horizons for Health through Mobile Technologies. Available online: https://www.who.int/goe/publications/goe_mhealth_web.pdf (accessed on 12 August 2021).
8. Marziniak, M.; Brichetto, G.; Feys, P.; Meyding-Lamade, U.; Vernon, K.; Meuth, S.G. The Use of Digital and Remote Communication Technologies as a Tool for Multiple Sclerosis Management: Narrative Review. *JMIR Rehabil. Assist. Technol.* **2018**, *5*, e5. [CrossRef]
9. Lavorgna, L.; Brigo, F.; Moccia, M.; Leocani, L.; Lanzillo, R.; Clerico, M.; Abbadessa, G.; Schmierer, K.; Solaro, C.; Prosperini, L.; et al. e-Health and multiple sclerosis: An update. *Mult. Scler.* **2018**, *24*, 1657–1664. [CrossRef]
10. Kern, R.; Haase, R.; Eisele, J.C.; Thomas, K.; Ziemssen, T. Designing an Electronic Patient Management System for Multiple Sclerosis: Building a Next Generation Multiple Sclerosis Documentation System. *Interact. J. Med. Res.* **2016**, *5*, e2. [CrossRef] [PubMed]
11. Haase, R.; Wunderlich, M.; Dillenseger, A.; Kern, R.; Akgun, K.; Ziemssen, T. Improving multiple sclerosis management and collecting safety information in the real world: The MSDS3D software approach. *Expert Opin. Drug Saf.* **2018**, *17*, 369–378. [CrossRef]
12. Matthews, P.M.; Block, V.J.; Leocani, L. E-health and multiple sclerosis. *Curr. Opin. Neurol.* **2020**, *33*, 271–276. [CrossRef]
13. Bundesministerium für Gesundheit. Available online: https://www.bundesgesundheitsministerium.de/digital-healthcare-act.html (accessed on 25 May 2021).
14. Lang, M.; Mayr, M.; Ringbauer, S.; Cepek, L. PatientConcept App: Key Characteristics, Implementation, and its Potential Benefit. *Neurol. Ther.* **2019**, *8*, 147–154. [CrossRef] [PubMed]
15. Lang, M.; ATTRv. Abstract Submitted to DGN Congress 2021. University of Luxembourg. CON-VINCE Study. Available online: https://wwwde.uni.lu/universitaet/aktuelles/diashow/erste_ergebnisse_der_con_vince_studie (accessed on 27 May 2021).
16. Klawonn, F.; Lechner, W.; Lechner, C.; Mayr, M.; Lang, M.; Grigull, L. Neuromuskuläre Erkrankungen: Mit künstlicher Intelligenz zur schnelleren Diagnose; Abstract Submitted to DGN Congress 2021. Available online: https://dgnkongress.org/home.html (accessed on 12 August 2021).
17. Cepek, L.; Guggenmoos, F.; Ringbauer, S.; Mayr, M.; Lang, M. Telemetrische Untersuchung des Augenhintergrunds; Abstract Sumitted to DGN Congress 2021. Available online: https://dgnkongress.org/home.html (accessed on 12 August 2021).
18. Reich, D.S.; Lucchinetti, C.F.; Calabresi, P.A. Multiple Sclerosis. *N. Eng. J. Med.* **2018**, *378*, 169–180. [CrossRef]
19. Giovannoni, G.; Butzkueven, H.; Dhib-Jalbut, S.; Hobart, J.; Kobelt, G.; Pepper, G.; Sormani, M.P.; Thalheim, C.; Traboulsee, A.; Vollmer, T. Brain health: Time matters in multiple sclerosis. *Mult. Scler. Relat. Disord.* **2016**, *9*, S5–S48. [CrossRef] [PubMed]

20. Akter, S.; Ray, P. mHealth—an Ultimate Platform to Serve the Unserved. *Yearb. Med Inform.* **2010**, *19*, 94–100. [CrossRef]
21. Tachakra, S.; Wang, X.H.; Istepanian, R.S.; Song, Y.H. Mobile e-health: The unwired evolution of telemedicine. *Telemed J. E Health* **2003**, *9*, 247–257. [CrossRef]
22. Ziemssen, T.; Thomas, K. Treatment optimization in multiple sclerosis: How do we apply emerging evidence? *Expert Rev. Clin. Immunol.* **2017**, *13*, 509–511. [CrossRef]
23. D'Amico, E.; Haase, R.; Ziemssen, T. Review: Patient-reported outcomes in multiple sclerosis care. *Mult. Scler. Relat. Disord.* **2019**, *33*, 61–66. [CrossRef]
24. Brichetto, G.; Zaratin, P. Measuring outcomes that matter most to people with multiple sclerosis: The role of patient-reported outcomes. *Curr. Opin. Neurol.* **2020**, *33*, 295–299. [CrossRef]
25. Scholz, M.; Haase, R.; Trentzsch, K.; Stoelzer-Hutsch, H.; Ziemssen, T. Improving Digital Patient Care: Lessons Learned from Patient-Reported and Expert-Reported Experience Measures for the Clinical Practice of MultidimensionalWalking Assessment. *Brain Sci.* **2021**, *11*, 786. [CrossRef]
26. Yeandle, D.; Rieckmann, P.; Giovannoni, G.; Alexandri, N.; Langdon, D. Patient Power Revolution in Multiple Sclerosis: Navigating the New Frontier. *Neurol. Ther.* **2018**, *7*, 179–187. [CrossRef]
27. Rieckmann, P.; Centonze, D.; Elovaara, I.; Giovannoni, G.; Havrdova, E.; Kesselring, J.; Kobelt, G.; Langdon, D.; Morrow, S.A.; Oreja-Guevara, C.; et al. Unmet needs, burden of treatment, and patient engagement in multiple sclerosis: A combined perspective from the MS in the 21st Century Steering Group. *Mult. Scler. Relat. Disord* **2018**, *19*, 153–160. [CrossRef]
28. Heesen, C.; Bruce, J.; Feys, P.; Sastre-Garriga, J.; Solari, A.; Eliasson, L.; Matthews, V.; Hausmann, B.; Ross, A.P.; Asano, M.; et al. Adherence in multiple sclerosis (ADAMS): Classification, relevance, and research needs. A meeting report. *Mult. Scler.* **2014**, *20*, 1795–1798. [CrossRef]
29. Col, N.F.; Solomon, A.J.; Springmann, V.; Garbin, C.P.; Ionete, C.; Pbert, L.; Alvarez, E.; Tierman, B.; Hopson, A.; Kutz, C.; et al. Whose Preferences Matter? A Patient-Centered Approach for Eliciting Treatment Goals. *Med. Decis. Mak.* **2018**, *38*, 44–55. [CrossRef]
30. Rieckmann, P.; Boyko, A.; Centonze, D.; Elovaara, I.; Giovannoni, G.; Havrdova, E.; Hommes, O.; Kesselring, J.; Kobelt, G.; Langdon, D.; et al. Achieving patient engagement in multiple sclerosis: A perspective from the multiple sclerosis in the 21st Century Steering Group. *Mult. Scler. Relat. Disord.* **2015**, *4*, 202–218. [CrossRef]
31. Treadaway, K.; Cutter, G.; Salter, A.; Lynch, S.; Simsarian, J.; Corboy, J.; Jeffery, D.; Cohen, B.; Mankowski, K.; Guarnaccia, J.; et al. Factors that influence adherence with disease-modifying therapy in MS. *J. Neurol.* **2009**, *256*, 568–576. [CrossRef]
32. Lugaresi, A.; Ziemssen, T.; Oreja-Guevara, C.; Thomas, D.; Verdun, E. Improving patient-physician dialog: Commentary on the results of the MS Choices survey. *Patient Prefer. Adherence* **2012**, *6*, 143–152. [CrossRef] [PubMed]
33. Ammenwerth, E.; Schnell-Inderst, P.; Hoerbst, A. The impact of electronic patient portals on patient care: A systematic review of controlled trials. *J. Med. Internet Res.* **2012**, *14*, e162. [CrossRef] [PubMed]
34. Cnossen, I.C.; van Uden-Kraan, C.F.; Eerenstein, S.E.; Rinkel, R.N.; Aalders, I.J.; van den Berg, K.; de Goede, C.J.; van Stijgeren, A.J.; Cruijff-Bijl, Y.; de Bree, R.; et al. A Participatory Design Approach to Develop a Web-Based Self-Care Program Supporting Early Rehabilitation among Patients after Total Laryngectomy. *Folia Phoniatr. Logop.* **2015**, *67*, 193–201. [CrossRef] [PubMed]
35. Goel, M.S.; Brown, T.L.; Williams, A.; Hasnain-Wynia, R.; Thompson, J.A.; Baker, D.W. Disparities in enrollment and use of an electronic patient portal. *J. Gen. Intern. Med.* **2011**, *26*, 1112–1116. [CrossRef] [PubMed]
36. Kruse, C.S.; Bolton, K.; Freriks, G. The effect of patient portals on quality outcomes and its implications to meaningful use: A systematic review. *J. Med. Internet Res.* **2015**, *17*, e44. [CrossRef] [PubMed]
37. Lang, M.; Ringbauer, S.; Mayr, M.; Cepek, L. How to improve disease management of chronically ill patients? Perception of telemetric ECG recording and a novel software application. *Clin. Res. Trials* **2019**, *5*, 1–6. [CrossRef]
38. Kornhuber, A.; Lang, M. Interne und externe Einflussfaktoren auf die Adhärenz bei Multipler Sklerose—eine retrospektive und prospektive Analyse mit der Medication Possession Ratio. In Proceedings of the 87. Kongress der Deutschen Gesellschaft für Neurologie, München, Germany, 15–19 September 2014.
39. Radić, M.; Donner, I.; Waak, M.; Brinkmann, C.; Stein, L.; Radić, D. Digitale Gesundheitsanwendungen: Die Akzeptanz steigern. *Dtsch. Arztebl.* **2021**, *118*, A-286–B-250.
40. BfArM. DiGa-Verzeichnis. Available online: https://diga.bfarm.de/de/verzeichnis (accessed on 12 August 2021).
41. Feys, P.; Giovannoni, G.; Dijssebloem, N.; Centonze, D.; Eelen, P.; Lykke Andersen, S. The importance of a multi-disciplinary perspective and patient activation programmes in MS management. *Mult. Scler.* **2016**, *22*, 34–46. [CrossRef]
42. Gallien, P.; Gich, J.; Sanchez-Dalmau, B.F.; Feneberg, W. Multidisciplinary management of multiple sclerosis symptoms. *Eur. Neurol.* **2014**, *72*, 20–25. [CrossRef] [PubMed]
43. Messmer, U.M.; Battaglia, M.A.; Zagami, P.; Solaro, C. The interdisciplinary approach to the treatment of multiple sclerosis patients in Italy: An aspiration or a reality? *Mult. Scler.* **2002**, *8*, 36–39. [CrossRef]
44. Birnbaum, F.; Lewis, D.; Rosen, R.K.; Ranney, M.L. Patient engagement and the design of digital health. *Acad. Emerg. Med.* **2015**, *22*, 754–756. [CrossRef] [PubMed]
45. Martínez-Pérez, B.; de la Torre-Díez, I.; López-Coronado, M. Privacy and Security in Mobile Health Apps: A Review and Recommendations. *J. Med. Syst.* **2015**, *39*, 181. [CrossRef]

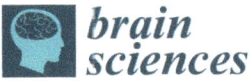

Article

A Novel Digital Care Management Platform to Monitor Clinical and Subclinical Disease Activity in Multiple Sclerosis

Wim Van Hecke [1,2,*,†], Lars Costers [1,2,†], Annabel Descamps [1], Annemie Ribbens [1], Guy Nagels [1,2,3], Dirk Smeets [1,2] and Diana M. Sima [1,2]

1. icometrix, 3012 Leuven, Belgium; lars.costers@icometrix.com (L.C.); annabel.descamps@icometrix.com (A.D.); annemie.ribbens@icometrix.com (A.R.); guy.nagels@vub.be (G.N.); dirk.smeets@icometrix.com (D.S.); diana.sima@icometrix.com (D.M.S.)
2. AI Supported Modelling in Clinical Sciences (AIMS), Vrije Universiteit Brussel, 1050 Brussels, Belgium
3. Department of Engineering, University of Oxford, Oxford OX1 3PJ, UK
* Correspondence: wim.vanhecke@icometrix.com
† The authors contributed equally to the manuscript.

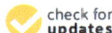

Citation: Van Hecke, W.; Costers, L.; Descamps, A.; Ribbens, A.; Nagels, G.; Smeets, D.; Sima, D.M. A Novel Digital Care Management Platform to Monitor Clinical and Subclinical Disease Activity in Multiple Sclerosis. *Brain Sci.* **2021**, *11*, 1171. https://doi.org/10.3390/brainsci11091171

Academic Editors: Tjalf Ziemssen and Rocco Haase

Received: 31 July 2021
Accepted: 1 September 2021
Published: 3 September 2021

Publisher's Note: MDPI stays neutral with regard to jurisdictional claims in published maps and institutional affiliations.

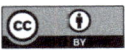

Copyright: © 2021 by the authors. Licensee MDPI, Basel, Switzerland. This article is an open access article distributed under the terms and conditions of the Creative Commons Attribution (CC BY) license (https://creativecommons.org/licenses/by/4.0/).

Abstract: In multiple sclerosis (MS), the early detection of disease activity or progression is key to inform treatment changes and could be supported by digital tools. We present a novel CE-marked and FDA-cleared digital care management platform consisting of (1) a patient phone/web application and healthcare professional portal (ico**mpanion**) including validated symptom, disability, cognition, and fatigue patient-reported outcomes; and (2) clinical brain magnetic resonance imaging (MRI) quantifications (ico**brain** ms). We validate both tools using their ability to detect (sub)clinical disease activity (known-groups validity) and real-world data insights. Surveys showed that 95.6% of people with MS (PwMS) were interested in using an MS app, and 98.2% were interested in knowing about MRI changes. The ico**mpanion** measures of disability ($p < 0.001$) and symptoms ($p = 0.005$) and ico**brain** ms MRI parameters were sensitive to (sub)clinical differences between MS subtypes. ico**brain** ms also decreased intra- and inter-rater lesion count variability and increased sensitivity for detecting disease activity/progression from 24% to 76% compared to standard radiological reading. This evidence shows PwMS' interest, the digital care platform's potential to improve the detection of (sub)clinical disease activity and care management and the feasibility of linking different digital tools into one overarching MS care pathway.

Keywords: multiple sclerosis; ico**mpanion**; ico**brain**; eHealth; digital health technology; mobile application; patient reported outcomes; magnetic resonance imaging

1. Introduction

Today, more than 2.8 million people are living with multiple sclerosis (MS), making it the most common progressive neurological condition in young people [1]. MS is characterized either by periods of relapses and remission or a progressive disability pattern. Currently, there are over 20 disease-modifying treatments (DMTs) available, aiming to slow down relapses and disease progression [2]. Thanks to these DMTs, the health of people with MS (PwMS), expressed in quality-adjusted life years (QALYs), has been estimated to have increased by 66% since the launch of the first drug in 1993 [3]. However, despite the increased availability of DMTs, 26% to 40% of PwMS are estimated to be on a suboptimal treatment [4,5].

These findings illustrate the challenge in MS care, which is providing individual PwMS with the right drug at the right time. Hence, in order to make informed treatment decisions, it is crucial to measure disease activity and progression in a standardized manner. In this context, disease activity and progression are typically evaluated by the clinical assessment of relapses and disability (measured by the Expanded Disability Status Scale (EDSS), and longitudinal changes on the brain magnetic resonance imaging (MRI) scans (looking at new/enlarging lesions and/or brain atrophy) [6].

However, it is known that clinical disease activity and progression often go unnoticed during clinical assessment, partly due to the problem that relapses are systematically underreported by around half of PwMS [6,7]. In addition, MS progression goes beyond relapses and physical disability worsening, as problems with memory but also linguistic and verbal fluency problems are known to be important components of MS-related disability [8,9]. These components are often not routinely assessed during the patient visit or are based on the PwMS' recollection on how they have been doing since the last visit. In addition, it has been demonstrated that there is a significant clinician-dependent variability in the assessment of MS patient disease activity [10].

The second component of evaluating disease activity is based on the assessment of subclinical progression on brain MRI scans. International guidelines recommend the acquisition of brain (and increasingly spinal cord) MRI scans for diagnosis and a yearly scan for follow-up [11]. However, in a clinical setting, brain MRI reading is known to be qualitative, based on a visual assessment, and radiologist-dependent, leading to discrepancies in the radiological reports [12]. Indeed, it has been reported that up to 24% of brain MRI reporting contains discrepancies when reviewed by a panel of radiologists [12].

There is great promise in implementing digital health solutions to standardize MS care, as they can improve efficiency and workflow, and complement clinical expertise. A recent study indicated healthcare professionals' (HCPs) most crucial problems in MS disease management to be the lack of forwarding of information by the patient, the need for the patient to visit on site for inquiries and poor reachability of PwMS, for which digital telemonitoring tools can be a solution [13].

Remote patient monitoring through medical health (mHealth) applications in MS care allows for a more continuous and data-driven monitoring of symptoms and disease progression [14,15]. Regular standardized check-ins through mHealth apps have the potential to mitigate the underreporting of important clinical events [7] and bridge the information gap between annual neurology visits. It has been estimated that personalized medicine tools in MS have the potential to increase the impact of treatments by more than 50% by quantifying both disease activity (clinical and subclinical) and the risk of side effects [3]. In addition to the value of mHealth tools for health-care professionals (HCPs), there is also the potential to further empower PwMS, resulting in an increased self-management and allowing more open and early conversations about disease progression [16,17].

In addition to mHealth applications, artificial intelligence (AI) solutions have been developed to detect and quantify disease activity on MRI scans, which play a central role in disease management. In the last decades, several software tools have been developed and applied for research and clinical trials. Examples of widely used neuroimage analysis packages for research purposes include Freesurfer (https://surfer.nmr.mgh.harvard.edu accessed on 27 August 2021), FMRIB Software Library (FSL; https//fsl.fmrib.ox.ac.uk/fsl, accessed on 27 August 2021), and Statistical Parametric Mapping (SPM; https://www.fil.ion.ucl.ac.uk/spm, accessed on 27 August 2021). However, only very few brain MRI solutions exist that have been thoroughly validated and cleared as a medical device for clinical use [18].

In this paper, we present a novel digital care management platform for MS that aims at standardizing MS patient care and allowing more data-driven clinical decisions in the MS care pathway. The platform includes a CE marked and FDA cleared mHealth application that collects patient-reported information in the period of time between neurology visits, a CE marked and FDA cleared solution that quantifies clinically relevant brain MRI changes in PwMS, and the necessary software solutions that guarantee a seamless integration of the digital MS care management platform into the clinical workflow. We investigate the needs and interests of PwMS concerning such solutions, and their potential to improve the detection of (sub-)clinical disease activity and care management of MS.

2. Materials and Methods

2.1. MS Care Management Platform

As illustrated in Figure 1, the care management platform consists of multiple components: (1) the ico**mpanion** patient mobile phone application (available on Android and iOS) and website (accessible via web browser: icompanion.ms), (2) the ico**mpanion** web portal for HCPs (accessible via web browser), (3) the ico**brain ms** volumetric brain reports and (4) integrations with hospitals' Picture Archiving and Communication System (PACS) and electronic medical record (EMR) systems.

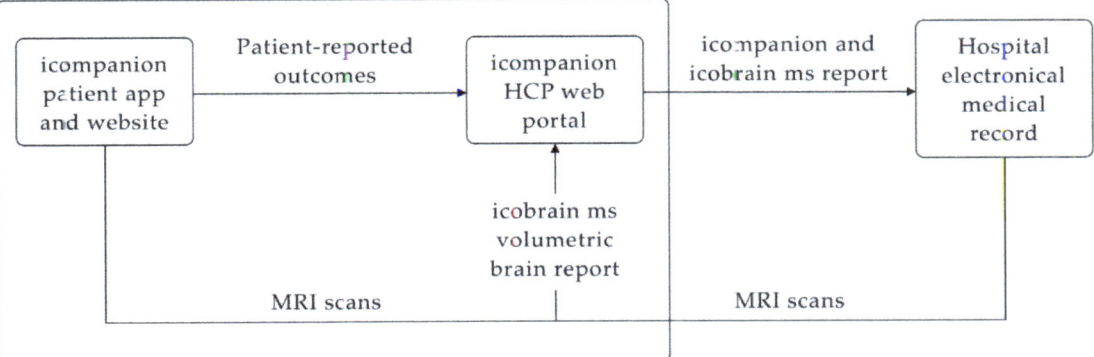

Figure 1. The MS care management platform consists of the ico**mpanion** patient app and website, ico**mpanion** HCP web portal, integration with ico**brain ms** volumetric brain reports and integration with hospital's electronic medical records.

Both ico**mpanion** and ico**brain ms** are registered medical devices and were developed by ico**metrix** (Leuven, Belgium). According to FDA regulation, ico**mpanion** is a class 1 medical device, and under EU MDD regulation a class 1 medical device. ico**brain ms** is an FDA class 2 medical device and MDD class 1m medical device. ico**metrix'** secure cloud is ISO13485 and ISO27001 certified and GDPR and HIPAA compliant regarding the Security and Privacy Rules. Incoming DICOM files of MRI scans are pseudonymized according to HIPAA standard and all fields containing private patient information are removed, except patient gender and birth date (transformed to YYYY-01-01) in order to be able to provide a correct analysis and compare the patient with a healthy population.

2.1.1. ico**mpanion** Patient App and Website

Using the ico**mpanion** app and website, PwMS can keep a diary, log symptoms, and perform tests for body function, cognitive function, and fatigue (Figure 2) based on clinically validated patient reported outcomes (PROs) described below [19–22], which can be shared with the patient's clinical team. In addition, PwMS can add treatment information, from DMTs to symptomatic and rehabilitation treatments, and set reminders on when to take or perform their treatment. Furthermore, PwMS can easily upload their MRIs (via the patient website) and view them (via patient website and app) as well as learn about topics related to MS (e.g., MS types, MRI, lesions). Finally, PwMS can prepare their consultations using a pre-visit checklist, the answers of which are also shared with the patient's clinical team (e.g., 'Do you need any new prescription, certificates or reimbursement documents?').

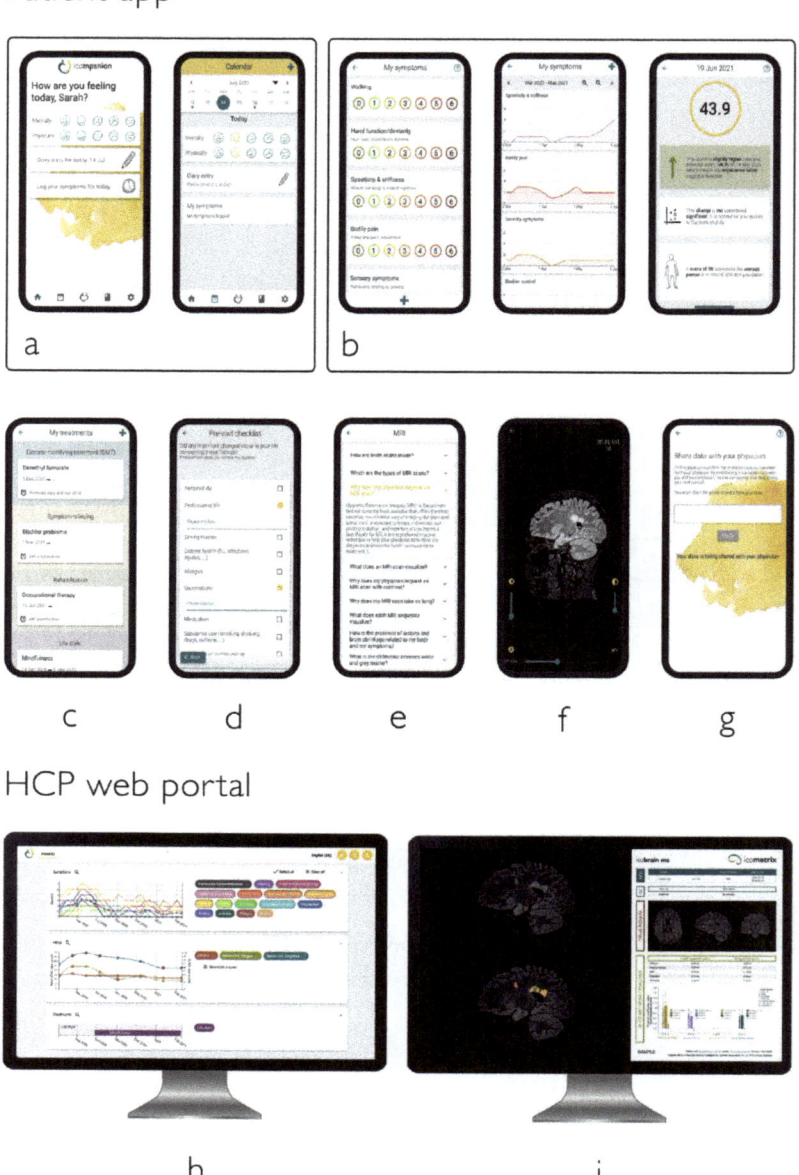

Figure 2. Overview of the ico**mpanion** patient app (**a–g**) and HCP platform features (**h,i**): (**a**) easy check-in and diary, (**b**) PROs for symptoms, EDSS, fatigue, cognition, . . . , (**c**) treatment logging and reminders, (**d**) preparation neurologist visit, (**e**) knowledge center, (**f**) MRI viewer, (**g**) linking with MS team, (**h**) interactive overview of PRO data and downloadable reports and (**i**) automatic import of MRI scans from hospital PACS system and integration with ico**brain ms** reports.

The clinically validated PROs included into icompanion are the SymptoMScreen, a patient-reported Expanded Disability Status Scale (prEDSS), Neuro-QoL (V1.0) Fatigue short-form, and the Neuro-QoL (V2.0) Cognitive Function short-form:

- The SymptoMScreen [21] is a 12-item battery for MS-related symptoms with a 7-point Likert scale per functional domain. Scores range from 'not affected at all' (score = 0) to 'total limitation' (score = 6). The SymptoMScreen composite is a score that summarizes general symptom severity by summing up the entered twelve symptom severities.
- The prEDSS is a patient-reported version of the Expanded Disability Status Scale (EDSS) which has shown to correlate well (Pearson's coefficient 0.85) with a neurologist-scored EDSS [22].
- The Neuro-QoL (V1.0) Fatigue and (V2.0) Cognitive short-forms are short questionnaires consisting of eight items scored on a five-point scale each [23], and have been clinically validated in MS [19,20]. The Neuro-QoL t-scores reported in this paper are standardized scores with a mean of 50 and standard deviation (SD) of 10 compared to a reference population (for Cognitive a US general reference sample, for Fatigue a clinical US sample; http://www.healthmeasures.net/images/neuro_qol/Neuro_QOL_Scoring_Manual_Mar2015.pdf accessed on 27 August 2021). As an example, a t-score of 60 means that a person scores 1 SD higher than the reference sample.

2.1.2. ico**brain ms** Volumetric MRI Analyses

ico**brain ms** is an AI software solution for brain magnetic resonance image analysis in MS, producing annotated images and pre-populated radiological reports (icometrix.com/services/icobrain-ms accessed on 27 August 2021). The main components of ico**brain ms** are the brain tissue segmentation and MS lesion segmentation on single-time point T1-weighted and FLAIR scans, as well as specific longitudinal volume change computations for establishing brain atrophy rates and lesion evolution. Whole brain and gray matter volumes, normalized for head size, are compared against age- and sex-matched reference controls populations. In Figure 3, an example of the ico**brain ms** output is shown, including the annotated images, the quantitative reports, and the pre-populated structured radiological report that are provided in the local PACS system and available by the time the radiological reading starts. In the top row of Figure 3, a sagittal slice of the annotated images (which are presented in the same space as the original scans) is shown, the bottom row includes the quantitative ico**brain ms** reports and an example of the pre-populated radiological report:

- top left = T1 overlaid with gray matter segmentation (blue) and T1 lesions (red);
- top middle = FLAIR overlaid with lesion segmentations color coded by location: periventricular (yellow), deep white matter (blue), juxtacortical (purple), and infratentorial (green)
- top right = FLAIR overlaid with color coded lesion changes compared to last available (or selected) scan: existing (green), enlarging (orange), new (red) lesions.
- bottom left = the quantitative report of whole brain and gray matter volume and atrophy (and comparison with healthy population).
- bottom middle = the quantitative report of existing, enlarging and, new FLAIR lesions and their location.
- bottom right = an example of a pre-populated radiological structured template, which already includes the ico**brain ms** measures and is available in the local language.

The technical details, validation, and clinical usefulness of the methodology have been published previously [24–28]. The software is seamlessly integrated in the clinical workflow via ico**bridge** (see Section 2.1.3 or https://icobridge.icometrix.com accessed on 27 August 2021). It includes direct and secure upload from the hospital's image archiving system to icometrix' servers, where the AI pipeline is run, and secure transfer of reports and annotated images back to the hospital's system in time for the radiological reading.

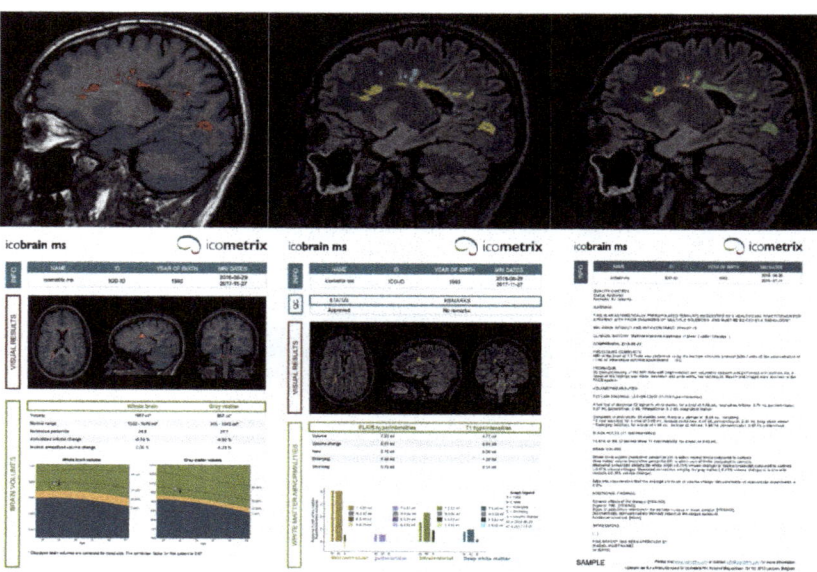

Figure 3. Output of the ico**brain ms** software, which is integrated with the local PACS. In the top row, a sagittal slice of the annotated images (which are presented in the same space as the original scans) is shown. The bottom row includes the quantitative ico**brain ms** reports and an example of the pre-populated radiological report.

2.1.3. ico**mpanion** HCP Portal

In the HCP portal, HCPs can access the entered ico**mpanion** PRO data from their linked PwMS as well as their MRI images and ico**brain ms** volumetric brain reports (Figures 1–3). Access to the data on this portal can be easily managed via the MS team functionality, which allows the set-up of a care team with different team members and roles. The entered ico**mpanion** PRO data can be viewed in an interactive plot with tools to help the interpretation, and HCPs can download pdf reports. HCPs can also view the PwMS' uploaded MRIs, and using ico**bridge** (https://icobridge.icometrix.com accessed on 27 August 2021), ico**metrix**' secure DICOM gateway, MRI scans can also be automatically imported from a hospital's PACS system. All imported MRI scans are analyzed using the ico**brain ms** volumetric analysis, after which a report can be downloaded from the HCP portal (Figure 3). The ico**mpanion** and ico**brain ms** reports (and raw data points or intermediate results) can be imported into a hospital's EMR system. Using the HL7 v2 protocol, these reports can be sent over to the EMR, either in their native pdf format, coded values or as simple text. From there on this data can for instance be shown in a radiologic report or attached to a study for future reference.

2.2. Patient Perspective

2.2.1. Patient Survey 1: Telemonitoring Tools for Monitoring Clinical Disease Activity

In order to develop a patient monitoring tool that responds to the needs of PwMS and fits PwMS' everyday life, a survey was sent out to PwMS with MS via local patient support groups without any randomization. In this survey, answered by 45 PwMS, the PwMS were asked about their knowledge about important topics such as MRI, EDSS, etc., which was used to develop educational content for ico**mpanion**. Next, the PwMS were asked about their attitude towards an app to monitor MS, different possible features, and their interest in using such an app.

2.2.2. Patient Survey 2: MR Imaging for Monitoring Subclinical Disease Activity

Together with ConquerMS (iConquerMS.org) a survey was sent out in June 2020 [29], with questions about MRI access, viewing and knowledge, which was answered by 876 PwMS. As an example, questions included (see Appendices A and B for the complete list of questions and possible answers in the survey):

- 'Would you like to view your MRI images on your own—Why or why not?'
- 'If you have or had access to your own MRIs, would you be interested in knowing whether there were any changes between one MRI and the next (such as new lesions or loss of brain volume)?'

2.3. Monitoring Clinical Disease Activity Using icompanion: Real-World Evidence

2.3.1. Study Synopsis-Characterizing MS Types with ico**mpanion**

The ico**mpanion** app and website were launched in July 2020. We describe the information entered into ico**mpanion** and investigate the validity of the real-world collected PRO data by looking at their sensitivity to clinical differences between MS types based on known-groups validity. These MS types include clinically isolated syndrome (CIS), relapsing-remitting MS (RRMS), secondary progressive MS (SPMS), and primary progressive MS (PPMS). The descriptions of the collected data and the analyses were based on an anonymized dataset of collected ico**mpanion** data. We performed a non-parametric Kruskal–Wallis H test (or a one-way analysis of variance (ANOVA) on ranks), with MS type as independent variable and the variable of interest as dependent variable (mental feeling, physical feeling, prEDSS, SymptoMScreen composite, Neuro-QoL Fatigue, and Neuro-QoL Cognitive Function). We used a significance level of 0.05 and p-values of the separate models were corrected for multiple comparisons using false discovery rate (FDR) correction [30]. For the variables that showed significant group effects, post-hoc multiple comparisons tests were carried out for pairwise differences between the different MS types with Dunn–Sidák correction, using a significance level of 0.05.

The percentage of PwMS with a statistically meaningful change in their Neuro-QoL Fatigue and Cognitive Function scores was evaluated based on the conditional minimal detectable change, specifically developed for the Neuro-QoL short-forms [31]. A statistically meaningful change can be interpreted as a difference of more than one standard error (SE). It was estimated from the average of the SEs from a normative dataset for any given pair of scores multiplied by the z score for a 95% confidence interval, or $([SE_{Score1} + SE_{Score2}]/2) \cdot 1.96 \cdot \sqrt{2}$ [31]. Solely PwMS with more than one result for these PROs were included

2.4. Monitoring Subclinical Disease Activity Using icobrain ms: Real-World Evidence

icc**brain ms** was launched in 2016 and has been adopted by more than 400 hospitals worldwide since then. In the context of standardizing MS care, in this manuscript, we evaluate how:

- ico**brain ms'** lesion annotations bring the performance of non-specialized radiologists closer to that of experienced neuroradiologists (Section 2.4.1)
- the availability of ico**brain ms** reports in MS follow-up refine the assessment of subclinical disease activity (Section 2.4.2)
- how the use of quantitative AI based brain MRI reporting can improve the radiological workflows (Section 2.4.2)
- ico**brain ms** volumetric brain biomarkers bring insights into the brain patterns of MS types (Section 2.4.3)

2.4.1. Study Synopsis-Reliability of Lesion Count with ico**brain ms**

ico**brain ms** lesion segmentations were compared with the assessment of two raters: one experienced radiologist and one assistant neurologist. The experiment consisted of marking and counting MS lesions on fluid-attenuated inversion recovery (FLAIR) and T1-weighted images acquired from 10 PwMS with a 3T MRI scanner (Achieva, Philips Medical Systems) at the University Hospital Brussels. Inclusion criteria were MS diagnosis according to McDonald Criteria 2010 and no MRI contraindication. For more details, see [27], from which a subset was used for this analysis. Two repeated acquisitions with patient repositioning were taken to assess test-retest reliability of the lesion count. The two raters independently assessed all images, which were presented in a shuffled order, first as original MRI scans, then with lesion annotations obtained by ico**brain ms**. In addition, the reporting time was recorded.

Intra-rater and inter-rater agreement of lesion counts was assessed. Of special interest was the question whether there is an improved agreement between the counts reported by the two raters after using ico**brain ms** segmentations, as opposed to the case when each rater counted lesions on the original images without ico**brain ms**.

2.4.2. Study Synopsis-Detecting Subclinical Disease Activity in MRI Follow-Up with ico**brain ms**

In this study, we evaluated how the availability of ico**brain ms** reports might change the findings of radiological reading when assessing follow-up brain MRI scans. Longitudinal MRI acquisitions from 25 PwMS approximately 1 year apart were randomly selected (and limited to 25 because of feasibility) from different institutions that use ico**brain ms** in clinical practice, ensuring that these centers obtained informed consent from their PwMS to use fully anonymized MRI scans for research. The inclusion criteria were (1) being diagnosed as RRMS or SPMS, (2) having 2 pairs of scans separated at least one or more years apart acquired at the same scanner, (3) Having MRI acquired at the 1.5T or 3T in which there is a presence of high-resolution 3D-T1 and 2D or 3D FLAIR sequence, (4) having Expanded Disability Status Scale (EDSS) assessment at baseline and at follow-up, and (5) not having steroid treatment or relapse 30 days prior to the MRI scan. Each MRI dataset was presented in random order to an experienced neuroradiologist: once without and once with an automatically generated ico**brain ms** report. In the latter case, besides color-coded lesion and brain segmentation overlays, the expert also had access to the structured ico**brain ms** reports. The two radiological reporting scenarios (without and with volumetric software results) were compared in terms of effect on diagnostic findings and reporting time.

2.4.3. Study Synopsis-Insights into the MS Brain Patterns Using ico**brain ms**

In this study, it was evaluated whether ico**brain ms** is able to reveal different brain or lesion volume patterns when comparing different MS clinical phenotypes. Multiple MR sessions from CIS ($n = 12$), RRMS ($n = 30$), PPMS ($n = 17$), and SPMS ($n = 28$) PwMS, with 3D T1w and 2D FLAIR images acquired on a 1.5T MR system (Sonata Siemens) at CERMEP in Lyon, were evaluated. EDSS was also available at each time point. For more details on the original dataset, see [32]. First, differences between MS groups were calculated in terms of longitudinal lesion evolution by location, where new and enlarging lesions were estimated between two time points at least 2 years apart for each patient. Secondly, we evaluated the known-groups validity or the sensitivity of ico**brain ms** to subclinical differences in brain volumetrics. This was done in the same way as for the ico**mpanion** data (see Section 2.3.1) using the Kruskal–Wallis H tests to look for a group effect, and pairwise post-hoc tests to look for differences between different MS type groups.

3. Results

3.1. Patient Perspective

3.1.1. Patient Survey 1: Telemonitoring Tools for Monitoring Clinical Disease Activity

45 PwMS completed the survey, of which 80% ($n = 36$) were women. The average age of participants was 45.6 (SD = 11.5). Of the sample, 55.6% ($n = 25$) were RRMS, 15.6% ($n = 7$) were SPMS, 11.1% ($n = 5$) PPMS while 17.8% ($n = 8$) did not know their MS type or did not want to disclose it. About one third of PwMS were diagnosed in the last three years (31.1%, $n = 14$) or had a disease duration of 3 to 10 years (31.1%, $n = 14$), while 22.2% ($n = 10$) and 15.5% ($n = 7$) had been diagnosed, respectively, 10 to 20 years ago and longer than 20 years ago. The larger part of participants thought of themselves to be very digitally

literate (33%, n = 15) or quite digitally literate (42.2%, n = 19) compared to neutral (22.2%, n = 10) and not quite digitally literate (2.2%, n = 1) while no PwMS indicated to be not very digitally literate.

We asked for PwMS' attitude about the use of an app to monitor the disease course, where only one person (2.2%) answered negatively (see Figure 4a). The most important features (see Figure 2 for an overview of the main functions) for this cohort were Knowledge center (97.8%, n = 44), Symptom logging (95.5%, n = 43), Treatment overview (88.9%, n = 40), and Test/PROs (88.9%, n = 40). These were also the features reported to be the most probable to be used by the PwMS. When asking whether PwMS had an intention to use the app, 68.9% (n = 31) answered yes, 26.7% (n = 12) answered maybe and 4.4% answered no (n = 2). When asking how frequently they would like to use the app, 26.7% (n = 12) answered daily, 31.1% (n = 14) multiple times per week, 22.2% once per week (n = 10), 2.2% (n = 1) once every two weeks and 13.3% (n = 6) once every month while 4.4% (n = 2) answered Other.

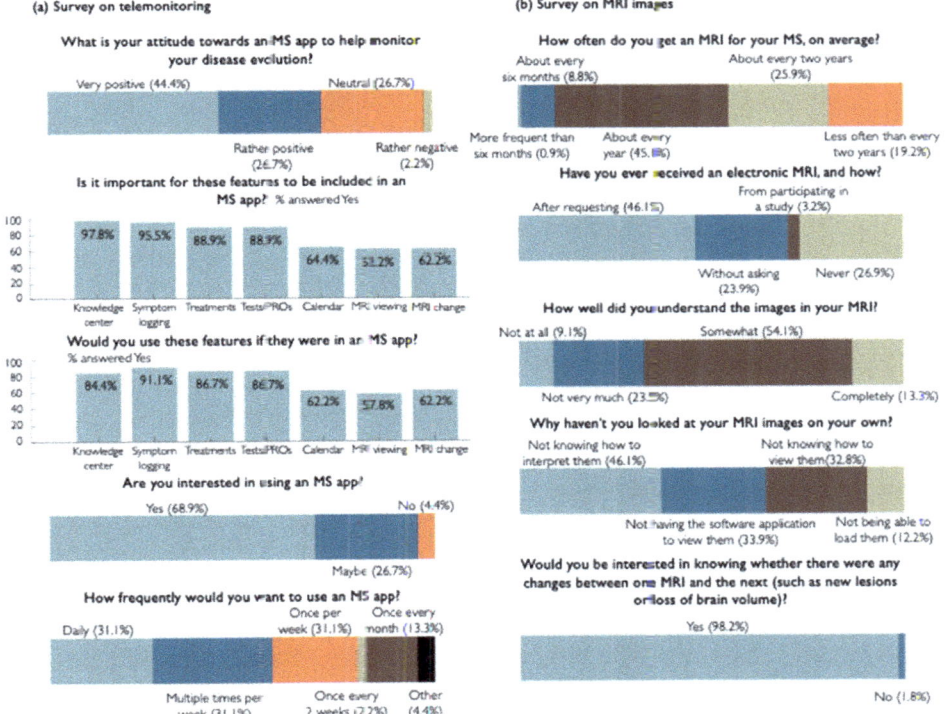

Figure 4. Visualization of answers for a selection of survey questions from the two surveys: (a) survey on telemonitoring tools for monitoring clinical disease activity, (b) survey on MR imaging for monitoring subclinical disease activity in collaboration with iConquerMS.

3.1.2. Patient Survey 2: MR Imaging for Monitoring Subclinical Disease Activity

The survey was answered by 876 PwMS, predominantly located in the U.S. and Canada (91.4%). Of the participants, 80% (n = 699) were female. 2.8% of PwMS were aged 75 to 84 years, 19.4% 65 to 74 years, 34.1% 55 to 64 years, 27.2% 45 to 54 years, 11.7% 35 to 44 years, and 4.9% 34 years or younger.

The results of the survey showed that only 0.6% (n = 5) of PwMS have never had an MRI performed for the purpose of diagnosing or treating. Only 54.9% (n = 474) undergo an MRI scan every year or more frequently (see Figure 4b). Almost 27% (26.9%, n = 228) of

PwMS have never received an electronic version of their MRI from their clinic or radiology lab. Of the PwMS that received an electronic version of their MRI, 79.9% ($n = 560$) got it on a CD-ROM, 15.6% ($n = 109$) through their clinic's patient portal, 4.0% ($n = 28$) through a direct download into their computer or other device and 0.6% ($n = 4$) on a USB-drive.

Of PwMS that received an electronic version of their MRI, 70. 5% ($n = 431$) looked at their MR images on their own. Of those people, only 13.3% ($n = 57$) claimed to completely understand their MR images. 70.2% ($n = 99$) of the PwMS that had access to an electronic MRI but have not looked at it on their own, would like to do so. Of the reasons for not viewing the MR images, 46.1% ($n = 83$) of PwMS indicated to not know how to interpret the images, while 33.9% ($n = 61$) did not have a software application to view them, 32.8% ($n = 59$) did not know how to view the images, and 12.2% ($n = 22$) failed to load the images onto their computer or software program.

Respectively 98.2% ($n = 836$) and 94.7% ($n = 767$) of PwMS answered to be interested in knowing about changes between their MRIs and whether their MRI scan was performed according to clinical MS guidelines. Finally, 96.6% ($n = 714$) of PwMS indicated that they would be willing to share their MRI scans with researchers.

3.2. icompanion MS Patient App Validation
Sensitivity to Clinical Differences between MS Types

Summary statistics of ico**mpanion** users' characteristics and entered data are presented in Table 1, including gender distribution, and average age and disease duration of the current user base. In Figure 5, the distribution of entered treatments per MS type is visualized, for PwMS on a DMT. For CIS, 28.6% were on glatiramer acetate, 42.9% on interferons, 14.3% on dimethyl fumarate, and 14.3% on teriflunomide. For people with RRMS, 12.5% indicated that they were on fingolimod, 13.8% on glatiramer acetate, 13.3% on interferons, 4.7% on cladribine, 17.8% on dimethyl fumarate, 9.4% on teriflunomide, 17.5% on ocrelizumab, 1.6% on alemtuzumab, and 9.4% on natalizumab. For people with SPMS, 8.3% indicated that they were on fingolimod, 8.3% on glatiramer acetate, 12.5% on interferons, 16.7% on dimethyl fumarate, 8.3% on teriflunomide, 33.3% on ocrelizumab, 8.3% on alemtuzumab and 4.2% on natalizumab. Finally, 4.4% of people with PPMS were on fingolimod, 4.3% on glatiramer acetate, 8.7% on cladribine, 4% on dimethyl fumarate or teriflunomide, 65.2% on ocrelizumab, and 9% on natalizumab.

Table 1. Descriptive statistics for the complete dataset of app users that indicated to know their MS type (82.8%, $n = 1301$). Except for gender, all variables are described as [average (standard deviation, n)]. Group effect column provides the results of the Kruskal–Wallis analyses to look for an effect of MS type on these variables. p-values have been corrected using FDR correction.

	CIS 3.1% $n = 42$	RRMS 78.4% $n = 1061$	SPMS 10.9% $n = 147$	PPMS 7.6% $n = 103$	Group Effect
Gender (female)	76.2%	75.7%	61.2%	63.1%	
Age	33.9 (10.2, 41)	39.7 (10.4, 1058)	47.7 (12.6, 144)	45.8 (12.6, 101)	
Disease duration	5.24 (6.87, 42)	7.98 (6.84, 1061)	16.5 (9.21, 147)	7.38 (6.25, 103)	
Mental feeling	0.17 (1.17, 33)	0.49 (0.91, 869)	0.37 (0.89, 114)	0.47 (0.91, 81)	$H(3) = 5.15$ $p = 0.193$
Physical feeling	0.12 (0.89, 33)	0.25 (0.88, 862)	−0.05 (0.81, 113)	0.06 (0.85, 80)	$H(3) = 10.85$ $p = 0.025$
prEDSS	2.87 (1.77, 16)	3.35 (1.57, 336)	5.13 (1.38, 41)	5.02 (1.62, 31)	$H(3) = 64.47$ $p < 0.001$
Sympto-MScreen composite	10.5 (13.2, 40)	12.8 (13.5, 1024)	17.0 (15.5, 140)	17.9 (15.9, 101)	$H(3) = 15.40$ $p = 0.005$
Neuro-QoL Fatigue	54.0 (11.91, 15)	55.1 (8.75, 319)	56.0 (7.74, 38)	55.1 (8.95, 30)	$H(3) = 0.31$ $p = 0.312$
Neuro-QoL Cognitive	48.5 (8.95, 15)	43.7 (8.87, 334)	42.0 (9.09, 41)	44.2 (7.97, 30)	$H(3) = 5.22$ $p = 0.193$

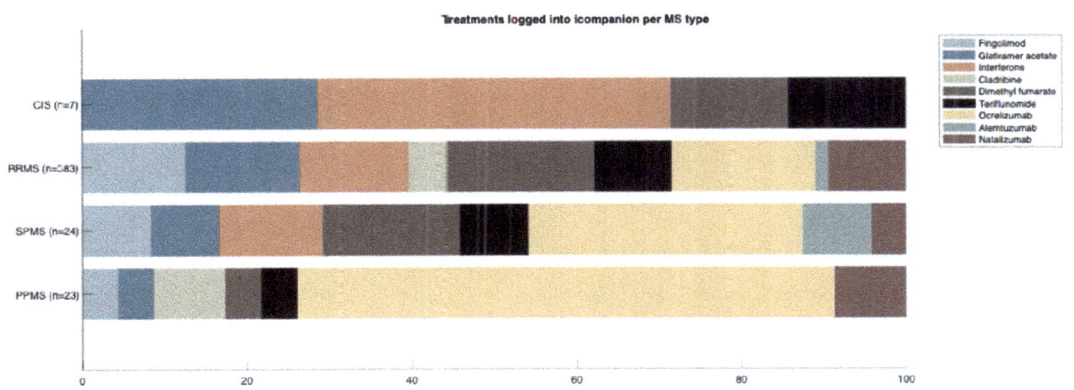

Figure 5. Treatments logged into icompanion by PwMS per MS type.

In context of the validation of icompanion through known-groups validity, we observed a group effect of MS type on physical feeling ($p = 0.025$) (see Table 1 and Figure 6C). We also observed a significant group effect of MS type on body function or prEDSS ($p < 0.001$ Figure 6D) and general symptom load or SymptoMScreen composite ($p = 0.005$) where progressive PwMS scored higher than people with CIS and RRMS (Table 1). For mental feeling ($p = 0.193$) and the Neuro-QoL Fatigue ($p = 0.312$), we observed no effect of MS type. For the latter, average scores for all MS types were worse than the average general US reference sample, but within the range of 1 SD (50 ± 10) [23]. The same was true for average scores on the Neuro-QoL Cognitive where lower scores indicate worse functioning, and where also no effect of MS type was observed ($p = 0.193$).

Post-hoc tests for the variables that showed significant effects of MS type were carried out, performing pairwise comparisons between the different MS types. For physical feeling, we observed a significantly higher or better physical feeling in people with RRMS compared to SPMS ($p = 0.014$). prEDSS scores for both PPMS and SPMS were each significantly higher than both people with RRMS and CIS (all $p < 0.001$). Average symptom load, or SymptoMScreen composite, was significantly higher in people with PPMS compared to RRMS ($v = 0.022$).

For the Neuro-QoL PROs, we were able to calculate whether two consecutive scores indicated a statistically meaningful change (based on conditional minimal detectable change, described in Section 2.3.1 and [31]). We observed such statistically meaningful change in 25.0% ($n = 36$) of PwMS with more than 1 logged Neuro-QoL Fatigue result score ($n = 118$) and 12.3% ($n = 18$) of PwMS with more than 1 logged Neuro-QoL Cognitive score ($n = 121$).

The scores for the separate 12 symptoms included in the SymptoMScreen are shown in Figure 7. Visually, a clear distinction could be made between CIS and RRMS and progressive MS types (SPMS, PPMS). Especially concerning Walking problems, SPMS (2.32) and PPMS (2.18) seem to score higher than CIS (0.86) and RRMS (1.13) on average, but also on Spasticity and stiffness (CIS: 0.89; RRMS: 1.20; SPMS: 1.96; PPMS: 1.84), Hand function and dexterity (CIS: 0.95; RRMS: 0.90; SPMS: 1.31; PPMS: 1.39) and Bladder control (CIS: 0.67; RRMS: 0.91; SPMS: 1.58; PPMS: 1.38).

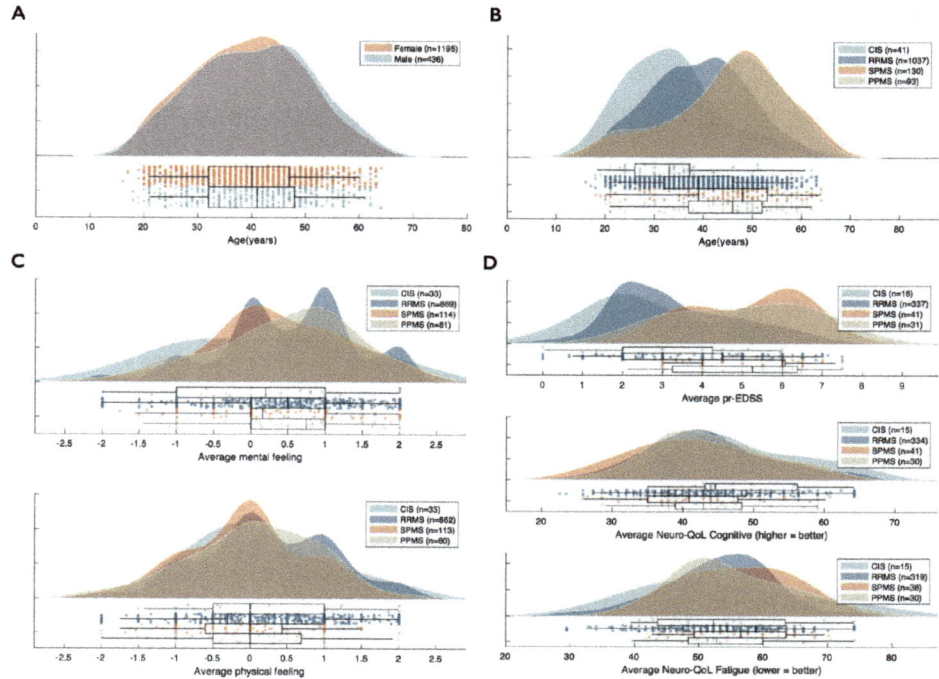

Figure 6. Summary statistics of ico**mpanion** users: (**A**) distribution of age based on sex, (**B**) distribution of age based on MS type, (**C**) distribution of average mental and physical feeling based on MS type, (**D**) distribution of average Neuro-QoL Cognitive and Fatigue score based on MS type.

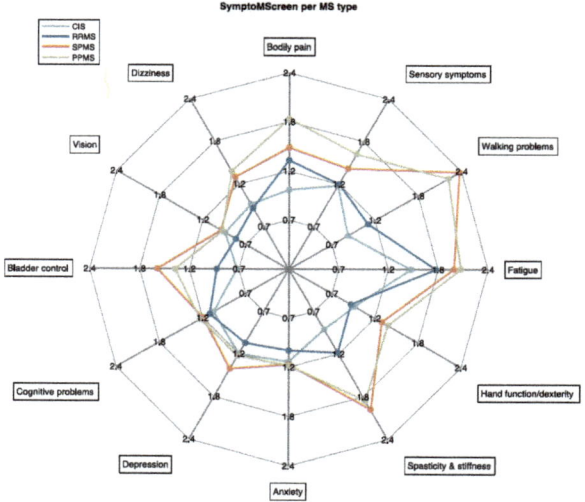

Figure 7. Average severity scored by ico**mpanion** users for all SymptoMScreen symptoms based on MS type. Severity is scored on a scale of 0–6.

3.3. icobrain ms Brain MRI Analysis Validation

3.3.1. Reliability of Lesion Count with icobrain ms

Intra-rater test-retest lesion count agreement on scan and rescan images was significantly improved for the assistant neurologist, from a standard deviation (SD) of the differences between test and retest lesion counts of 28.1 without icobrain ms to 22.0 with icobrain ms (improvement of 21.7%) but was constant for the experienced radiologist (SD = 7.3 in both scenarios). Larger changes were observed in the case of inter-rater agreement: without icobrain ms annotations, inter-rater lesion count agreement between experienced radiologist and assistant neurologist was significantly worse (SD = 20.8) than with icobrain ms (SD = 15.7), indicating an improvement of 32.5% by using icobrain ms. Figure 8 presents all intra- and inter-rater comparisons as Bland–Altman plots, annotated with bias and standard deviation of the lesion count differences, including the raters' comparisons with the automated lesion count obtained from the icobrain ms lesion annotations. It can be observed that the assistant neurologist consistently overestimated the counts of icobrain ms and of the experienced radiologist. Similar trends were observed when repeating the analysis for T1 hypointensities (blackholes) and lesions per location, see [33].

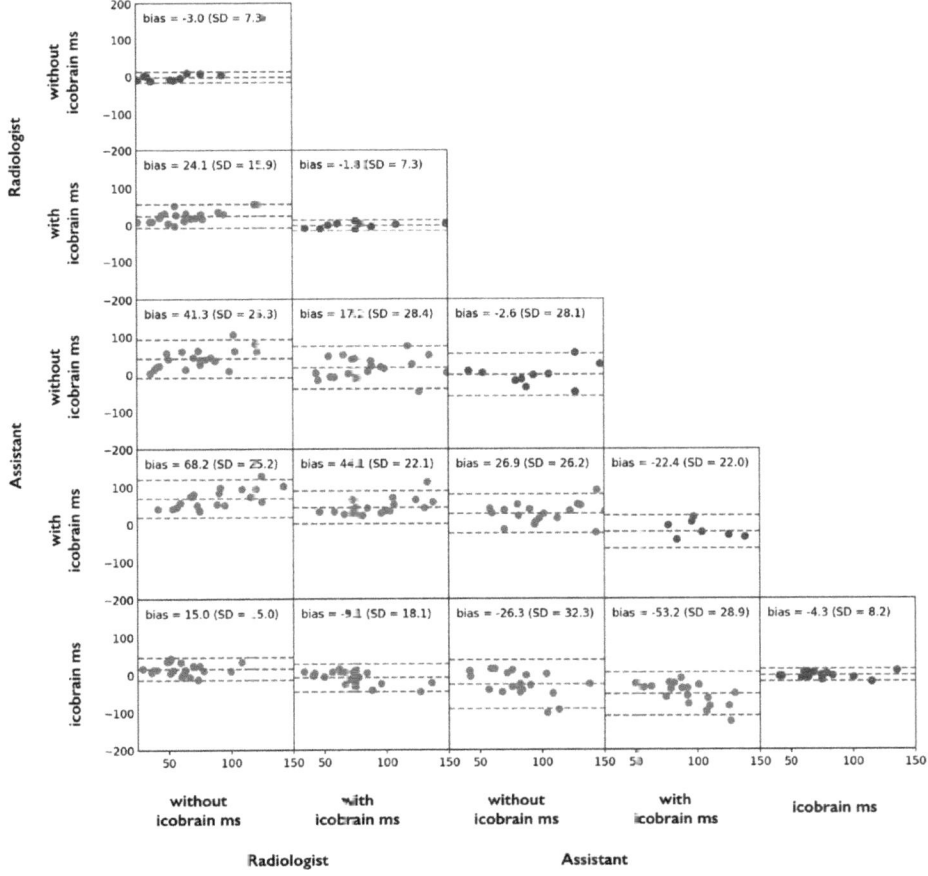

Figure 8. Bland–Altman plots of total FLAIR lesion counts on scan-rescan MRI data from 10 PwMS for 2 different raters (expert radiologist and assistant neurologist) and different scenarios per rater (without and with icobrain ms). The main diagonal depicts the intra-rater test-retest agreement over the 10 repeated MRI scans. Non-diagonal plots represent inter-rater or inter-scenario comparisons using the complete dataset of 20 MRI scans.

The timing also differed significantly between the task of performing lesion count without (mean ± SD: 54.3 ± 11.8 min), or with ico**brain ms** (mean ± SD: 26.7 ± 19.8 min).

3.3.2. Detecting Subclinical Disease Activity in MRI Follow-Up with ico**brain ms**

Radiological findings were compared between the scenario when the radiologist examined the raw MRI follow-up scans and the scenario when ico**brain ms** annotations and reports were also available. The PwMS were considered stable, slightly active, and active, as follows [34]:

- stable: if they had no new or enlarging lesions and had normal rate of brain atrophy compared to controls (within 0.2% from normal atrophy rate of sex- and age-matched healthy controls in the case of ico**brain ms** measurements);
- slightly active: if they had enlarging lesions or slightly abnormal atrophy rate compared to controls (further than 0.2% but within 0.4% from normal atrophy rate of sex- and age-matched healthy controls in the case of ico**brain ms** measurements);
- active: if they had new lesions or severe progression of brain atrophy (further than 0.4% from the normal atrophy rate of sex- and age-matched healthy controls in the case of ico**brain ms** measurements).

Conventional radiological reporting indicated 19 out of 25 stable PwMS (no lesion activity, no apparent atrophy) and 6 active PwMS (new lesion formation or lesion enlargement). The radiological findings with access to ico**brain ms** indicated 7 out of 25 PwMS as stable (normal atrophy, no lesion activity), 7 PwMS with slight disease activity (slightly abnormal atrophy rate and/or enlarging lesions), and 11 active PwMS (5 with new lesions, 10 with abnormal atrophy rate for their age). All stable PwMS identified by ico**brain ms** were also deemed stable by conventional radiological reading. All active PwMS identified by conventional reading were also identified as active or slightly active when using ico**brain ms**. However, the automatic brain MRI measurements indicated several other PwMS as (slightly) active, even if these were part of the stable group according to conventional radiological reading. As such, the percentage of PwMS deemed as having (slight) disease activity or progression grew from 24% in conventional reading to 76% (44% active, 32% slightly active, according to the definitions above) with the ico**brain ms** assisted reading.

With respect to timing, radiological reporting took on average 7 min 28 s (SD: 3 min 6 s) without ico**brain ms** and 5 min 49 s (SD: 2 min 15 s) with ico**brain ms**. In other words, computer-aided radiological reporting with ico**brain ms** was faster than conventional reporting, with approximately 8 conventional reports per hour versus 13 computer-aided reports per hour, which is an improvement by about 40%.

3.3.3. Insights into the MS Brain Patterns: Sensitivity to Subclinical Differences between MS Types

In a two-year MRI follow-up study, new and enlarging lesions assessed with ico**brain ms** were evaluated in different MS subtypes of CIS ($n = 12$), RRMS ($n = 30$), PPMS ($n = 17$), and SPMS ($n = 28$) PwMS, with average age at baseline 31.8, 33.2, 39.5, and 41.1 years and average disease duration 2.9, 8.3, 7.5, and 14.9, respectively [35]. The largest volume of new lesion formation (i.e., lesions not touching any older lesion) was observed in CIS, with approximately 0.1ml new lesion volume over 2-year follow-up, without a preferred location (juxtacortical, periventricular, deep white matter). Further, it was also observed that people with RRMS exhibited more deep white matter (WM) lesions (either new or pre-existing) in comparison to other MS types. PPMS and SPMS had virtually no new periventricular lesions, but a significant amount of enlargement in that region, consistent with a longer disease duration. Figure 9 illustrates the location-dependent evolution patterns for new and enlarging lesions obtained with ico**brain ms** in the 4 MS clinical phenotypes.

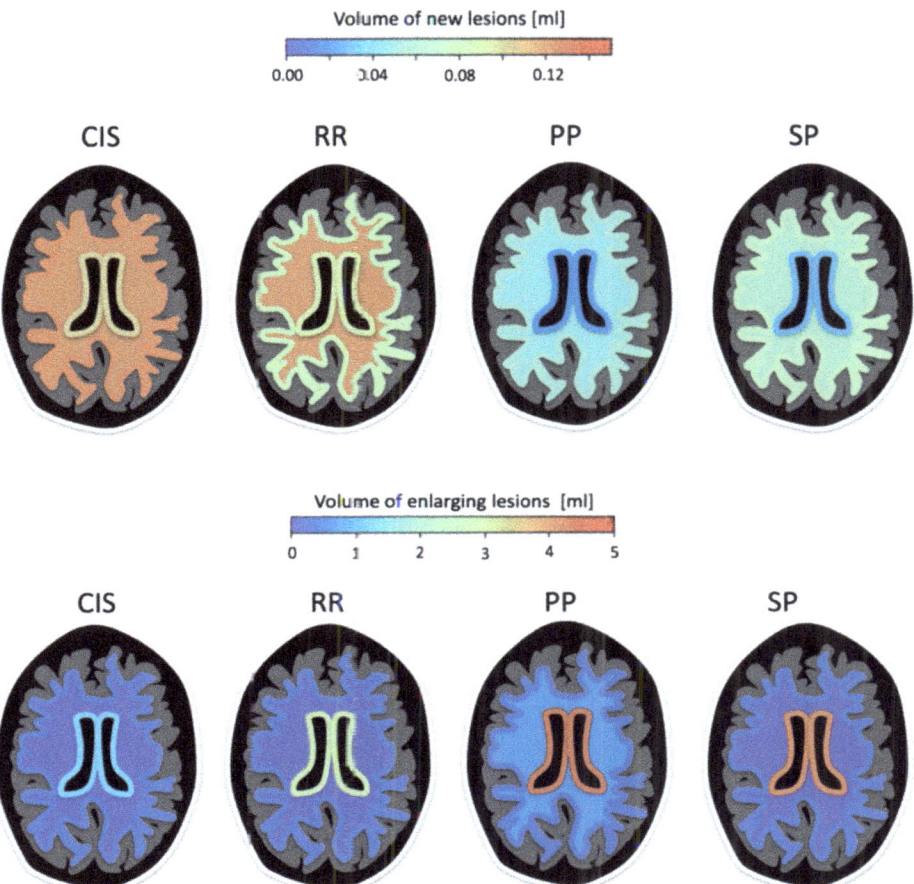

Figure 9. Location prevalence and average volumes for new and enlarging lesions in subjects with CIS, RRMS, PPMS, and SPMS. The schematic representation shows three colored layers, where colors represent new or enlarging lesion volumes in the given scales (mL). For each brain slice, the innermost contour represents periventricular lesions; the outermost contour represents juxtacortical lesions; and middle region represents deep white matter lesions.

When examining brain and lesion volumes simultaneously (whole brain volume, gray matter volume, lateral ventricles volume, total FLAIR lesion volume, and T1 blackholes volume), very distinct group patterns were observed for the MRIs corresponding to all time points for which EDSS was lower than or equal to 4 (Figure 10a), with all volumes significantly different between groups according to a non-parametric Kruskal–Wallis H test with MS type as independent variable ($p < 0.001$) (Table 2). The CIS and RRMS groups showed significantly higher whole brain and gray matter volumes and lower ventricular volumes compared to the PPMS and SPMS groups (Table 2). Highest volumes of FLAIR hyperintensities and T1 blackholes were evident in SPMS. At higher EDSS (greater than 4), the patterns corresponding to PPMS and SPMS groups were almost indistinguishable with no significant volume differences observed for whole brain, gray matter, lateral ventricles and T1 blackholes (Table 2). In contrast, the RRMS group with EDSS > 4 showed higher whole brain volume and lower ventricles volume compared to the progressive groups.

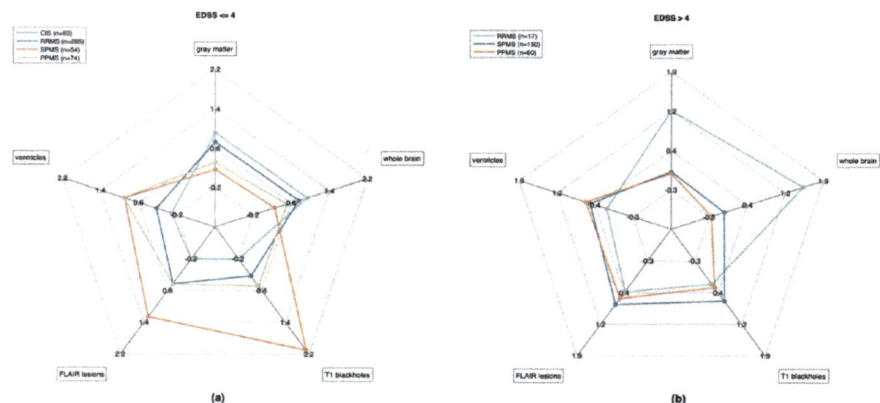

Figure 10. Volumetric patterns observed with ico**brain ms** are illustrated for (**a**) EDSS lower than or equal to 4 and (**b**) greater than 4 (right). For each considered volume (whole brain, gray matter, lateral ventricles, FLAIR lesions, T1 blackholes), the represented radius goes from low volume in the center to high volume on the exterior (each volume being re-scaled based on 1st and 3rd quartiles in the four groups combined). Solid lines link the median volumes per group.

Table 2. Results from statistical analysis of differences in ico**brain ms** volumetrics between MS types. The group effect rows provide the results of the Kruskal–Wallis analyses looking for an effect of MS type on these variables. Other rows indicate the group differences as observed via post-hoc pairwise tests. *p*-values have been corrected for multiple comparisons.

	Whole Brain	Gray Matter	Lateral Ventricles	FLAIR Lesions	T1 Blackholes
EDSS ≤ 4					
Group effect	$p < 0.001$	$p < 0.001$	$p < 0.001$	$p < 0.001$	$p < 0.001$
CIS vs. RRMS	$p = 0.008$	$p = 0.258$	$p = 0.029$	$p < 0.001$	$p < 0.001$
CIS vs. SPMS	$p < 0.001$	$p < 0.001$	$p < 0.001$	$p < 0.001$	$p < 0.001$
CIS vs. PPMS	$p < 0.001$	$p < 0.001$	$p < 0.001$	$p < 0.001$	$p < 0.001$
RRMS vs. SPMS	$p < 0.001$	$p < 0.001$	$p < 0.001$	$p < 0.001$	$p < 0.001$
RRMS vs. PPMS	$p < 0.001$	$p < 0.001$	$p < 0.001$	$p < 0.001$	$p = 0.173$
SPMS vs. PPMS	$p = 0.935$	$p = 1.000$	$p = 1.000$	$p = 0.902$	$p < 0.001$
EDSS > 4					
Group effect	$p = 0.013$	$p = 0.072$	$p = 0.014$	$p = 0.013$	$p = 0.054$
RRMS vs. SPMS	$p = 0.005$	$p = 0.073$	$p = 0.006$	$p = 0.034$	$p = 0.101$
RRMS vs. PPMS	$p = 0.007$	$p = 0.094$	$p = 0.027$	$p = 0.716$	$p = 0.662$
SPMS vs. PPMS	$p = 0.992$	$p = 1.000$	$p = 0.955$	$p = 0.033$	$p = 0.251$

4. Discussion

Digital solutions have the potential to assist clinicians to further standardize MS clinical decision making, to allow for an early detection of disease activity and inform therapeutic decisions. As these solutions are now available with the necessary regulatory clearances and hospital integrations, they can be used in a routine clinical setting.

In this paper, we present the initial real-world evidence results of such a novel regulatory cleared and workflow-integrated MS care path solution. It was demonstrated that the ico**mpanion** mHealth application is a response to clear patient needs and that it is a sensitive tool to capture clinically relevant information about MS symptoms and patient wellbeing, as well as significant longitudinal changes in cognition and fatigue over time. In addition, it was shown that ico**brain ms**' MRI volumetric brain reports save radiologists 40% time while also detecting subclinical MRI activity with a significantly higher sensitivity.

4.1. Patient Perspective

In order to gain insight into the PwMS' perspective on digital telemonitoring solutions we carried out a survey which was answered by 45 PwMS of which the larger part (75.2%) indicated to see themselves as digitally literate. Only one patient (2.2%) indicated to have a negative attitude towards using an app to monitor their disease course, which is in line with previous reports about positive attitudes of PwMS [13].

Patients reported the most important features to be a knowledge center, symptom logging, tests/PROs and treatment overviews (88–98%), but more than 60% also found having an appointment calendar, viewing their own MRI scans, and viewing the evolution of their MRI scan important. The features that PwMS thought they would actually use were symptom logging, performing tests/PROs, treatment overviews and a knowledge center were found to be most popular (84–91%). This is in line with recent research indicating a patient demand for medication schedules and reminders [13]. This study also indicated a strong interest for visit overviews, which has been implemented into icompanion's calendar and visit preparation feature recently. What differentiates icompanion from other MS apps available is that icompanion integrates all the features mentioned above and, at the same time, is a CE-marked and FDA-cleared medical device.

From PwMS in our cohort, 68.9% indicated to intend to start using an MS app like icompanion, and 80.1% intended to start using it daily or weekly which is in line with a previous study [36]. While our survey suggests that PwMS are interested in telemonitoring apps and their features, and actually using them, it must be noted that the sample size of this survey was relatively small and potentially biased due to the relatively small number of non-digitally literate PwMS.

A second survey was carried out to gain insight into PwMS' perspective on MRI scans in collaboration with iConquerMS. The survey investigated PwMS' experiences with MRI scans as well as their knowledge and viewing behavior and was answered by a total of 876 PwMS. Responses indicated that about 45% of PwMS did not have a yearly brain MRI scan, as advised by the MAGNIMS-CMSC-NAIMS recommendations [11]. Of the PwMS who received an electronic version of their MRI, 70.5% looked at their images on their own, but only 13.3% of PwMS reported to completely understand these MR images, in line with previous studies [37]. Considering the key role that MRI plays in clinical decisions in MS care, and the positive outcomes related to an increased patient involvement in clinical decisions [38,39], it is important to include an MRI-focused knowledge center and MRI viewer in medical apps for MS.

Relevant to the latter, our survey showed that many technological limitations prevented PwMS from looking at their MRI scans on their own. 33.9% of PwMS reported not having a software application to view the images, 32.8% not knowing how to view the images, and 12.2% failing to load the images onto their computer or software program. 94.7% of PwMS indicated to be interested in knowing about whether their MRI scan was performed according to clinical guidelines. This is relevant to PwMS, providers and payers, as it has been demonstrated that less than 10% of the MRI scans for PwMS were acquired according to the local guidelines [40]. Finally, almost all PwMS (98.2%) indicated their interest in knowing about changes between their MRIs. This information is provided to PwMS' care teams via icobrain ms in the MS care platform.

4.2. icompanion MS Patient App Validation

In a first exploratory analysis aimed at investigating the validity and clinical relevance of the real-world collected icompanion data, we assessed the sensitivity of icompanion PROs (mental and physical feeling, prEDSS, SymptoMScreen composite, Neuro-QoL Fatigue and Neuro-QoL Cognition) to clinical differences between MS types, so-called known-groups validity. A significant effect of MS type on physical feeling, prEDSS and SymptoMScreen composite was observed. We found physical feeling to be significantly worse in people with SPMS compared to RRMS, while prEDSS scores for both RRMS and CIS showed to be significantly lower than both PPMS and SPMS. These results are in line with previous studies that described a significant effect of MS type on EDSS [38,39,41]. Average symptom load or SymptoMScreen composite was found to be significantly higher in people with PPMS compared to RRMS, which is in line with a previous study [39] that found that scores for symptoms associated with spinal cord abnormalities were significantly higher for SPMS and PPMS than for RRMS. These symptoms were included in the SymptoMScreen as Spasticity and stiffness, Sensory symptoms, and Bladder control, and consequently also in the SymptoMScreen composite [21]. While these findings are expected, and in line with the literature described above, they indicate that the prEDSS [22] and SymptoMScreen [21] PROs included in the ico**mpanion** mobile app are able to pick up important clinical differences between MS types.

In addition, we observed statistically meaningful changes, based on conditional minimal detectable change [31], for the Neuro-QoL (V1.0) Fatigue in 25.0% of PwMS with more than one datapoint, and in 12.3% of PwMS with more than one datapoint for the Neuro-QoL (V2.0) Cognitive. This is the first time that this measure, aimed at providing a clinically useful way of interpreting individual change in the Neuro-QoL short-forms, is employed in MS, and this suggests that ico**mpanion** is able to pick up statistically meaningful and consequently clinically relevant changes in cognition and fatigue in PwMS. In the HCP portal, HCPs can easily evaluate whether changes in the data entered by linked PwMS for these PROs are statistically meaningful based on this measure. This provides them with an indication of changes in clinical symptoms that are large enough to help motivate treatment changes [31].

In summary, we provide real-world data obtained by a medical device app which are in line with other published studies and provide initial evidence that it is feasible to obtain reliable real-world data which can potentially be used for clinical decision making. Further in-depth analyses will be needed on how mHealth app telemonitoring data can help PwMS, inform clinicians, and impact clinical decision making and outcomes.

4.3. icobrain ms Brain MRI Analysis Validation

The use of follow-up brain MRI scans to detect disease activity in PwMS is recommended by all international guidelines. Typically, changes in terms of new and enlarging lesions and brain volume compared to the previous brain scan are evaluated visually. However, especially because many lesions can be present in an MS patient's brain and subtle but significant brain atrophy is almost impossible to visually assess, it is known that visual MRI reading is prone to inter-rater variability and potential discrepancies [12]. This was confirmed by the results reported in this paper, which demonstrate a significant inter-rater lesion count difference, which can in part be explained by a subjective rater's preference for merging certain nearby lesions into one connected lesion, or for indicating separate nearby lesion foci as distinct lesions. It should be mentioned here that in the presented experiment the raters were asked to provide the best possible lesion count as possible, not to perform a brain MRI reading they would do in a clinical setting. Given the time pressure and distractions in a clinical context, it can be expected that the variability in detecting (new) lesions can be even higher. In this study, it was demonstrated that ico**brain ms** has an excellent test-retest lesion count agreement, and that the expert raters improved their test-retest lesion count agreement when the software annotations were made available. Such results are in line with previous studies that used various other assistive research software approaches [42–45] although we must note that one limitation of this analysis was the small number of raters.

As detecting brain MRI based disease activity is an essential part of the current MS treatment guidelines, it is important to assess to what extent AI augmented radiological reading can impact clinical decision making. In this context, it was demonstrated that the use of ico**brain ms** together with the radiological reading detected a significantly higher number of PwMS with disease activity when compared to the visual radiological assessment alone. This is in line with the results reported by [46], where the proportion of PwMS who were found as having evidence of disease activity/progression grew from around 35% based on clinical criteria alone to around 54% based on conventional radiological reading (with lesion activity and/or visually estimated brain atrophy), to 61% and 80% when employing radiological reading assisted by icobrain ms (only lesion activity, and lesion activity and estimated annual atrophy thresholded at 0.4%, respectively). In addition, and as crucial to implement new technologies in the clinical setting, it was observed that the radiological reading workflow was improved by 40%, which is significant given the increasing time pressure on radiologists [47].

Finally, known-groups validity was also demonstrated for icobrain ms (Table 2) as significant group differences were observed between MS phenotypes for the different icobrain ms volumetric measures (Figure 10). These findings, albeit based on limited sample sizes, indicated that lesion evolution and brain volumetry, as well as cognitive performance and symptoms, have distinct patterns in the relapsing and progressive types/phases of MS, but that the patterns seem to become more indistinguishable once the disease is more advanced. Indeed, there is more heterogeneity in brain atrophy and lesion burden patterns among different MS groups (relapsing-remitting, primary progressive, secondary progressive) at low EDSS, and, conversely, brain atrophy and lesion burden patterns converge to a common pattern when EDSS gets higher (Figure 10). The RRMS group is clearly distinct from the progressive forms of MS. This divergence, followed by unification of clinical and subclinical findings, is in line with the unifying concept of MS [48]. This highlights the importance of not allowing the disease to progress beyond a certain stage, by addressing the earliest signs of disease activity before irreversible damage sets in.

The results from these analyses demonstrate that it is feasible to implement brain MRI AI solutions in a clinical routine setting and that they can improve the radiological workflow. In addition, it is shown that the icobrain ms software, as an assistive tool for radiological reading, decreases the intra- and inter-rater radiological reading variability. Finally, it was demonstrated that icobrain ms results can help differentiate between MS subtypes, in line with the literature, and that they allow for a significantly higher detection rate of MS disease activity.

In further research, we aim to provide the combined icompanion and icobrain ms results to clinicians to evaluate the potential impact of these technologies on clinical decision making and standardization of care.

5. Conclusions

Given the heterogeneity of the disease, the increasing number of available treatment options, and the long-term outcome effects of early clinical decisions in chronic disorders such as MS, there is a clear need to move towards more personalized decision making in MS. Hence, MS care pathways need to become more data-driven and standardized. In this paper, real-world evidence on how new digital/AI technologies can impact MS patient care was presented, and the feasibility of linking different digital tools into one overarching MS care pathway was demonstrated.

Author Contributions: Conceptualization, W.V.H.; Methodology, W.V.H., L.C., A.D., A.R., D.S. and D.M.S.; Software, L.C., A.D. and D.M.S.; Validation, W.V.H., L.C., A.D. and D.M.S.; Formal analysis, L.C., A.D. and D.M.S.; Investigation, W.V.H., L.C., A.D. and D.M.S.; Resources, W.V.H., A.R., D.S. and D.M.S.; Data curation, L.C., A.D. and D.M.S.; Writing—original draft, W.V.H., L.C. and D.M.S.; Writing—review & editing, W.V.H., L.C., A.D., A.R., G.N., D.S. and D.M.S.; Visualization, L.C., A.D. and D.M.S.; Supervision, W.V.H., A.R., G.N. and D.S.; Project administration, W.V.H., A.R., D.S. and D.M.S.; Funding acquisition, W.V.H. All authors have read and agreed to the published version of the manuscript.

Funding: This research did not receive specific funding.

Institutional Review Board Statement: All reported studies were conducted according to the guidelines of the Declaration of Helsinki and approved by the relevant Institutional Review Boards and/or Ethics Committees except for the survey studies as these were considered market research studies and did not require specific ethical approval.

Informed Consent Statement: Informed consent was obtained from all subjects involved in the reported studies, except for the iConquerMS survey as it was considered market research and all data was collected anonymously. All ico**mpanion** users approved a Terms of Use (https://files.icometrix.com/icompanion/Terms-of-use/Terms-of-use-short-en-GB.pdf, accessed on 27 August 2021) and a Privacy Policy (https://files.icometrix.com/icompanion/Privacy-policy/Privacy-policy-en-GB.pdf, accessed on 27 August 2021) in which they confirm that ico**metrix** can use their data for research.

Data Availability Statement: The data presented in this study are not publicly available due to PwMS' privacy rights.

Acknowledgments: The authors would like to thank all the colleagues who contributed to the implementation of the described platform and who assisted in the execution of the surveys (in particular, Hollie Schmidt, Sara Loud, Robert McBurney, and David Gwynne from iConquerMS and the Accelerated Cure Project for Multiple Sclerosis, and Eva de Roey, Liese Steenwinckel, Aske Vloebergs, and Katrien Verhoeven for the survey on MS app patient preferences) validation studies (in particular, Guido Wilms who performed expert radiological reading, Dominique Sappey-Marinier, and Françoise Durand-Dubief (CERMEP-Imagerie du vivant and CREATIS (UMR5220 CNRS & U1294 INSERM), Université de Lyon) for the long-standing collaboration on the analysis of their longitudinal MRI data, as well as to Andreas Lysandropoulos, Than Vân Phan, Thijs Vande Vyvere, and Nathan Torcida for their contribution to the reported MRI studies). Special thanks are due to all the persons with multiple sclerosis who participated in the surveys and studies reported in this paper.

Conflicts of Interest: The following authors are employed by icometrix: Lars Costers, Annabel Descamps, Annemie Ribbens, Dirk Smeets, Diana M. Sima. Guy Nagels is medical director neurology at icometrix and minority shareholder; he or his institution (VUB/UZ Brussel) have received research, educational and travel grants from Biogen, Roche, Genzyme, Merck, Bayer and Teva. Wim Van Hecke is CEO, founder, shareholder and member of the board of icometrix.

Appendix A

Note that these questions are part of a broader questionnaire that surveyed PwMS' expectations of an MS app.

General

- What is your sex?
    - ○ Male
    - ○ Female
    - ○ Other
- What is your age?
- When were you diagnosed with MS?
    - ○ Less than 6 months ago
    - ○ 6 months–1 year ago
    - ○ 1–3 years ago
    - ○ 3–5 years ago
    - ○ 5–10 years ago
    - ○ 10–15 years ago
    - ○ 15–20 years ago
    - ○ Over 20 years ago
    - ○ I don't know
    - ○ I prefer not to share this information
- Which type of MS do you have?
    - ○ Primary Progressive MS or PPMS
    - ○ Secondary Progressive MS or SPMS

- ○ Relapsing Remitting MS or RRMS
- ○ I don't know
- ○ I prefer not to share this information

Attitude towards MS application

- What is your attitude towards an MS app to help monitor your disease evolution?
  - ○ Very negative
  - ○ Rather negative
  - ○ Neutral
  - ○ Rather positive
  - ○ Very positive

Features

- Is it important that a knowledge center is included in an MS app?
  - ○ Yes
    - Would you use this feature?
      - Yes
      - No
  - ○ No
- Is it important that symptom logging is included in an MS app?
  - ○ Yes
    - Would you use this feature?
      - Yes
      - No
  - ○ No
- Is it important that an overview and analysis of your MRI scans is included in an MS app?
  - ○ Yes
    - Would you use this feature?
      - Yes
      - No
  - ○ No
- Is it important that the evolution of your MRI scans is included in an MS app?
  - ○ Yes
    - Would you use this feature?
      - Yes
      - No
  - ○ No
- Is it important that tests are included in an MS app?
  - ○ Yes
    - Would you use this feature?
      - Yes
      - No
  - ○ No
- Is it important that a calendar to plan your doctor's visits is included in an MS app?
  - ○ Yes
    - Would you use this feature?
      - Yes

- No
  - ○ No
- Are you interested in an MS app?
  - ○ Yes
  - ○ Maybe
  - ○ No
- How frequently would you use an MS app?
  - ○ Daily
  - ○ Multiple times per week
  - ○ Once per week
  - ○ Once every two weeks
  - ○ Once per month
  - ○ Other

Appendix B

In case of fixed possible answers, see italic.

- Have you ever had an MRI performed for the purpose of diagnosing or treating your MS?
- How often do you get an MRI for your MS, on average? Please disregard any recent delays in getting an MRI that you may have experienced due to the COVID-19 pandemic.
- When did you last get an MRI of your brain?
- When did you last get an MRI of your neck or spinal column?
- Have you ever received or been given access to an electronic copy of your MRI? Check all that apply.
  - ○ *Yes, my clinic or radiology lab gave it to me without my requesting it*
  - ○ *Yes, my clinic or radiology lab gave it to me after I requested it*
  - ○ *Yes, I got one from participating in a research study*
  - ○ *No*
  - ○ *Not sure/prefer not to say*
- Have you ever received or been given access to an electronic copy of your MRI? Check all that apply.
  - ○ *CD/disc*
  - ○ *USB drive/thumb drive*
  - ○ *Direct download into my computer or other device*
  - ○ *Access through my clinic's patient portal*
  - ○ *Other—Write In*
  - ○ *Not sure/prefer not to say*
- Have you ever looked at your own MRI images on your own, without your healthcare provider present?
  - ○ [in case of Yes] Did you find it helpful in any way to view your MRI images on your own? If so, how?
  - ○ [in case of Yes] Did you find it unhelpful in any way to view your MRI images on your own? If so, how?
  - ○ [in case of Yes] How well did you understand the images on your MRI?
  - ○ [in case of No] Why haven't you looked at your MRI images on your own? Check all that apply.
    - *I wasn't sure how to view the images*
    - *I didn't have a software program or application for viewing the files*
    - *I couldn't load the images onto my computer or another device where I could view them*
    - *I didn't know how to interpret the images*

- I wasn't interested in viewing my MRI images on my own
- Not sure/prefer not to say:
- Other—Write In

○ [in case of No] Would you like to view your MRI images on your own? Why or why not?

- Would you be interested in having your own copy of your MRI images to view? Why or why not?
- If you have or had access to your own MRIs, would you be interested in knowing whether the MRI was performed according to the current clinical guidelines for MS? Why or why not?
- If you have or had access to your own MRIs, would you be interested in knowing whether there were any changes between one MRI and the next (such as new lesions or loss of brain volume)? Why or why not?
- If you have or had access to your own MRIs, would you be willing to share your electronic MRI with a researcher, if asked? Why or why not?
- If you have or had access to your own MRIs, would you be willing to share them with iConquerMS, if asked, and allow iConquerMS to share them with researchers? Why or why not?

References

1. Coetzee, T.; Thompson, A.J. Atlas of MS 2020: Informing Global Policy Change. *Mult. Scler.* **2020**, *26*, 1807–1808. [CrossRef]
2. National MS Society (Medications). Available online: https://www.nationalmssociety.org/Treating-MS/Medications (accessed on 29 July 2021).
3. Hult, K. *Measuring the Potential Health Impact of Personalized Medicine: Evidence from MS Treatments*; National Bureau of Economic Research, Inc.: Cambridge, MA, USA, 2017.
4. Sá, M.J.; de Sá, J.; Sousa, L. Relapsing–Remitting Multiple Sclerosis: Patterns of Response to Disease-Modifying Therapies and Associated Factors: A National Survey. *Neurol. Ther.* **2014**, *3*, 89–99. [CrossRef]
5. Daugherty, K.K.; Butler, J.S.; Mattingly, M.; Ryan, M. Factors Leading Patients to Discontinue Multiple Sclerosis Therapies. *J. Am. Pharm. Assoc.* **2005**, *45*, 371–375. [CrossRef]
6. Giovannoni, G.; Butzkueven, H.; Dhib-Jalbut, S.; Hobart, J.; Kobelt, G.; Pepper, G.; Sormani, M.P.; Thalheim, C.; Traboulsee, A.; Vollmer, T. Brain Health: Time Matters in Multiple Sclerosis. *Mult. Scler. Relat. Disord.* **2016**, *9* (Suppl. 1), S5–S48. [CrossRef]
7. Duddy, M.; Lee, M.; Pearson, O.; Nikfekr, E.; Chaudhuri, A.; Percival, F.; Roberts, M.; Whitlock, C. The UK Patient Experience of Relapse in Multiple Sclerosis Treated with First Disease Modifying Therapies. *Mult. Scler. Relat. Disord.* **2014**, *3*, 450–456. [CrossRef]
8. Amato, M.P.; Ponziani, G.; Siracusa, G.; Sorbi, S. Cognitive Dysfunction in Early-Onset Multiple Sclerosis: A Reappraisal after 10 Years. *Arch. Neurol.* **2001**, *58*, 1602–1606. [CrossRef] [PubMed]
9. Magnano, I.; Aiello, I.; Piras, M.R. Cognitive Impairment and Neurophysiological Correlates in MS. *J. Neurol. Sci.* **2006**, *245*, 117–122. [CrossRef] [PubMed]
10. Kürtüncü, M.; Tuncer, A.; Uygunoğlu, U.; Çalişkan, Z.; Paksoy, A.K.; Efendı, H.; Kocaman, A.S.; Özcan, C.; Terzı, M.; Turan, Ö.F.; et al. Differences Between General Neurologists and Multiple Sclerosis Specialists in the Management of Multiple Sclerosis Patients: A National Survey. *Noro psikiyatri arsivi* **2017**, *56*. [CrossRef]
11. Wattjes, M.P.; Ciccarelli, O.; Reich, D.S.; Banwell, B.; de Stefano, N.; Enzinger, C.; Fazekas, F.; Filippi, M.; Frederiksen, J.; Gasperini, C.; et al. 2021 MAGNIMS–CMSC–NAIMS Consensus Recommendations on the Use of MRI in Patients with Multiple Sclerosis. *Lancet Neurol.* **2021**. [CrossRef]
12. Rosenkrantz, A.B.; Duszak, R.; Babb, J.S.; Glover, M.; Kang, S.K. Discrepancy Rates and Clinical Impact of Imaging Secondary Interpretations: A Systematic Review and Meta-Analysis. *J. Am. Coll. Radiol.* **2018**, *15*. [CrossRef] [PubMed]
13. Haase, R.; Voigt, I.; Scholz, M.; Schlieter, H.; Benedict, M.; Susky, M.; Dillenseger, A.; Ziemssen, T. Profiles of eHealth Adoption in Persons with Multiple Sclerosis and Their Caregivers. *Brain Sciences* **2021**, *11*, 1087. [CrossRef]
14. Ziemssen, T.; Thomas, K. Treatment Optimization in Multiple Sclerosis: How Do We Apply Emerging Evidence? *Expert Rev. Clin. Immunol.* **2017**, *13*, 509–511. [CrossRef] [PubMed]
15. D'Amico, E.; Haase, R.; Ziemssen, T. Review: Patient-Reported Outcomes in Multiple Sclerosis Care. *Mult. Scler. Relat. Disord.* **2019**, *33*, 61–66. [CrossRef] [PubMed]
16. Celius, E.G.; Thompson, H.; Pontaga, M.; Langdon, D.; Laroni, A.; Potra, S.; Bharadia, T.; Yeandle, D.; Shanahan, J.; van Galen, P.; et al. Disease Progression in Multiple Sclerosis: A Literature Review Exploring Patient Perspectives. *Patient Prefer. Adherence* **2021**, *15*, 15–27. [CrossRef] [PubMed]
17. Hamann, J.; Neuner, B.; Kasper, J.; Vodermaier, A.; Loh, A.; Deinzer, A.; Heesen, C.; Kissling, W.; Busch, R.; Schmieder, R.; et al. Participation Preferences of Patients with Acute and Chronic Conditions. *Health Expect.* **2007**, *10*, 358–363. [CrossRef] [PubMed]

18. van Leeuwen, K.G.; Schalekamp, S.; Mjcm, R.; van Ginneken, B.; de Rooij, M. Artificial Intelligence in Radiology: 100 Commercially Available Products and Their Scientific Evidence. *Eur. Radiol.* **2021**, *31*. [CrossRef]
19. Medina, L.D.; Torres, S.; Alvarez, E.; Valdez, B.; Nair, K.V. Patient-Reported Outcomes in Multiple Sclerosis: Validation of the Quality of Life in Neurological Disorders (Neuro-QoL™) Short Forms. *Mult Scler J Exp Transl Clin* **2019**, *5*, 2055217319885986. [CrossRef]
20. Miller, D.M.; Bethoux, F.; Victorson, D.; Nowinski, C.J.; Buono, S.; Lai, J.-S.; Wortman, K.; Burns, J.L.; Moy, C.; Cella, D. Validating Neuro-QoL Short Forms and Targeted Scales with People Who Have Multiple Sclerosis. *Mult. Scler.* **2016**, *22*, 830–841. [CrossRef]
21. Green, R.; Kalina, J.; Ford, R.; Pandey, K.; Kister, I. SymptoMScreen: A Tool for Rapid Assessment of Symptom Severity in MS Across Multiple Domains. *Appl. Neuropsychol. Adult* **2017**, *24*, 183–189. [CrossRef]
22. Leddy, S.; Hadavi, S.; McCarren, A.; Giovannoni, G.; Dobson, R. Validating a Novel Web-Based Method to Capture Disease Progression Outcomes in Multiple Sclerosis. *J. Neurol.* **2013**, *260*, 2505–2510. [CrossRef]
23. Cella, D.; Lai, J.-S.; Nowinski, C.J.; Victorson, D.; Peterman, A.; Miller, D.; Bethoux, F.; Heinemann, A.; Rubin, S.; Cavazos, J.E.; et al. Neuro-QOL: Brief Measures of Health-Related Quality of Life for Clinical Research in Neurology. *Neurology* **2012**, *78*, 1860–1867. [CrossRef] [PubMed]
24. Jain, S.; Sima, D.M.; Ribbens, A.; Cambron, M.; Maertens, A.; Van Hecke, W.; De Mey, J.; Barkhof, F.; Steenwijk, M.D.; Daams, M.; et al. Automatic Segmentation and Volumetry of Multiple Sclerosis Brain Lesions from MR Images. *NeuroImage Clin.* **2015**, *8*, 367–375. [CrossRef]
25. Rakić, M.; Vercruyssen, S.; Van Eyndhoven, S.; de la Rosa, E.; Jain, S.; Van Huffel, S.; Maes, F.; Smeets, D.; Sima, D.M. Icobrain Ms 5.1: Combining Unsupervised and Supervised Approaches for Improving the Detection of Multiple Sclerosis Lesions. *Neuroimage Clin* **2021**, *31*, 102707. [CrossRef]
26. Smeets, D.; Ribbens, A.; Sima, D.M.; Cambron, M.; Horakova, D.; Jain, S.; Maertens, A.; Van Vlierberghe, E.; Terzopoulos, V.; Van Binst, A.-M.; et al. Reliable Measurements of Brain Atrophy in Individual Patients with Multiple Sclerosis. *Brain Behav.* **2016**, *6*, e00518. [CrossRef] [PubMed]
27. Lysandropoulos, A.P.; Absil, J.; Metens, T.; Mavroudakis, N.; Guisset, F.; Van Vlierberghe, E.; Smeets, D.; David, P.; Maertens, A.; Van Hecke, W. Quantifying Brain Volumes for Multiple Sclerosis Patients Follow-up in Clinical Practice—Comparison of 1.5 and 3 Tesla Magnetic Resonance Imaging. *Brain Behav.* **2016**, *6*, e00422. [CrossRef] [PubMed]
28. Beadnall, H.N.; Wang, C.; Van Hecke, W.; Ribbens, A.; Billiet, T.; Barnett, M.H. Comparing Longitudinal Brain Atrophy Measurement Techniques in a Real-World Multiple Sclerosis Clinical Practice Cohort: Towards Clinical Integration? *Ther. Adv. Neurol. Disord.* **2019**, *12*, 175628641882346. [CrossRef]
29. Costers, L.; Schmidt, H.; Loud, S.; McBurney, R.; Gwynne, D.; Van Vlierberghe, E.; Descamps, A.; Smeets, D.; Van Hecke, W. MRI in MS Survey—Insights into Access, Understanding and Interest by People with MS. *Mult. Scler. J.* **2021**, *27*, 70.
30. Benjamini, Y.; Hochberg, Y. Controlling the False Discovery Rate: A Practical and Powerful Approach to Multiple Testing. *J. R. Stat. Soc.* **1995**, *57*, 289–300. [CrossRef]
31. Kozlowski, A.J.; Cella, D.; Nitsch, K.P.; Heinemann, A.W. Evaluating Individual Change with the Quality of Life in Neurological Disorders (Neuro-QoL) Short Forms. *Arch. Phys. Med. Rehabil.* **2016**, *97*, 650–654.e8. [CrossRef]
32. Ion-Mărgineanu, A.; Kocevar, G.; Stamile, C.; Sima, D.M.; Durand-Dubief, F.; Van Huffel, S.; Sappey-Marinier, D. Machine Learning Approach for Classifying Multiple Sclerosis Courses by Combining Clinical Data with Lesion Loads and Magnetic Resonance Metabolic Features. *Front. Neurosci.* **2017**, *11*, 398. [CrossRef]
33. Sima, D.M.; Podevyn, F.; Torcida, N.; Wilms, G.; Lysandropoulos, A.; Van Hecke, W.; Smeets, D. Impact of MSmetrix Automatic Lesion Segmentation on the Visual Count of Multiple Sclerosis Lesions. In Proceedings of the 2018 European Congress of Radiology, Vienna, Austria, 28 February–4 March 2018; p. C-2472.
34. Sima, D.M.; Wilms, G.; Vyvere, T.V.; Van Hecke, W.; Smeets, D. On the Use of Icobrain's Prepopulated Radiology Reporting Template for Multiple Sclerosis Follow-Up. In Proceedings of the 2020 European Congress of Radiology, Vienna, Austria, 15–19 July 2020; p. C-11342.
35. Sima, D.M.; Jain, S.; Roura, E.; Maertens, A.; Smeets, D.; Sappey-Marinier, D.; Durand-Dubief, F.; Van Hecke, W. New and Enlarging Lesion Location for Different MS Clinical Phenotypes. In Proceedings of the MSParis2017—7th Joint ECTRIMS-ACTRIMS, Paris, France, 25–28 October 2017; p. EP1559.
36. Potemkowski, A.; Brola, W.; Ratajczak, A.; Ratajczak, M.; Zaborski, J.; Jasińska, E.; Pokryszko-Dragan, A.; Gruszka, E.; Dubik-Jezierzańska, M.; Podlecka-Piętowska, A.; et al. Internet Usage by Polish Patients with Multiple Sclerosis: A Multicenter Questionnaire Study. *Interact. J. Med. Res.* **2019**, *8*, e11146. [CrossRef]
37. Brand, J.; Köpke, S.; Kasper, J.; Rahn, A.; Backhus, I.; Poettgen, J.; Stellmann, J.-P.; Siemonsen, S.; Heesen, C. Magnetic Resonance Imaging in Multiple Sclerosis–Patients' Experiences, Information Interests and Responses to an Education Programme. *PLoS ONE* **2014**, *9*, e113252. [CrossRef]
38. Ruano, L.; Portaccio, E.; Goretti, B.; Niccolai, C.; Severo, M.; Patti, F.; Cilia, S.; Gallo, P.; Grossi, P.; Ghezzi, A.; et al. Age and Disability Drive Cognitive Impairment in Multiple Sclerosis across Disease Subtypes. *Mult. Scler.* **2017**, *23*, 1258–1267. [CrossRef] [PubMed]
39. Nijeholt, G.J.; van Walderveen, M.A.; Castelijns, J.A.; van Waesberghe, J.H.; Polman, C.; Scheltens, P.; Rosier, P.F.; Jongen, P.J.; Barkhof, F. Brain and Spinal Cord Abnormalities in Multiple Sclerosis. Correlation between MRI Parameters, Clinical Subtypes and Symptoms. *Brain* **1998**, *121 Pt 4*, 687–697. [CrossRef] [PubMed]

40. Vercruyssen, S.; Brys, A.; Verheijen, M.; Steach, B.; Van Vlierberghe, E.; Sima, D.M.; Smeets, D. Conformance to CMSC Magnetic Resonance Imaging (MRI) Guidelines in a Real-World Multicenter MRI Dataset. *Int. J. MS Care* **2020**, *22*, 47.
41. Tsagkas, C.; Magon, S.; Gaetano, L.; Fezold, S.; Naegelin, Y.; Amann, M.; Stippich, C.; Cattin, P.; Wuerfel, J.; Bieri, O.; et al. Preferential Spinal Cord Volume Loss in Primary Progressive Multiple Sclerosis. *Mult. Scler. J.* **2019**, *25*, 947–957. [CrossRef]
42. Dahan, A.; Wang, W.; Gaillard, F. Computer-Aided Detection Can Bridge the Skill Gap in Multiple Sclerosis Monitoring. *J. Am Coll. Radiol.* **2018**, *15*, 93–96. [CrossRef]
43. Wang, W.; van Heerden, J.; Tacey, M.A.; Gaillard, F. Neuroradiologists Compared with Non-Neuroradiologists in the Detection of New Multiple Sclerosis Plaques. *AJNR Am. J. Neuroradiol.* **2017**, *38*, 1323–1327. [CrossRef]
44. van Heerden, J.; Rawlinson, D.; Zhang, A.M.; Chakravorty, R.; Tacey, M.A.; Desmond, P.M.; Gaillard, F. Improving Multiple Sclerosis Plaque Detection Using a Semiautomated Assistive Approach. *AJNR Am. J. Neuroradiol.* **2015**, *36*, 1465–1471. [CrossRef]
45. Zopfs, D.; Laukamp, K.R.; Paquet, S.; Lennartz, S.; Pinto Dos Santos, D.; Kabbasch, C.; Bunck, A.; Schlamann, M.; Borggrefe, J. Follow-up MRI in Multiple Sclerosis Patients: Automated Co-Registration and Lesion Color-Coding Improves Diagnostic Accuracy and Reduces Reading Time. *Eur. Radiol.* **2019**, *29*, 7047–7054. [CrossRef]
46. Beadnall, H.N.; Ly, L.; Wang, C.; Billiet, T.; Ribbens, A.; Van Hecke, W.; Zivadinov, R.; Barnett, M.H. 103 Exploring the Influence of Quantitative Magnetic Resonance Imaging on Decision-Making in Multiple Sclerosis Clinical Practice. *J. Neurol. Neurosurg. Psychiatry* **2018**, *89*, A41.
47. Lexa, F.J. Duty Hour Limits for Radiologists: It's About Time. *J. Am. Coll. Radiol.* **2021**, *18*, 208–210. [CrossRef] [PubMed]
48. Confavreux, C.; Vukusic, S. Natural History of Multiple Sclerosis: A Unifying Concept. *Brain* **2006**, *129*. [CrossRef] [PubMed]

MDPI
St. Alban-Anlage 66
4052 Basel
Switzerland
Tel. +41 61 683 77 34
Fax +41 61 302 89 18
www.mdpi.com

Brain Sciences Editorial Office
E-mail: brainsci@mdpi.com
www.mdpi.com/journal/brainsci

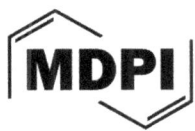

www.ingramcontent.com/pod-product-compliance
Lightning Source LLC
LaVergne TN
LVHW070748100526
838202LV00013B/1329